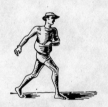

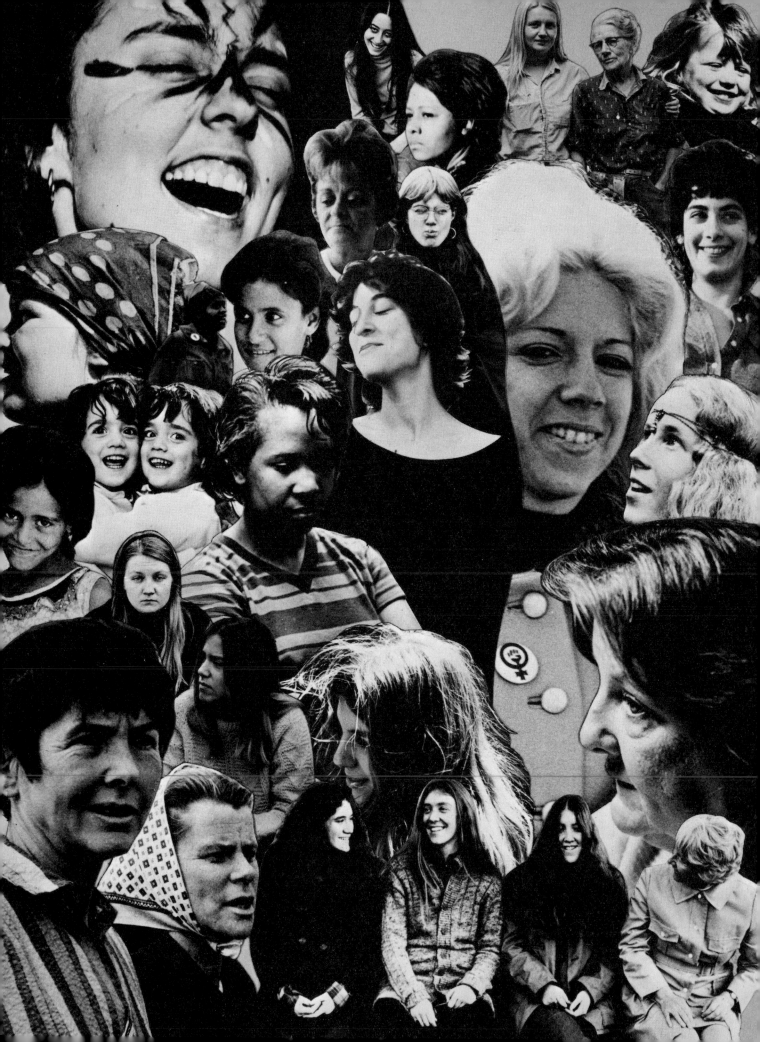

Our Bodies, Ourselves
A Book By and For Women

by
The Boston Women's Health Book Collective

SIMON AND SCHUSTER

New York

SBN 671-21434-9 Casebound edition
SBN 671-21435-7 Touchstone paperback edition
Library of Congress Catalog Card Number: 72-83220
Manufactured in the United States of America

2 3 4 5 6 7 8 9 10 11 12 13 14 15

Clinic Discount: OUR BODIES, OURSELVES is available to clinics and other groups providing health-counseling services, at a 70% discount (88.5¢ per paperback copy) plus shipping costs. Orders must be for 12 or more copies with payment and a document verifying health service status enclosed. The document must be a copy of a statement filed with a state or federal agency indicating health services or health education as a primary purpose of your group. Address orders to Clinic Copies, *Our Bodies, Ourselves,* Simon and Schuster, 630 Fifth Ave., New York, N.Y. 10020.

Copies so purchased may not be offered for resale.

Thanks to the following people for their information, advice and support:

Judy Alland
Kathee Allen
Elayne Archer
Kathy Babel
Diane Balser
Ruth Balser
Don Bell
Trude Bennett
Madelene Berkowitz
Andrea Black
Liz Blum
Cathy Booth
Women in the Boston Association for
    Childbirth Education, Inc.
Edward Brecher
Thomas Brewer
Geraldine Bridgeman
Nancy Brigham
Jan Bumstead
Hester Butterfield
Mary Jane Campbell
Joanna Caplan
Peggy Carlson
Michelle Clark
Peggy Clark
Betsy Cole
Beverly Coleman
Joanne Collins
Cynthia Cook
Lee Cooke
Laurie Crumpacker
Pauline D'Allesandro
Irene Davidson
Bruce Ditzion
Irvin Doress
Mary Elizabeth

Judy Folkmanis
Rachel Fruchter
Marsha Gerstein
Louise Glück
Miriam Goodman
Linda Gordon
Emily Graeser
Helen L. Gray
Marian Johnson Gray
Roger W. Gray
Mary Greeley
John W. Grover
Sara Hale
Pat Haseltine
Andy Hawley
Gina Hawley
Joshua Hawley
The Health Organizing Collective of the
    New York Women's Health and
    Abortion Project
Ellin Hirst
Linda Hunt
Susan Katz
Jane Kaufman
Jamie Kelem
Claire Keough
Joseph Kerrins
Grace Kleinbach
Carol Koury
Louise Lander
Wini Lawrence
Jane Levy
Jancis Long
Robert Margulis
Joan Matheson
Mercedes Mattsen

Barbara McHugh
Lynne Morgan
Robin Morgan
Merry Muscato
Linda Neville
The Staff of the *New England Free Press*
Cookee Paul
Ed Pincus
Ann Popkin
Gina Prenowitz
Janet Press
Kathy Queer
Jean Raisler
Alberta Richmond
Nathan Rome
Kris Rosenthal
Betsey Sable
Ted Schocken
Marzi Schorin
Leonard Schwartz
Kathy Segal
Nancy Shaw
Marilyn Slotkin
Linda Slotnik
Somerville Hospital School of Nursing
    Library
Roland Stern
Nancy Stokely
Dorothy Tennov
Dorothy Termos
Ruth D. Terzaghi
Ann Walsh
Jane Knowles Webb
Thayer Williams
Marliese Wior
Carol Yarmosky

AUTHORSHIP LIST

Preface   Wilma Diskin and Wendy Coppedge Sanford

Our Changing Sense of Self   Joan Sheingold Ditzion

The Anatomy and Physiology of Reproduction   Esther R. Rome and Nancy Press Hawley based on work by Abby Schwartz with the help of Gina Prenowitz

Sexuality   Nancy Press Hawley based on work by Jane de Long, Ginger Goldner and Nancy London with help from Wendy Sanford and Judy Norsigian

Living with Ourselves and Others: Our Relationships   Nancy Press Hawley with help from Wendy Sanford and Judy Norsigian

In Amerika They Call Us Dykes   A Boston gay collective

Nutrition and the Food We Eat   Judy Norsigian

Women in Motion   Janet Jones and Carol McEldowney

Rape   Gene Bishop and Roxane Hynek

Self-Defense   Janet Jones and Carol McEldowney

Venereal Disease   Esther R. Rome and Fran Ansley

Birth Control   Wendy Sanford based on work by Abby Schwartz and Pamela Berger, with the help of Thayer Williams, Betsey Sable, and Joanna Caplan

Abortion   Pamela Berger and Wendy Sanford based on work by Carol Driscoll, Nancy Press Hawley, and Betsey Sable

Deciding Whether to Have Children   Jane Kates Pincus and Wendy Sanford with help from Mary Rollston Stern, Cathy Booth, and Judy Norsigian

Childbearing: Pregnancy   Jane Kates Pincus with help from Ruth Davidson Bell, Norma Swenson, and Paula Brown Doress

Childbearing: Prepared Childbirth   Ruth Davidson Bell with help from Norma Swenson, Nancy Press Hawley, Paula Brown Doress, and Jane Kates Pincus

Childbearing: Postpartum—After the Baby Is Born   Paula Brown Doress with the help of Esther R. Rome, Wendy Sanford, and Norma Swenson

Menopause   Meg Hickey and Irene Davidson with help from Marliese Wior, Carol Koury, Jane Kates Pincus, and Wendy Sanford

Women and Health Care

The American Health Care System   Mary Rollston Stern based on work by Barbara Perkins, Lucy Candib, and Nancy Todd

Choosing and Using Medical Care   Norma Swenson with help from Mary Rollston Stern, Jane Kates Pincus, and the Seattle Health Collective

Common Medical Problems and Practices   Terry Thorsos, Judy Norsigian, and Meg Hickey

Contents

Preface, 1

1 Our Changing Sense of Self, 5

Changing Our Internalized Sexist Values, 6
Rediscovering Activity, 8

Rediscovering Anger, 10
Rediscovering Our Separateness, 10

2 The Anatomy and Physiology of Reproduction and Sexuality, 12

Our Feelings—Finding Out About Ourselves, 12
Description of Reproductive Organs—Anatomy (Structure) and Physiology (Function), 14
  Outer Organs—Vulva: Pubis, Outer Lips, Clitoris, Inner Lips, Urinary Opening, Vaginal Opening, Perineum, Hymen, 14
  Inner Organs—Bartholin Glands, Vagina, Fornix, Pelvic Floor Muscles, Uterus (Womb), Cervix, Fallopian Tubes, Ovaries, 15
  Schematic Description, 17
  Development of the Sexual Organs, 17
Stages in the Reproductive Cycle, 17
  The Ovarian Cycle—Ovulation: Follicles, Hormones
(Estrogen and Progesterone), Ovulation, Mittelschmerz, Corpus Luteum, Fertilization, 17
  The Uterine Cycle—Menstruation, 18
    The Menstrual Discharge, 19
    Feelings About Menstruation, 20
    Menstrual Problems: Painful Periods (Dysmenorrhea); Premenstrual Depression; Lack of Periods (Amenorrhea), 20
Appendix: Hormones of the Menstrual Cycle, 21
  Negative Feedback Mechanism, FSH, LH, Estrogen, Progesterone, 21
  Cervical Cycle, 22
Further Readings, 22

3 Sexuality, 23

A Cultural Orientation, 23
Sexual Feelings, 24
Growing Up, 26
Virginity, 27

Fantasies, 29
Masturbation, 30
Lovemaking, 31
Further Readings, 39

4 Living with Ourselves and Others: Our Relationships, 42

Feelings About Celibacy, 43
Feelings About Homosexuality, 44
Our Experiences, 45
1. Laura: Family, Marriage and Separation, 45
2. Mathilde: A Deepening Relationship, 47
3. Sarah: Thoughts and Feelings About Monogamy, 48

4. The Experience of Being Single: Many Voices, 48
5. Abigail: Search for New Forms—Excerpts from the Diary of an Eleven-Year Marriage, 52
6. Lesbian Relationships: A Few Words, 52
7. Elena: Marriage and Multiple Relationships, 53
8. Anger and Relationships, 55

5 In Amerika They Call Us Dykes: A Boston Gay Collective, 56

1. Introduction, 56
2. Out of the Closet and into the Frying Pan, 61
3. The—rapists: Lesbians and Psychiatry, 63
4. The Bars, 65

5. Loving, 66
6. "Blessed Are the Poor," 70
7. Lesbian Mothers, 71

6 Nutrition and the Food We Eat, 74

The Necessary Nutrients, 74
About Protein, 77
Fats and Oils, 78

Carbohydrates, 79
Problems with the Food and Agriculture Industries, 80
Some Valuable Suggestions, 81
Further Readings, 82

7 Women in Motion, 83

Why We Don't Get the Exercise We Need, 83
Things Are Beginning to Change, 85

Choosing an Exercise: Some Guidelines and Some Benefits, 87
Some Final Advice, 90

8 Rape and Self-Defense, 92

Rape, 92
 Whose Fault Is Rape?, 92
 Rape and Race, 93
 Rape and the Law, 93
 What We Can Do as Women, 93

What to Do if You Have Been Raped, 93
Self-Defense, 94
 Learning to Protect Ourselves, 94
 Self-Defense Training, 95
 Some Things You Can Do, 95

9 Venereal Disease, 98

The Problem, 98
 Syphilis and Gonorrhea—How They Spread, 98
 Prevention—General, 98
 Treatment—General, 99
Syphilis, 100
 Symptoms, 100
 Diagnosis, 100
 Treatment and Test for Cure, 100
 Syphilis and Pregnancy, 100
Gonorrhea, 101
 Symptoms, 101

Testing and Diagnosis, 101
Treatment, 102
Test for Cure, 102
Pregnancy and Gonorrhea, 102
Other Venereal Diseases, 103
The Politics of Venereal Disease, 103
Protect Yourself—Protect Others, 104
Summary Chart on Syphilis and Gonorrhea, 105
Important Information About Penicillin Treatment, 105
Further Readings, 105

10 Birth Control, 106

Introduction: Factors affecting our decision about birth control and our ability to choose and use a birth control method that is good for us, 106
Conception. The process to be interrupted. How pregnancy happens. Some facts about sperm, 110
Birth Control Pills, 111
IUD, or Intrauterine Device: Coil, Loop, and Shield, 120
The Diaphragm, 123
The Cervical Cap, 127
The Condom (Rubber, Prophylactic, "Safe"), 127
Foam—Aerosol Vaginal Spermicide, 129
Jellies and Creams for Use Alone, 131
Birth Control Methods That Don't Work Very Well, 132
 Withdrawal. Rhythm Method (Safe Period). Vaginal

Tablets and Suppositories, 132
Nonmethods—Attempts at Birth Control That Don't Work at All, 134
 Douching, Avoidance of Orgasm by the Woman. Avoiding Actual Intercourse. Norforms and Other Feminine Hygiene Products, 134
After Unprotected Intercourse—"The Morning-After Pill," 135
When You Are All Done: Sterilization, 135
 Tubal Ligation. Laparoscopy. Vasectomy (for the man), 135
Future Methods of Birth Control, 136
 Male Contraceptive Research. Female Contraceptive Research, 136
Helpful Organizations, 137
Further Readings, 137

11   Abortion, 138

History, 139
Abortion Practices in Some Other Countries, 140
Abortion Law Reform, Repeal and the Medical Community, 141
If You Think You Are Pregnant, 143
Where to Go for Counseling and Referral, 143
The New York Abortion, 144
Having the Abortion, 144
    Timing, 144
    Medical Techniques for Abortion, 144
        Up to Three Days After Unprotected Intercourse, 144
        Up to 12 Weeks. Vacuum Suction or Dilation and Curettage, 145
        12–16 Weeks, 145
        After 16 Weeks: Saline Injection, 146

After 20 Weeks: Hysterotomy, 146
Medical Preliminaries: The Importance of the Woman's Medical History and Blood Type, 146
Anesthesia, 146
Complications: Hemorrhage, Infection, Incomplete Abortion, 146
Aftercare, 147
Birth Control After an Abortion, 147
Abortion Counseling, 147
Illegal Abortion, 148
    The Doctor-Performed Illegal Abortion, 148
    Methods of the Unskilled Abortionist, 149
    Self-Induced Abortion, 149
Future Prospects, 149
Two Personal Experiences, 151
Further Readings, 153

12   Deciding Whether to Have Children, 154

13   Childbearing, 157

Introduction: Moving Toward Understanding and Control of Our Childbearing Experience, 157
Section One: Pregnancy, 159
    A. A Preventive Program: What You Can Do to Prepare Yourself, 159
        Taking Care of Yourself: Choice, Commitment, Preparation, Feelings, Emotional Needs, 159
        Taking Care of Your Physical Needs, 160
        Nutrition, 161
        A Good Diet for Your Pregnancy, 161
        Why These Foods Are Important, 161
        Controversy About Nutrition, 162
        Gaining Weight, 162
        Toxemia, 162
        Edema, 163
        Diuretics, 163
        Diet Pills, 163
        Salt, 163
        Effect of Medication, 164
        Nutrition—a Political Issue, 164
    B. The Pregnancy Itself, 164
        First Trimester, 165
        Physical Changes, 165
        Procedures for Detecting Pregnancy, 166
        Pelvic Exam, 166
        Some Women Just Know They Are Pregnant, 166
        Exam Schedule, 166
        Your Feelings About Yourself and Your Pregnancy, 167
        Growth of the Fetus, 168
        Second Trimester, 168
        Physical Changes, 168
        Your Feelings About Yourself, 170
        Your Feelings About Your Baby, 170
        Men's Feelings About You, Your Pregnancy, 172
        Intercourse, 172

Medical Fact and Fiction, 172
    Your Feelings About Making Love, 173
    If You Are Living with a Group of People, 173
Third Trimester, 174
    Physical Changes, 174
    Your Feelings About Yourself and Your Pregnancy, 175
Appendices: 177
    Miscarriage (Natural Abortion), 177
    Ectopic Pregnancy, 178
    Rh Factor in Blood, 179
    Early Diagnosis of Birth Defects, 180
    Infertility, 180
Section Two: Prepared Childbirth, 182
    Introduction: Why Preparation?, 182
    Home or Hospital?, 183
    What Is Labor?, 185
    Less Usual Presentations, 187
    Some Signs of Abnormal Labor and Delivery, 189
    Premature Labor, 191
    Induction of Labor, 191
    Drugs, 192
    Exercises, 195
    Being in Labor, 198
    The Immediate Postpartum Period, 205
    Appendix:
        Associations Concerned with Childbirth Education, 206
        How to Choose a Childbirth Class, 206
Section Three: Postpartum—After the Baby Is Born, 207
    Kinds of Postpartum Emotional Problems, 207
    Possible Causes of Postpartum Disturbances, 209
        The Childbearing Year as Maturational Crisis, 209
        Life Changes of Becoming a Parent, 210
        The Physical Context—Fatigue, 211
        The Social Context, 212

Education and Preparation for Child Care, 213
The Family Context, 213
The Medical Context, 215
Theories of Contributing Factors and Some Clinical
    Research, 215
Physical-Stress Theories, 215
Possible Connections Between Physical and Social
    Factors, 216

Social Stress Theories and Prevention, 216
Some Proposals for Change, 218
Appendices:
    Feelings When the Baby Dies, 219
    Physical Aspects of Postpartum, 220
    Infant Care, 223
Further Readings, 225

14   Menopause, 224

What Is Menopause?, 230
What Are the Symptoms?, 231
What You Can Do About It, 232
Depression and Menopause, 233

Pregnancy and Menopause, 234
Sex and Menopause, 234
Further Readings, 235

15   Women and Health Care, 236

Section One: The American Health Care System, 236
    Problems of Inadequate Care for Women, 237
    The Organization and Control of Health Care, 238
    The Capitalist Theory of Disease Causation, 238
    The Power and Role of Male Doctors, 239
    Women as Workers in the Health System, 240
    The Profit Motive in Health Care, 241
Section Two: Choosing and Using Medical Care, 242
    Introduction—The Myths of Choice and Quality, 242
    Choosing the Doctor, 244
        The General Practitioner—The Specialist—Group
            Practice, 244
        What to Look For, 246
        The Doctor-Patient Relationship, 248
        Managing the Obstetrician-Gynecologist, 249
        Doctors: Summary, 252
    The Clinic, 253
    The Hospital, 255
        Hospital Maternity Care, 256
        Hospitals: Summary, 257
Section Three: Common Medical Problems and Proce-
    dures, 259
    Glossary of Common Medical Terms, 259
    Hygiene, 259
        Douches, 260

Vaginal Infections (Vaginitis), 260
    Yeast Infection (Candidiasis or Moniliasis), 260
    Trichomoniasis, 261
    Nonspecific Vaginitis, 261
    Atrophy or Senile Vaginitis, 261
Crabs, 261
Endometriosis, 261
Cervical Erosion, 261
Cystitis, 262
Cancer, 263
    Breast Cancer, 263
    Breast Self-Exam, 263
    Treatment of Breast Cancer, 264
    Cervical Cancer, 265
    Other Female Cancers, 265
The Gynecological Exam, 266
Dilation and Curettage (D & C), 267
Hysterectomy, 267
Section Four: How to Cope and Organize, 267
    Future Demands, 269
    Some New Beginnings, 270
    Appendix A: Preamble to the 1970 Accreditation
        Manual for Hospitals, 271
    Appendix B: Guidelines for NEIGHBORS, 273
Further Readings, 275

ILLUSTRATION CREDITS

(All are photo credits except as indicated.)

Preface

I

A GOOD STORY

The history of this book, *Our Bodies, Ourselves*, is lengthy and satisfying.

It began at a small discussion group on "women and their bodies" which was part of a women's conference held in Boston in the spring of 1969. These were the early days of the women's movement, one of the first gatherings of women meeting specifically to talk with other women. For many of us it was the very first time we got together with other women to talk and think about our lives and what we could do about them. Before the conference was over some of us decided to keep on meeting as a group to continue the discussion, and so we did.

In the beginning we called the group "the doctor's group." We had all experienced similar feelings of frustration and anger toward specific doctors and the medical maze in general, and initially we wanted to do something about those doctors who were condescending, paternalistic, judgmental and non-informative. As we talked and shared our experiences with one another, we realized just how much we had to learn about our bodies. So we decided on a summer project—to research those topics which we felt were particularly pertinent to learning about our bodies, to discuss in the group what we had learned, then to write papers individually or in small groups of two or three, and finally to present the results in the fall as a course for women on women and their bodies.

As we developed the course we realized more and more that we were really capable of collecting, understanding, and evaluating medical information. Together we evaluated our reading of books and journals, our talks with doctors and friends who were medical students. We found we could discuss, question and argue with each other in a new spirit of cooperation rather than competition. We were equally struck by how important it was for us to be able to open up with one another and share our feelings about our bodies. The process of talking was as crucial as the facts themselves. Over time the facts and feelings melted together in ways that touched us very deeply, and that is reflected in the changing titles of the course and then the book—from *Women and Their Bodies* to *Women and Our Bodies* to, finally, *Our Bodies, Ourselves*.

When we gave the course we met in any available free space we could get—in day schools, in nursery schools, in churches, in our homes. We expected the course to stimulate the same kind of talking and sharing that we who had prepared the course had experienced. We had something to say, but we had a lot to learn as well; we did not want a traditional teacher-student relationship. At the end of ten to twelve sessions—which roughly covered the material in the current book—we found that many women felt both eager and competent to get together in small groups and share what they had learned with other women. We saw it as a never-ending process always involving more and more women.

After the first teaching of the course, we decided to revise our initial papers and mimeograph them so that other women could have copies as the course expanded. Eventually we got them printed and bound together in an inexpensive edition published by the New England Free Press. It was fascinating and very exciting for us to see what a constant demand there was for our book. It came out in several editions, a larger number being printed each time, and the time from one printing to the next becoming shorter. The growing volume of requests began to strain the staff of the New England Free Press.* Since our book was clearly speaking to many people, we wanted to reach beyond the audience who lived in the area or who were acquainted with the New England Free Press. For wider distribution it made sense to publish our book commercially.

You may want to know who we are. We are white, our ages range from 24 to 40, most of us are from middle-class backgrounds and have had at least some college education, and some of us have professional degrees. Some of us are married, some of us are separated, and

*New England Free Press publications cover a wide range of topics. Contact them for a free literature list at 791 Tremont Street, Boston, Mass. 02118.

some of us are single. Some of us have children of our own, some of us like spending time with children, and others of us are not sure we want to be with children. In short, we are both a very ordinary and a very special group, as women are everywhere. We are white middle-class women, and as such can describe only what life has been for us. But we do realize that poor women and non-white women have suffered far more from the kinds of misinformation and mistreatment that we are describing in this book. In some ways, learning about our womanhood from the inside out has allowed us to cross over the socially created barriers of race, color, income and class, and to feel a sense of identity with all women in the experience of being female.

We are twelve individuals and we are a group. (The group has been ongoing for three years and some of us have been together since the beginning. Others came in at later points. Our current collective has been together for one year.) We know each other well—our weaknesses as well as our strengths. We have learned through good times and bad how to work together (and how not to as well). We recognize our similarities and differences and are learning to respect each person for her uniqueness. We love each other.

Many, many other women have worked with us on the book. A group of gay women got together specifically to do the chapter on lesbianism. Other papers were done still differently. For instance, along with some friends the mother of one woman in the group volunteered to work on menopause with some of us who have not gone through that experience ourselves. Other women contributed thoughts, feelings and comments as they passed through town or passed through our kitchens or work-rooms. There are still other voices from letters, phone conversations, a variety of discussions, etc., that are included in the chapters as excerpts of personal experiences. Many women have spoken for themselves in this book, though we in the collective do not agree with all that has been written. Some of us are even uncomfortable with part of the material. We have included it anyway, because we give more weight to accepting that we differ than to our uneasiness. We have been asked why this is exclusively a book about women, why we have restricted our course to women. Our answer is that we are women and, as women, do not consider ourselves experts on men (as men through the centuries have presumed to be experts on us). We are not implying that we think most twentieth-century men are much less alienated from their bodies than women are. But we know it is up to men to explore that for themselves, to come together and share their sense of themselves as we have done. We would like to read a book about men and their bodies.

We are offering a book that can be used in many dif-ferent ways—individually, in a group, for a course. Our book contains real material about our bodies and ourselves that isn't available elsewhere, and we have tried to present it in a new way—an honest, humane, and powerful way of thinking about ourselves and our lives. We want to share the knowledge and power that comes with this way of thinking and we want to share the feelings we have for each other—supportive and loving feelings that show we can indeed help one another grow.

From the very beginning of working together, first on the course that led to this book and then on the book itself, we have felt exhilarated and energized by our new knowledge. Finding out about our bodies and our bodies' needs, starting to take control over that area of our life, has released for us an energy that has overflowed into our work, our friendships, our relationships with men and women, for some of us our marriages and our parenthood. In trying to figure out why this has had such a life-changing effect on us, we have come up with several important ways in which this kind of body education has been liberating for us and may be a starting point for the liberation of many other women.

First, we learned what we learned equally from professional sources—textbooks, medical journals, doctors, nurses—and from our own experiences. The facts were important, and we did careful research to get the information we had not had in the past. As we brought the facts to one another we learned a good deal, but in sharing our personal experiences relating to those facts we learned still more. Once we had learned what the "experts" had to tell us, we found that we still had a lot to teach and to learn from one another. For instance, many of us had "learned" about the menstrual cycle in science or biology classes—we had perhaps even memorized the names of the menstrual hormones and what they did. But most of us did not remember much of what we had learned. This time when we read in a text that the onset of menstruation is a normal and universal occurrence in young girls from ages ten to eighteen, we started to talk about our first menstrual periods. We found that, for many of us, beginning to menstruate had not felt normal at all, but scary, embarrassing, mysterious. We realized that what we had been told about menstruation and what we had not been told, even the tone of voice it had been told in—all had had an effect on our feelings about being female. Similarly, the information from enlightened texts describing masturbation as a normal, common sexual activity did not really become our own until we began to pull up from inside ourselves and share what we had never before expressed—the confusion and shame we had been made to feel, and often still felt, about touching our bodies in a sexual way.

Learning about our bodies in this way really turned

us on. This is an exciting kind of learning, where information and feelings are allowed to interact. It has made the difference between rote memorization and relevant learning, between fragmented pieces of a puzzle and the integrated picture, between abstractions and real knowledge. We discovered that you don't learn very much when you are just a passive recipient of information. We found that each individual's response to information is valid and useful, and that by sharing our responses we can develop a base on which to be critical of what the experts tell us. Whatever we need to learn now, in whatever area of our life, we know more how to go about it.

A second important result of this kind of learning has been that we are better prepared to evaluate the institutions that are supposed to meet our health needs—the hospitals, clinics, doctors, medical schools, nursing schools, public health departments, Medicaid bureaucracies, and so on. For some of us it was the first time we had looked critically, and with strength, at the existing institutions serving us. The experience of learning just how little control we had over our lives and bodies, the coming together out of isolation to learn from each other in order to define what we needed, and the experience of supporting one another in demanding the changes that grew out of our developing critique—all were crucial and formative political experiences for us. We have felt our potential power as a force for political and social change.

The learning we have done while working on *Our Bodies, Ourselves* has been such a good basis for growth in other areas of life for still another reason. For women throughout the centuries, ignorance about our bodies has had one major consequence—pregnancy. Until very recently pregnancies were all but inevitable, biology *was* our destiny—that is, because our bodies are designed to get pregnant and give birth and lactate, that is what all or most of us did. The courageous and dedicated work of people like Margaret Sanger started in the early twentieth century to spread and make available birth control methods that women could use, thereby freeing us from the traditional lifetime of pregnancies. But the societal expectation that a woman above all else will have babies does not die easily. When we first started talking to each other about this we found that that old expectation had nudged most of us into a fairly rigid role of wife-and-motherhood from the moment we were born female. Even in 1969 when we first started the work that led to this book, we found that many of us were still getting pregnant when we didn't want to. It was not until we researched carefully and learned more about our reproductive systems, about birth-control methods and abortion, about laws governing birth control and abortion,

not until we put all this information together with what it meant to us to be female, did we begin to feel that we could truly set out to control whether and when we would have babies.

This knowledge has freed us to a certain extent from the constant, energy-draining anxiety about becoming pregnant. It has made our pregnancies better, because they no longer happen to us; we actively choose them and enthusiastically participate in them. It has made our parenthood better, because it is our choice rather than our destiny. This knowledge has freed us from playing the role of mother if it is not a role that fits us. It has given us a sense of a larger life space to work in, an invigorating and challenging sense of time and room to discover the energies and talents that are in us, to do the work we want to do. And one of the things we most want to do is to help make this freedom of choice, this life space, available to every woman. That is why people in the women's movement have been so active in fighting against the inhumane legal restrictions, the imperfections of available contraceptives, the poor sex education, the highly priced and poorly administered health care that keeps too many women from having this crucial control over their bodies.

There is a fourth reason why knowledge about our bodies has generated so much new energy. For us, body education is core education. Our bodies are the physical bases from which we move out into the world; ignorance, uncertainty—even, at worst, shame—about our physical selves create in us an alienation from ourselves that keeps us from being the whole people that we could be. Picture a woman trying to do work and to enter into equal and satisfying relationships with other people—when she feels physically weak because she has never tried to be strong; when she drains her energy trying to change her face, her figure, her hair, her smells, to match some ideal norm set by magazines, movies, and TV; when she feels confused and ashamed of the menstrual blood that every month appears from some dark place in her body; when her internal body processes are a mystery to her and surface only to cause her trouble (an unplanned pregnancy, or cervical cancer); when she does not understand nor enjoy sex and concentrates her sexual drives into aimless romantic fantasies, perverting and misusing a potential energy because she has been brought up to deny it. Learning to understand, accept, and be responsible for our physical selves, we are freed of some of these preoccupations and can start to use our untapped energies. Our image of ourselves is on a firmer base, we can be better friends and better lovers, better *people,* more self-confident, more autonomous, stronger, and more whole.

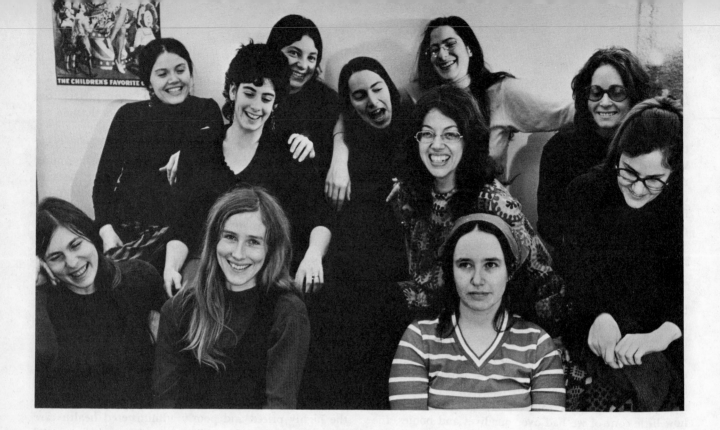

II

OUR FACES BELONG TO OUR BODIES*

Our faces belong to our bodies.
Our faces belong to our lives.

Our faces are blunted.
Our bodies are stunted.
We cover our anger with smiles.

Our faces belong to our bodies.
Our faces belong to our lives.

Our anger is changing our faces, our bodies.
Our anger is changing our lives.

Women who scrub have strong faces
Women who type have strong faces
Women with children have strong faces
Women who love have strong faces
Women who laugh have strong faces

Women who fight have strong faces
Women who cry have strong faces
Women who die have strong faces.

Our love is changing our faces, our bodies.
Our love is changing our lives.

Our sisters are changing our faces, our bodies.
Our sisters are changing our lives.

Our anger is changing our faces, our bodies.
Our anger is changing our lives.

Our power is changing our faces, our bodies.
Our power is changing our lives.

Our struggle is changing our faces, our bodies.
Our struggle is changing our lives.

*Please use this song only with permission of the It's All Right
to Be a Woman Theatre, 318 West 101 Street, New York, New York
10025.

1
Our Changing Sense of Self

THIS book was written by many women. Those responsible for seeing its completion form the Boston Women's Health Book Collective. This, in part, is who we are: we are in our mid-twenties and early thirties, mostly married or in (or have been in) some long-term relationship with a man. Some of us have had children recently. We are college educated (some of us have gone to graduate school), and all of us have spent a number of years living away from home either with female roommates, with men, alone, or in some varying combination. We have worked or are working. Most of us feel that unlike what we were promised in childhood, we were not totally fulfilled by marriage (a man), and/or motherhood (a child), and/or a (typically feminine) job. This is not to say that we have not grown a lot within marriages and with our children or in our work. Most of us see these relationships as continuing. But just being wife or wife and mother and viewing our work as secondary was too limiting for us. We needed space to do our own work or find out what work we wanted to do. We also needed space to discover who we were separate from these primary relationships so that we could become autonomous adult people as well as have important relationships with others.

We can talk only for ourselves, although we consider ourselves part of a larger movement of women in the Boston area—a group of great variety. We realize that the development of the ideas presented in this book comes from many women we know from other women's collectives as well as our own.

Coming together with women was exciting. We were individual women coming together out of choice and strength. Since we had patterned and focused much of our life around men, this was liberating. It was also liberating because we were legitimizing our need for one another. Most of us had gone to college, had lived with women, and so had had close female friendships with women, but viewed this as a transitional stage leading up to a male-centered life. That was the traditional pattern, and that is what we expected of our lives. We felt that as young adult women we had missed close female friendships. Traditionally, the extended family provided close female contacts—women in unself-conscious ways providing support, sharing experience and wisdom with each other. Most of us were not living in cities where our families lived, and needed to create for ourselves a place and occasion for women to come together.

Coming together to do something about our lives was scary. It was admitting that we were not completely satisfied with the lives we were leading. We knew we would be standing back and taking a hard look at ourselves, and this aroused anxiety, fear of the unknown. Some of us fantasized that commitment to the women's movement and pressure from the group would weaken our ties with our men, children, jobs, life styles—we would lose control over our lives. We came to realize that this fear was unrealistic. No one could take from us what we did not want to give up. We were coming together out of choice. Our hope was to come to feel ourselves to be fuller, more integrated female persons.

Like most early women's groups, we talked to each other about what life was like for us, growing up female. The underlying purpose of this introspection and analysis of our past was to have some basis to figure out how we wanted to change the ways we thought and felt about ourselves. We could act on this new sense of self in our lives to create a broader sense of what it means to be female. To do this very personal work we made an accepting environment for ourselves—a place where we could talk and work together and think out loud. Probably the most valuable learning for each of us was learning to feel good about speaking for ourselves and being ourselves.

At first we feared disclosing personal information. We

each thought we might be ridiculed, rejected, misunderstood, gossiped about by the others. Many of us were friends before the group began and we were shy about getting into personal discussions about our relationships with men. Our fears of other women were exaggerated. We turned out to have a lot in common as women. And as we related to each other in more direct and honest ways, more genuine relationships were possible. On the other hand, we found it takes a long time to feel comfortable and trusting in a group. If we do not feel comfortable and trusting, there is probably some basis for it.

We also feared rejecting each other. We would see traits in others we did not want to see in ourselves, which were different from our own or which we did not like. We realized that as women we had been raised to be nice to everyone, to please everyone, and that we had not allowed ourselves to experience ambivalent feelings about ourselves and others. Facing this allowed us to be more honest with ourselves and others.

One thing that came out in talking together about growing up was that most of us felt we had spent a lot of time and energy in inner conflict during adolescence —trying to become selfless, sweet, passive, dependent children so that our princes would find us and we would live happily ever after. By the end of adolescence most of us had resolved the conflict by learning to conform to the feminine role, while suppressing qualities within

us inappropriate to that role—independence, activity, anger and pride. These human qualities which would have got in the way of our "femininity" were, logically enough, labeled by our culture "male."

From our beginning conversations with each other we discovered four cultural notions of femininity which we had in some sense shared: woman as inferior, woman as passive, woman as beautiful object, woman as exclusively wife and mother. In our first discussions we discovered how severely those notions had constricted us, how humanly limited we felt at being passive, dependent creatures with no identities of our own. As time passed, with each other's support we began to rediscover ourselves. The passion with which we did this came from getting in touch with human qualities in ourselves that had been taboo.

We all went through a time when we rejected our old selves and took on the new qualities exclusively. For a while we became distortions, angry all the time or fiercely independent. It was as though we had partly new selves and we had to find out what they were like. But ultimately we came to realize that rejecting our "feminine" qualities was simply another way of going along with our culture's sexist values. So with our new energy came a desire to assert and reclaim that which is ours.

In no way do we want to become men. We are women and we are proud of being women. What we do want to do is reclaim the human qualities culturally labeled "male" and integrate them with the human qualities that have been seen as "female" so that we can all be fuller human people. This should also have the effect of freeing men from the pressure of being masculine at all times—a role as equally limiting as ours has been. We want, in short, to create a cultural environment where all qualities can come out in all people.

Changing Our Internalized Sexist Values

When we started talking to each other we came to realize how deeply ingrained was our sense of being less valuable than men.

* * *

In my home I always had a sense that my father and brother were more important than my mother and myself. My mother and I shopped, talked to each other, and had friends over—this was considered silly. My father was considered more important—he did the real work of the world.

* * *

In my home I got a complicated message. On the one hand I was told I was as important and as competent as men. In other ways I was told this was not true. Money was set aside for my brother to go to college but not for me.

* * *

In school we learned that we were expected to do well, but our real vocation was to be wife and mother. Boys were being trained for the important work in society. We learned that what our culture labeled important work was not for us, and what we did was not seen as important.

* * *

I wanted to be a doctor, but I was told in direct and indirect ways that my ultimate ambition should be marrying a doctor and raising a family. I gave up my dream.

* * *

I wanted to be an elementary school teacher, mostly because I had hated going to elementary school and I wanted to make it better for others. Although at first I thought this was important work, I learned not to value it because it was considered second-rate in this culture.

* * *

The few of us who did *not* stay out of "male" work suffered the consequences. We had to choose between being a "brain" or being a woman.

* * *

For me the evidence of my mental competence was unavoidable, and I never had any trouble defending or voicing my opinion with men, because I beat them in all the tests. Consequently, none of them would come near me in my first seventeen years of life.

* * *

It was as if to be considered women we had to keep in our inferior place. If we challenged this we were treated badly and came to think of ourselves in negative ways.

Our learned sense of inferiority affected the way we thought about our bodies—our physical selves.

* * *

I remember coming home from high school every day and going over my body from head to toe. My forehead was too high, my hair too straight, my body too short, my teeth too yellow, and so on.

* * *

And when we evaluated our present situations we found that we still thought in sexist terms. Among our male peers we always found ourselves valuing what men said over what we said, and what men did over what we did.

* * *

Every time my husband has free time he sits down and reads a book. We both have a sense that that is really important. When I have free time I sit and crochet or read, and it feels as if I am doing nothing.

* * *

I genuinely enjoy loving and raising kids and setting up a home, but I have always felt that it was not important.

* * *

I have a lot of talents. I like to paint, dance, and am sensitive to people and their needs, but whenever I demonstrate this I think, Anyone could do this.

* * *

I look at the way we have divided up the space in our house. My husband has a little space that is considered his own, and I have no space that is mine. It is as if I exist everywhere and nowhere.

* * *

We lived our lives as if there was something intrinsically inferior about us.

What was exciting through all this talking together was learning that what each of us had thought was a personal sense of inferiority was in fact shared by many women. This reflected a larger cultural problem: that power is unequally distributed in our society; men, having the power, are considered superior and we, having less power, are considered inferior. What we have to change are the power relationships between the sexes, so that each sex has equal power and people's qualities can be judged on their own merits rather than in terms of power. Although this problem is not easily solvable, at least the situation is changeable, since it is not based on biological facts. We know we will feel daily tension in recognizing the gap between our ideology and the realities of our everyday life caused by our resistance to change, male resistance, and external social structures not supportive of our ideology. Still, we have a direction we want to move in.

We looked at our present lives and realized how we were perpetuating unequal power relationships between ourselves and men. Many of the instances, which are numerous, are explored in this book. We never expected enough time and pleasure in sex, we never respected the questions we asked our doctors, we never expected men to adjust their lives to parenthood as we bore the child for both of us, we never expected men to take on some of the worry about birth control, we didn't take care of our bodies as if they/we mattered, we never respected the support and comfort other women gave us when we needed it. The list is endless. We began to see our relationships with ourselves, men, other women, and the social institutions in this country in a new way. To be able to see and feel the strength, beauty and potential in women was exhilarating. We began to feel prouder and prouder of ourselves.

We started considering what we had thought of as our weaknesses as our strengths. At the same time we were trying to become separate people. We began to really appreciate our capacity to empathize, to nurture, to be passive, and to be dependent. By empathy we mean the ability to identify emotionally with other people and be sensitive to what their life events mean to them. Although this can be bad for us if we only identify with others and have no sense of self, this capacity of ours is valuable and ours to use when we choose. By nurturing we mean taking care of the emotional and physical needs of others—maintaining life. Although in the past we only maintained life and depended on men to do and act and build, this capacity to maintain life is valuable and ours to use. By passivity we mean the ability to sit back. Although in our past we were passive and not able to act when we wanted, now we realize that we can act, but it is nice to choose not to at times. By dependency we mean the capacity to depend on and rely on another person. Previously we had had no sense of self and *had* to depend on someone else. Now we can choose to be dependent, and we see this as a strength, because intimate relationships are dependent relationships. The list could go on. We are really coming to enjoy our talents and our abilities, who we are and what we do.

Still, as we grow and change we discover things about ourselves that we don't like—our limitations, our imperfectness, our mistakes—but we realize that these do not reflect our inferiority, but are part of being human. We are learning to tolerate parts of ourselves that we don't like and build on what we do.

Rediscovering Activity

Talking to each other, we realized that many of us shared a common perception of men—that they all seemed to be able to turn themselves on and to do things for themselves. We tended to feel passive and helpless and to expect and need men to do things for us. We were trained to give our power over to men. We had reduced ourselves to objects. We remained children, helpless and giving other people power to define us and objectify us.

As we talked together we realized that one of our central fantasies was our wish to find a man who could turn us on, to do for us what we could not do for ourselves, to make us feel alive and affirm our existence. It was as if we were made of clay and man would mold us, shape us, and bring us to life. This was the material of our childhood dreams: "Someday my prince will come." We were always disappointed when men did not accomplish this impossible task for us. And we began to see our passive helpless ways of handing power over to others as crippling to us. What became clear to us was that we had to change our expectations for ourselves. There was no factual reason why we could not assert and affirm our own existence and do and act for ourselves.

There were many factors that affected our capacity to act. For one, the ideal woman does less and less as her class status rises. Most of us, being middle-class, were brought up not to do very much. Also, the kind of activity that is built into the traditional female role is different in quality from masculine activity. Masculine activity (repairing a window, building a house) tends to be sporadic, concrete, and have a finished product. Feminine activity (comforting a crying child, preparing a meal, washing laundry) tends to be repetitive, less tangi-

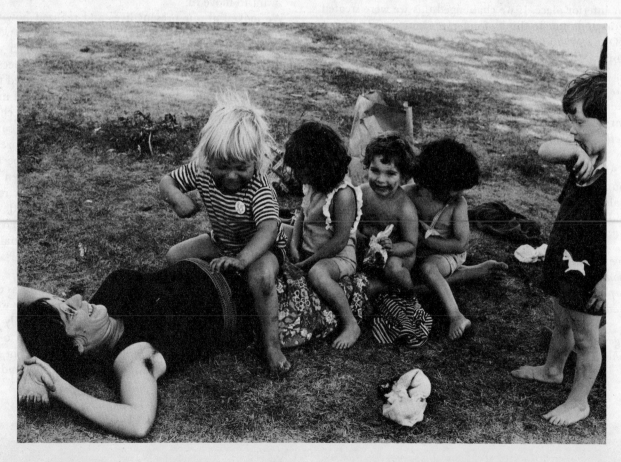

ble, and have no final durable product. Here again our sense of inferiority came into play. We had come to think of our activity as doing nothing—although essential for maintaining life—and of male activity as superior. We began to value our activity in a new way. We and what we did were as valuable as men and what they did.

On the other hand, we tried to incorporate within us the capacity to do more "male" product-oriented activity. Our motivation to write this book falls into that category. To be more specific: what began as conversation was translated into written papers, was extended into a course based on informal discussion and the presentation of some of the material we had learned, and culminated in the publishing of our papers as a book. During this slow evolution we became more and more motivated to work hard on our ideas—to refine them, to clarify them, and to present them in a form that would be accessible to other women. This sustained work on a tangible product is exciting to us. But throughout this process we have in no way sacrificed the quality of our relationships with each other, as men often do when they work together. We have genuinely collaborated with each other, which meant having good communication as we worked together. We devised our own form of working and doing within the social context we created.

Along with our more task-oriented activity comes a new sense of wanting to succeed. By wanting to succeed we mean getting recognition for what we do. By success we also mean an inner sense of having done something well. This ties in with our new sense of pride—feeling proud of what we do.

This is new for us. As women we have been taught to want to fail, or if not to fail, to walk a fine line between success and failure. We were never encouraged to use the full strength of ourselves. This new motivation to do and do things well is more risky. It involves taking and accepting responsibility because others are counting on us to come through with what we can do.

* * *

I am aware that I am responsible to other human beings —my parents, my husband, my children, my friends. What greater responsibility is there?

* * *

It also means that we have to maintain a rather consistent performance, according to our own standards. It also involves the strength to stand up for ourselves and what we can do while realizing that others may reject what we do, do it differently, or put us down. Still, it is worth these risks, because these are the risks of living.

With our new sense of strength and activity comes a new sense that it is all right to be passive as long as we choose to be.

* * *

In lovemaking I have come to take great pleasure in taking a passive role as long as I actively choose it. I also know that I can be active. It is wonderful to know there is time to both give and receive love and caresses.

* * *

We have also come to enjoy physical activity as well as mental and emotional activity. Again, the realm of physical strength is traditionally male. Once again we realized that we were active in our own ways, but we did not value them. As we looked at the details of our lives— the shopping and the cleaning—we realized that we used up a lot of physical energy every day but that we had taken it for granted and thought of it as nothing. We did avoid heavy, strenuous activity.

* * *

I thought that girls did not have to be physically strong. They could do everything they needed with their heads. The fact is that some mental work involves a back-up of physical strength. For example, engineers and architects can become more experienced in their trades if they are physically able and have the strength and stamina to build machines and structures. I now feel that all desirable qualities and abilities are neither male nor female, but rather human, and I am trying to get the most out of my body, mind, and feelings.

* * *

We are learning to do new things—mountain climbing, canoeing, karate, auto mechanics.

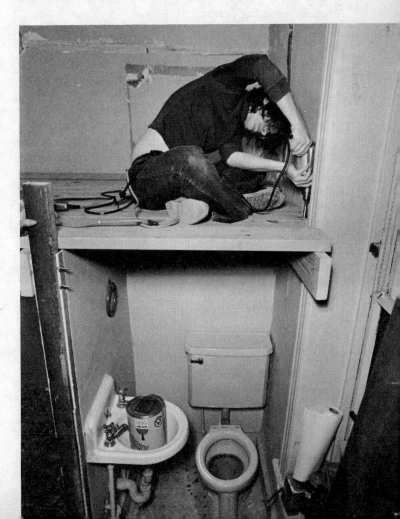

Rediscovering Anger

As we were changing we found we were frequently feeling angry. This surprised us and embarrassed us. We had grown up feeling that we needed to love everyone and be loved by everyone. If we got angry at someone, or they at us, we felt in some sense that we were failures.

We shared memories of our pasts. Nearly all of us had had a hard time expressing anger verbally or physically.

* * *

In my family my mother expressed love and my father spanked me. My mother was super-uncritical of me and my father hypercritical. I learned that women are never disapproving or angry.

* * *

I have very few memories of fighting. Each time I did I felt guilty and embarrassed.

* * *

We did fight a lot at home, but I never made a public display of any anger or aggression. That was unladylike.

* * *

We shared perceptions of our current situations.

* * *

My husband has this habit of not listening to me when I talk. I get angry at him, but I don't tell him.

* * *

I seem to put up with a lot of nonsense from people. It is as if I am always being the accepting, forgiving, and accommodating person.

* * *

We began to admit that we had felt angry during our lives, but we had been using the anger against ourselves in hating ourselves. There were many ways we had learned to cover up our anger. It had built up for so long inside us that we were afraid we would explode if we let it out. We have come to realize that there are many aspects of our lives and our relationships that make us angry. Until we know and feel our own oppression we are not motivated to try to create constructive alternative ways of being and living. Many have accused us of being shrill. Our mood is far more complex. Our critics hear only the anger, and anger separated from real issues is a distortion. The anger that is in us is a starting point for creative change and growth.

Rediscovering Our Separateness

In our early discussions it became clear that we did not really feel ourselves to be separate, independent people. The men in our lives embodied or felt they were supposed to embody, freedom and independence. The women in our lives stayed at home, needed company, and were always dependent on those near them. They embodied, or felt they should, dependency, need and connection. As we talked to each other we realized that as children and even as young adults we had never thought it would be possible to live without someone else, particularily a man. We trembled at the thought of being alone. But we realized that we were no longer powerless, helpless children. We realized that we could survive on our own and that until we felt confident of our ability to feel like separate people and take on the freedom and responsibility of being adults, we were not free to live with another out of choice. We wanted our coming together with another to result from choice and joy and not fear and necessity.

This is not to say that we do not seek relationships out of need and loneliness as well. Some of us who are married have tried to develop the capacity to feel like separate persons within the context of the marriage. Others of us in marriage or long-term relationships have decided to end the relationships or separate. Those of us who were not involved in relationships built up our own strengths. Each of us found her own way to become a separate person. The point was not that one way was better than another, but that it was freely chosen.

During this period of building up our own sense of ourselves we tried to find out what we were like on our own, what we could do on our own. We discovered resources we never thought we had. Either because we had been dependent on men to do certain things for us or because we had been so used to thinking of ourselves as helpless and dependent, we had never tried.

It is hard. We are forever fighting a constant, inner struggle to give up and become weak, dependent, and helpless again.

* * *

I started making batiks again and have become very seriously involved in this craft. It still surprises me that I can create something other than a child. Each time I complete one by myself I feel alone and trembling. Also, each time I have to fight inner voices saying, You are not going to do it.

* * *

I went with other women on a trip south almost two years ago. That was the first time I had gone on a trip without my husband. Several things went wrong with the car on the trip. When I came back to Boston I decided that I really wanted to learn how to take care and be in control of a car myself. I learned about auto mechanics. It required a lot of work and discipline. In a way I identify with the car. There is a connection between my feelings of wanting to take care and control of my life and the feelings of wanting to take care and control of my car.

* * *

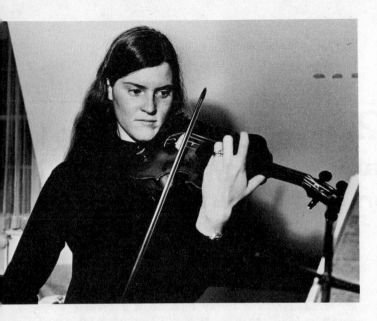

It feels so good not to have to walk around all the time worrying about what my husband, friends, other people are thinking about me.

* * *

Although during the last five years of marriage I have worked in a variety of jobs, my major commitment is to teaching and teacher training. Although I got great pleasure from this work, I never acknowledged to myself that throughout my life I wanted some work that is my own. I have come to realize that in my marriage my husband and I need separate time and space for ourselves to do our own work as well as time to be together. This would be more complicated if we had children.

* * *

My husband and son have always been important to me, but I found that when my son was a few months old I was feeling unfocused and had low energy a lot of the time and was very unself-confident in relating to people outside my family. I joined with some friends who felt the same way and started a play group (cooperative child care) and began to learn to be a birth-control counselor. Over the past two years I have found the energy and talent to do this work, and the good people I work with have affirmed me as a person and a counselor. When I am home I am glad to be there. I still feel some conflict between my home-family self and my work self. But hard as it is sometimes, I do not want to give up one for the other.

* * *

As we have come to feel separate we try to change old relationships and/or try to enter new relationships in new ways. We now also feel positive about our needs to be dependent and connect with others. We have come to value long-term commitments, which we find increasingly rare in such a changing society, just as we value our new separateness.

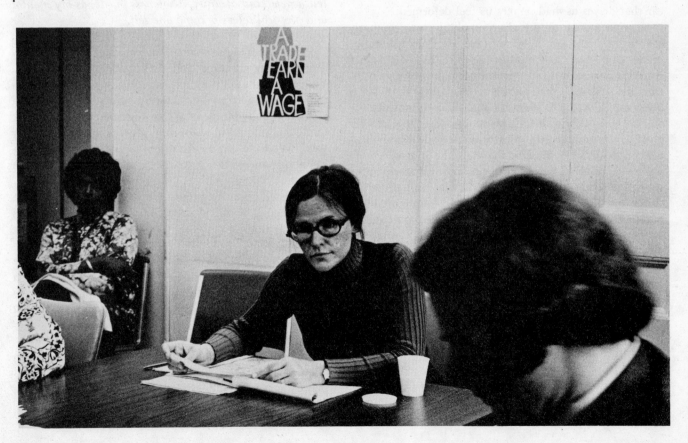

2
The Anatomy and Physiology of Reproduction and Sexuality

OUR FEELINGS

Our feelings about our anatomy have often been very negative. Our hair is too straight or too curly, our noses too small or too large, our breasts too big or too small. We don't like our body hair or body odors. Our stomachs are too fat. We are too bony. Our genitals—well, we just try to ignore those parts (our "privates"). They are slightly smutty and unmentionable. And there are those tiny things too, like the mole two inches below the left ear that drives us mad, makes us feel deformed.

In other words, we are always making some comparison, we're never okay the way we are. We feel ugly, inadequate. And it's no wonder! The ideal woman in America is something very specific. She may change over time (for instance, small breasts are "in" these days, large ones "out"), yet there is always something to measure up to. We are "down" and have to measure "up" to be good. Unfortunately, this ideal is not *our* ideal, not what *we* created. It's the ideal of the men, the judges, whom we are supposed to please and win approval from. Family, friends, school, church, TV, movies all tell us to fulfill this image, to blend together and hide our differences. There is little encouragement to love our bodies as they are.

Sometimes it's hard to like our bodies, because we feel so far away from our physical selves. As we grow up we are taught to relate more to our minds ("be smart," "use your head," "mind over matter") than our bodies. We are supposed to think rationally and not respond to feelings.

* * *

Having my first child was the first experience in my life in which I felt my physical being was as important as
my mind. I related to my total body. I became very unself-conscious. I felt my body as a fantastic machine!

* * *

Taking yoga was like opening up a whole new world to me. I became aware of parts of my body that I didn't feel existed and conscious that those parts were made of many other parts. I also discovered mental and physical processes working together. I realized that my scalp began to hurt when I thought too much, and could consciously begin to focus on relaxing those muscles. Gradually I felt a new kind of unity, wholeness in me, as my mental and physical selves became one self.

* * *

Experiences in the women's movement have drastically changed our thinking and feelings about our bodies. We've shared such common experiences as going to doctors and not getting satisfactory medical advice about a particular body problem. We've described to one another the ways in which we've felt physically and sexually weak. We have given each other support to begin learning about our bodies so that we could act to make some changes.

Until we began to prepare this material for a course for women many of us didn't know the names of parts of our anatomy.

* * *

The first month I was at college some of my friends were twittering about a girl down the hall. She was having a painful time trying to learn to put in a tampon. Finally someone helped her and found she was trying to put it in her anus.

* * *

Some of us had learned bits and pieces of information about specific body functions (menstruation, for example), but it was not permissible to find out too much.

12

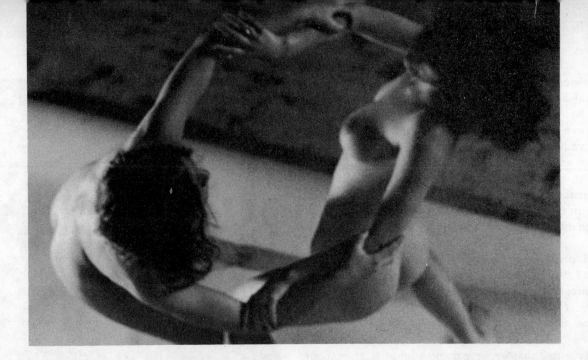

The taboos were strongest in the areas of reproduction and sex, which is why our course and our book concentrate on them.

Four of us were working on the anatomy chapter one morning. We developed an outline, filled in a lot of the details: menstruation; naming parts of our anatomy, especially genitals. In preparation for this section, we discussed how we were feeling about our bodies. Then a marvelous thing happened. We had been sitting, talking, and thinking for an hour or so. We were feeling stiff. One woman said, "Hey, let's do some exercises together, let's use our bodies." We went into the next room, showed each other our favorite exercises, did some mime, exercises, gave each other back rubs. . . . The anatomy paper was complete for the day!

It will take time to become more aware, to use our bodies better. (For more on strengthening our bodies see the chapter, "Women in Motion.") A growing confidence in our ability to change and our growing awareness of new feelings is flowing through us. Knowing that we're coming to feel our bodies as ourselves feels great!

Finding Out About Ourselves

Knowing facts about our anatomy and physiology helps us to become more familiar with our bodies. Learning this information has been very exciting for us. It's exhilarating to discover that the material was not so difficult as we had first thought. Understanding the medical terminology now meant that we could understand the things the doctor said. Learning their language makes medical people become less mysterious and frightening. We now feel more confident when asking questions. Sometimes a doctor was startled to find us speaking "his" language. "How do you know that? Are you a medical student?" we heard again and again. "A pretty woman like you shouldn't be concerned about that."

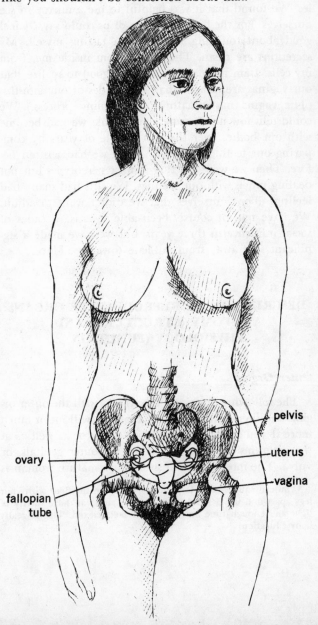

pelvis
uterus
vagina
ovary
fallopian tube

But we were. Out of our concerns we gained specific medical knowledge: names of body parts, bodily processes, how to recognize certain medical problems, when to go to a doctor and when we could handle a situation ourselves. Equally important, we were sharing our experiences with one another. From this sharing we developed an awareness of difference as well as similarity in our anatomy and physiology. We started to have confidence in our knowledge, and that confidence helped us change our feelings about ourselves.

* * *

I used to wonder if my body was abnormal even though I didn't have any reason to believe it was. I had nothing to compare it with until I started to talk with other women. I don't feel anymore that I might be a freak and not know it.

* * *

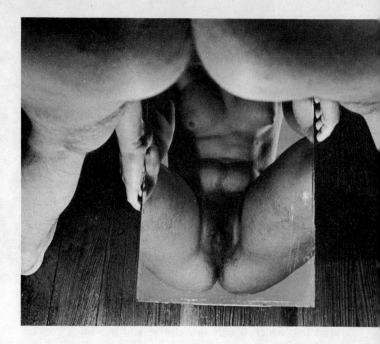

We realized that we were doing a lot of talking about our sexual organs but that we were not as familiar with their appearance as we were with other parts of our bodies. We found that it was helpful to use a mirror to see ourselves. For the first time some of us could say, "I feel good about touching myself, even tasting myself. My secretions are clean. They come from inside me, from my cells. I am not obscene." It was good to realize that our vaginas are cleaner than the insides of our mouths. (The vagina has a natural self-cleaning process.) We could tell how much more comfortable we had become with our bodies over the past couple of years by comparing our feelings now with what we had written before. Then we were reacting against stereotypes but not dealing much with our feelings. We still had many bad feelings about ourselves that we didn't want to admit. We have not, of course, been able to erase decades of social influence in three years, but we have made a significant step away from self-hate toward self-love.

DESCRIPTION OF REPRODUCTIVE ORGANS: ANATOMY (STRUCTURE) AND PHYSIOLOGY (FUNCTION)

Outer Organs

The following description deals first with the outer organs and then with the inner organs. It will mean much more if you look at yourself with a mirror as well as at the diagrams.* First you will see the outer genitals, or vulva. The most obvious feature on a mature woman is

*You can squat over a large mirror or sit on the floor with your legs apart and use a hand mirror. Make sure you have plenty of light and enough time and privacy to feel relaxed. This is really body education!

the pubic hair. This grows out of the pubis and the outer lips (labia majora). The pubis (mons veneris, or "mountain of Venus") is the rounded, fatty, hair-covered mass in front of the pubic symphysis. (The pubic bones are part of the hip girdle; the point at which one meets the other is called a symphysis.)

As you look more closely you will see the clitoris (klit'-or-is), a small organ of erectile tissue that plays an important role in every female orgasm. The clitoris can range in different women from less than $\frac{1}{4}$ inch to 1 inch in length. It is composed of shaft (from root to tip) and glans, just like its larger counterpart, the male penis

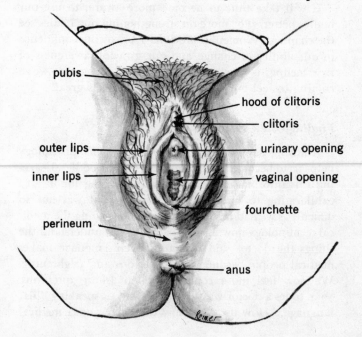

pubis

hood of clitoris

clitoris

outer lips

urinary opening

inner lips

vaginal opening

fourchette

perineum

anus

SOME HYMEN VARIATIONS

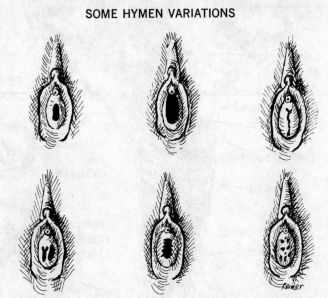

(the glans clitoridis is the tip of the clitoris, from the Latin *glans,* or "acorn"; the glans penis is the acorn-shaped tip of the penis). In a woman the shaft is hidden under a hood like the male foreskin, but the glans protrudes, looking like a small bump. The erectile tissue of the clitoris, like that of the penis, has hollow areas (corpora cavernosa) which, during sexual arousal, fill with blood, making the clitoris become stiff or erect. If you are not sure of the location of your clitoris, feel your genitals until you hit upon the most sensitive spot. This is pretty sure to be the clitoris, since it is richly supplied with nerves. Generally the outer organs have more nerve endings than the inner organs, which often respond only to strong pressure, if at all.*

The hood which covers the shaft of the clitoris is part of the inner lips (labia minora), which extend from the clitoris to frame the sides of the vaginal opening. The inner lips, composed partly of erectile tissue, become swollen during sexual arousal. The vestibule is the cleft between the inner lips which extends from the clitoris toward the anus, stopping at the perineum. It contains the urinary and vaginal openings (orifices). The urinary opening (urethral meatus), which is much smaller than the vaginal opening, is just between the clitoris and the vagina, and its position accounts for the occasional irritation felt when you urinate after extremely vigorous or prolonged intercourse. The vaginal opening is between the urinary opening and the perineum. The perineum, or perineal region, is the area between the vagina and the anus.

*For a discussion of the history of society's attitude toward the clitoris we refer you to Ruth and Edward Brecher's excellent summary of the Masters and Johnson findings: *An Analysis of Human Sexual Response.*

The hymen ("cherry," "maidenhead") is seen in a virgin as a thin fold of membrane situated at the vaginal opening. Normally it has some openings; it rarely completely blocks the vaginal opening. The hymen may be entirely absent even in a virgin; however, when present, it can have one of many shapes and degrees of thickness. There are little folds of tissue that remain after it has been broken or stretched.

Inner Organs

Bartholin's glands are two small, rounded bodies on either side of the vaginal opening, in contact with the posterior end of the inner lips. They are not easy to see. They produce mucous but contribute very little to vaginal lubrication during intercourse, although this function has been commonly attributed to them in the past. Bartholin's glands are important to know about because they occasionally become infected.

The vagina (frequently called the birth canal) extends inward from the outer genitals up beyond the cervix toward the small of the back. The part beyond the cervix, sometimes as much as one-third of the vagina, is called the fornix. The vagina lies between the bladder and the rectum at a 45-degree angle to the floor when you are standing. It is like a flexible tube with the walls ordinarily in contact; its volume is potential, not actual. Women are not a series of holes. The length of the relaxed vagina averages three and a half inches, but is capable of considerable stretching. This elasticity of the vaginal skin is due to the folds, which flatten out as the vagina expands in intercourse or childbirth.* When you

*There is an illustration of this elasticity on p. 185 of the "Childbearing" chapter.

FEMALE REPRODUCTIVE
ORGANS
(SIDE VIEW)

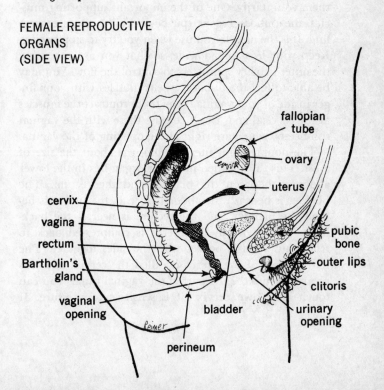

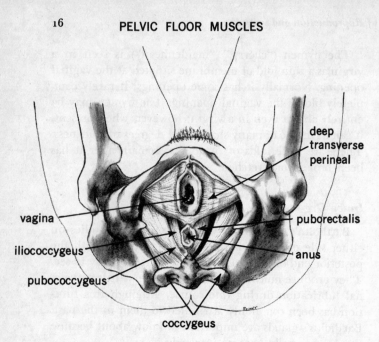

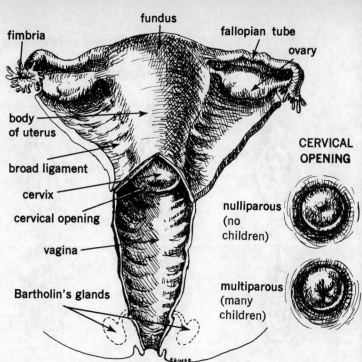

feel your own vagina with your fingers you can also tell that the outer third is sensitive when you touch it. The rest of the vagina has almost no nerve endings.

Surrounding the vagina, urethra, and anus is a series of muscles called the pelvic floor muscles. These muscles are important for supporting the lower organs. If these muscles are weak, are stretched unduly, or are cut during an improperly done episiotomy (see "Childbearing" chapter), complications such as a rectocele (lower colon falling into the vagina), cystocele (bladder falling into the vagina), prolapsed uterus (uterus falling into the vagina), or urinary incontinence (uncontrollable urinating) can eventually occur. These complications are often corrected surgically, but could probably be prevented by knowing where the muscles are and strengthening them by contracting them voluntarily. One of the important supporting muscles, the pubococcygeus (pū'-bō-cock-sij'-ē-us), is easy to find. It is the muscle you use when you try to stop peeing. Keep your legs spread wide, so that you are not using the outer urinary sphincters to control the flow. You may be able to feel the pubococcygeus muscles with your finger inside of your vagina if you try to contract the muscles at the cervical end. Don't confuse these with the vaginal sphincters, which are right at the opening of the vagina.

The nonpregnant uterus (womb) is about the size of a fist. This thick-walled muscular organ lies in the lower abdomen between the bladder and the rectum. The bladder is beneath the abdominal wall, the uterus is behind the bladder, and the rectum is nearest the backbone. The cavity of the uterus is compressed back to front into a small pocket with the sides together. The narrow part of the uterus is called the cervix, and this protrudes into the top part of the vaginal canal. You can touch your own cervix. It is sensitive to pressure. If

you've never had a baby, it feels like the end of your nose with a small dimple (entrance to uterus) in its center. If you've had a baby it may feel more like a chin. The uterus changes position during the menstrual cycle, so the place where you feel the cervix one day may be slightly different from the place where you feel it the next. Some days you can barely reach it, so you won't always be able to feel the dimple. The entrance into the uterus through the cervix is very small, about the diameter of a very thin straw, and is called the *os*.

Extending outward and back from the sides of the upper end of the uterus are the two fallopian tubes (oviducts, literally "egg tubes"). They look like four-inch (approximately) ram's horns facing backward. The opening from the inside of the uterus to the fallopian tube is so small that only a fine needle can penetrate it. The other end of the tube is fimbriated (fringed) and funnel-shaped. The wide end of the funnel wraps part way around the ovary but does not actually connect to it.

The ovaries are organs about the size and shape of unshelled almonds, located on either side and somewhat behind the uterus. They are held in place by connecting tissue and are protected by a surrounding mass of fat. They have a twofold function: to produce germ cells (eggs) and to produce female sex hormones (estrogen and progesterone). The small gap between the ovary and the end of the corresponding tube allows the egg to float freely after it bursts from the ovary. The fingerlike ends of the fallopian tube move to set up currents which wave the egg into the tube. In rare cases when the egg is not "caught" by the tube, it can be fertilized outside the tube, resulting in an abdominal pregnancy. (See ectopic pregnancy appendix to "Childbearing" chapter for more on this.)

Schematic Description

If you have difficulty visualizing your organs, think of them in terms of familiar objects about the same size and shape. Imagine your vagina to be a cardboard tube from a toilet-paper roll. The sides are squashed together. Coming into that at right angles two-thirds or more of the way from the "front" is an upside-down pear. The part sticking into the tube is the cervix. The rest is the body of the uterus. From each side of the pear come short lengths of telephone cord (fallopian tubes) which end in unshelled almonds (ovaries). Of course the body has muscles, ligaments and other connecting tissues to hold the organs in place in relation to other parts of the body.

Development of Sexual Organs

Men and women seem to be very different, but in fact many of their reproductive organs are similar in origin, developing from the same embryonic tissue (homologous), and are similar in function (analogous).

Organ	Homologous	Analogous
ovaries/testes	X	X
labia majora/scrotum	X	
clitoris/penis	X	X
bulb of the vestibule/bulb of corpus spongiosum	X	X
Bartholin's glands/bulbourethral glands (Cowper's glands)	X	X

The embryonic gonad (sex gland) is "indifferent"; that is, it will become male or female depending on the chromosomes and hormones present during fetal development.

MALE REPRODUCTIVE ORGANS

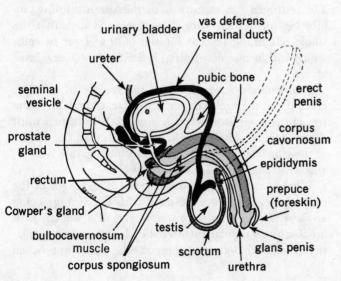

STAGES IN THE REPRODUCTIVE CYCLE

In childhood our bodies are immature. During puberty we make the transition from childhood to maturity. In the woman, puberty is characterized by decreased bone growth, by growth of breasts, pubic and axillary (armpit) hair, starting of menstruation (menarche) and ovulation, increase of the sexual urge, and emotional changes. Women have a third stage, in which they are no longer able to reproduce. The climacteric is the transition between the reproductive and postreproductive stages. (Although "menopause" is commonly used to mean the whole transition period, medically this is incorrect.) Menstruation stops (menopause) and ovulation stops. At this time women frequently experience hot flashes, decrease in skin tone, vaginal discharge, painful intercourse, headaches, and emotional changes. Menopause brings positive changes as well: freedom from fear of pregnancy, from cyclical moods, and from the monthly menstrual flow; and these freedoms often bring a heightened sexuality. (See "Menopause" chapter.)

This entire reproductive cycle is regulated by hormones. Hormones function as chemical messengers and initiators in the body. Women have high levels of sex hormones (estrogen and progesterone) during their reproductive period and low levels during childhood and after menopause. The signs and symptoms of the transitional periods are thought to be caused by the changing levels of hormones.

Within the lifelong fluctuations there are hormone-caused cycles of approximately one month's duration. These monthly fluctuations of hormones determine the timing of ovulation and menstruation. This cycle, the menstrual cycle, prepares a woman's body for the possibility of pregnancy every month.

The Ovarian Cycle—Ovulation

The ovaries at birth contain 40,000–300,000 follicles, which are spherical arrangements of cells with an immature egg in the center. Only about 300–400 of these will develop, producing mature eggs. The other follicles degenerate before completing development.

Each month one follicle (occasionally more than one) matures under the influence of hormones. (See Appendix for fuller description of hormones.) One of the cell layers in the follicle secretes estrogen. The follicle, with the maturing egg, moves toward the surface of the ovary. Ovulation is the process of the follicle rupturing and

THE MENSTRUAL CYCLE

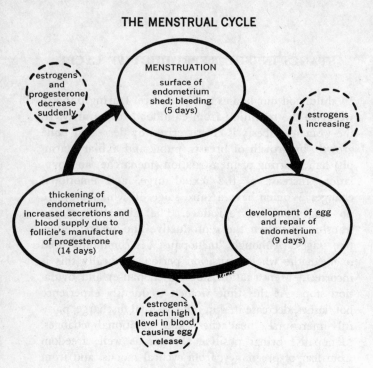

estrogens and progesterone decrease suddenly

MENSTRUATION
surface of endometrium shed; bleeding (5 days)

estrogens increasing

thickening of endometrium, increased secretions and blood supply due to follicle's manufacture of progesterone (14 days)

development of egg and repair of endometrium (9 days)

estrogens reach high level in blood, causing egg release

releasing the egg from the ovary. Sometimes this can be felt as a cramp on the left or right side of the lower abdomen and/or there is some bloody discharge from the vagina. The cramp is sometimes painful enough to be confused with appendicitis. However, there is no nausea or abdominal tenderness. The phenomenon is called mittelschmerz (literally "middle pain").

After ovulation another cell layer in the follicle starts secreting progesterone. The follicle is now called a corpus luteum (literally "yellow body," referring to the yellowish fat in it when it is almost completely degenerated). If the woman becomes pregnant, the hormones produced by the corpus luteum help to maintain the pregnancy.

The released egg is trapped by the funnel-shaped end of the oviduct (fallopian tube) and begins its six-and-a-

FOLLICLE CHANGES DURING MONTHLY CYCLE

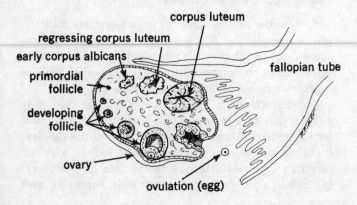

corpus luteum
regressing corpus luteum
early corpus albicans
primordial follicle
developing follicle
fallopian tube
ovary
ovulation (egg)

half-day journey to the uterus, moved along by peristaltic (wavelike) contractions of the oviduct. Fertilization, the process of union of an egg and sperm, takes place in the outer third of the oviduct (nearest the ovaries), and therefore occurs within one day of ovulation. There is a slight possibility that the fertilized egg may implant in the oviduct while en route to the uterus. This is an ectopic pregnancy and requires surgery before the tube ruptures. If the egg is not fertilized, it disintegrates or is sloughed off in the vaginal secretions. This usually happens before menstruation.

Uterine Cycle—Menstruation

Estrogen, made by the maturing follicle, causes the uterine lining (endometrium) to proliferate (to grow, thicken, and form glands that will secrete embryo-nourishing substances). Progesterone, made by the ruptured follicle after ovulation, causes the uterine glands to begin secreting the nourishing substances and also increases the uterine blood supply. An egg can implant only in a secretory lining, not in a proliferative one. The lining is proliferative until the egg is ovulated; after ovulation the corpus luteum starts secreting progesterone, which changes the character of the lining to secretory. If all goes well, the egg, after its six-and-a-half-day journey, should find a well-developed lining.

The ruptured follicle will produce estrogen and progesterone for only about twelve days, with the amount dwindling in the last few days if pregnancy has not occurred. As the estrogen and progesterone levels drop, the lining cannot be maintained and it is shed. This is menstruation. It is possible to menstruate without ovulating (anovulatory period), but this usually occurs only around the time of puberty or the climacteric. Menstruation lasts only a week or less, because a new follicle starts growing and starts secreting estrogen to begin the cycle again. This estrogen causes growth of the uterine lining, inhibiting further shedding. The timing is such that the whole old lining (except for the bottom layer of cells, which will form a new lining) is shed before a new layer grows.

Menstruation starts in about the middle of puberty, generally at the age of eleven or twelve, though any time from nine to eighteen years is normal. It continues until the average age of forty-eight or forty-nine, in the middle of the climacteric. The age range for menopause is somewhere between ages forty and fifty-five.

What is a normal menstrual cycle? The length of the cycle ranges from 20 to 36 days, with the average being 28 days. There is no record, however, of a woman with an absolutely regular menstrual cycle. There are spontaneous small changes and there can be major ones when

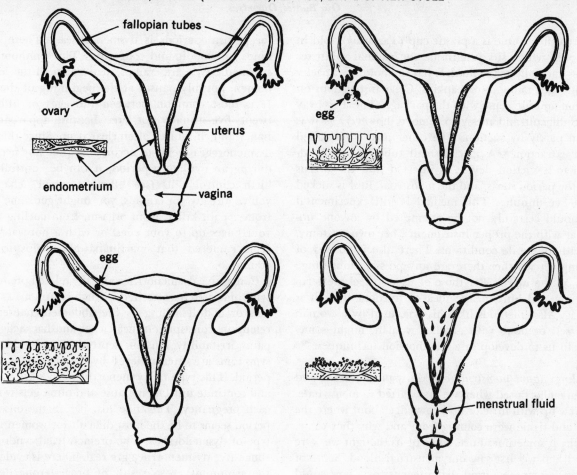

a woman is under a great deal of stress (such as a pregnancy scare). A normal period lasts 2–8 days, with 4–6 days being the average. During long periods the flow may stop and start again. A usual discharge for a menstrual period is about 4–6 tablespoons, or 2–3 ounces. Each woman has her own normal cycle, which really is a more important guideline than the statistics, since the acceptable ranges vary from one medical source to another. Many women feel an increased sexual urge during one part of the cycle. For some it comes around ovulation, for others it comes right before or during the period.

Should you do anything special or avoid anything special during your period? There is no evidence to indicate that you should stay in bed, avoid exercise, refrain from sexual intercourse, or observe any of the other taboos surrounding menstruation. However, if doing something makes you feel bad, it is only common sense to avoid doing it. Myths have endowed menstruating women with everything from supernatural healing powers to supernatural destructive powers. Too bad they aren't true.

The menstrual discharge. The menstrual discharge contains cervical and vaginal mucus and degenerated endometrial particles as well as blood (sometimes clotted), but this mixed content is not obvious since the blood stains everything red. This regular loss of blood, even though small, can cause anemia. (See chapter on "Nutrition and the Food We Eat" for ways to avoid this.) The discharge does not smell until it makes contact with the bacteria in the air and starts to decompose.

The most common method of absorbing menstrual fluid is through the use of tampons and sanitary napkins. In a pinch there are clean rags and toilet paper. Tampons are a convenience to many women. If you are just starting to menstruate or have not used a tampon before, you can find clear instructions in any package of them. If you have any trouble inserting the tampon into your vagina, wait until you don't have your period if you want to, then use a mirror to help you find the entrance to your vagina, and try lubricating the tampon with some lubricating jelly (K-Y jelly, not vaseline, which is not sterile). There is a myth that says you can't use tampons until you've had intercourse. If the hymen didn't have openings in it, the menstrual fluid couldn't come out. (In rare cases this happens.) However most girls and women have hymens with large enough openings to accommodate at least a small-sized tampon.

There are at least two other methods of dealing with

menstrual fluid. One is a plastic cup (Tassaway), sold in drugstores, which sits just inside the vaginal sphincter muscles and collects the fluid. It has the holding capacity of about four tampons or napkins. Clear instructions on insertion and use come with the package. The Tassaway can be difficult and messy to remove, however, as it is held in partly by suction. The other method is called period extraction.* A special small tube (cannula), attached to a suction device, is inserted into the uterus when the period starts, and the menstrual fluid is sucked out in five minutes. This method is still experimental and should certainly not be attempted by anyone unfamiliar with the proper instruments, her own anatomy, and without sterile conditions. There also is no way of knowing yet whether there are any possible long-range effects on the uterus. For those of us who feel menstruating is a real burden, the idea of freedom from it is exciting. Also, methods like this one, used by a woman on herself or done with another woman, might someday help us to develop safe self-abortion techniques.

Feelings about menstruation. Many of us were scared or even embarrassed when we first started to menstruate. We grew up with little or no knowledge about where the blood and tissue were coming from and why they came, and why it sometimes hurt. Some of us thought we were dying when we first saw our menstrual blood. Some of us were desperately afraid that a teacher or a boy would notice when we had our period. On the other hand some of us felt inadequate somehow if we didn't menstruate.

* * *

I used to worry about having my period. It seemed that all my friends had gotten it already, or were just having it. I felt left out. I began to think of it as a symbol. When I got my period, I would become a woman.

* * *

Starting to menstruate will always be different for each person—welcome to some, just the beginning of inconvenience for others. What we want to be sure to do is to tell both our sons and daughters about menstruation so that they can be comfortable with it and open about it in a way that we were not. We feel we can help our daughters to celebrate a new part of life.

Menstrual problems. Uncomfortable or painful periods are among the most common problems that women have. Most women experience at least some menstrual-connected discomfort sometime in their lives. Yet very little is known about why it happens. The medical term

*See Ellen Frankfort, "Vaginal Politics."

for painful periods is dysmenorrhea.* There are two kinds, spasmodic and congestive. The symptoms of the spasmodic type are cramps, acute pain in the lower abdomen, possibly nausea at the beginning of the period. It is most common between the ages of fifteen and twenty-five—usually not later, because apparently pregnancy and childbirth often clear it up. Since this type of dysmenorrhea seems to occur only (but not necessarily) during an ovulatory period, it can be controlled with birth control pills (see "Birth Control" chapter). If you've already got cramps, you might get some comfort from a pain killer, from orgasm, from curling up with your knees up to your chest or with a hot-water bottle. It is rumored that marijuana also helps to relieve cramps.

Congestive dysmenorrhea and the related premenstrual syndrome are characterized by such symptoms as a heaviness or a dull aching in the abdomen, nausea, water retention, constipation, headaches and backaches, breast pains, irritability, tension, depression, and lethargy. The symptoms are often relieved by the heaviest flow of the period. This type of dysmenorrhea can start at puberty and continue until menopause and often gets worse with each pregnancy. The time just before the onset of the period seems to be the most difficult for women with this type of dysmenorrhea. The premenstrual syndrome and congestive dysmenorrhea are real. There is evidence that the symptoms are a result of progesterone deficiency. Depression, particularly, may be caused by sodium retention and potassium depletion in the cells resulting from a lowered progesterone level.†

Some women have no menstrual difficulties. Among those who do, the problems are not uniform throughout their lives, nor are they necessarily severe. For those of us who have problems either occasionally or even fairly regularly, it is important to recognize that they exist and to deal with them—arranging schedules so we can get more rest if we need it at that time, planning exams or critical meetings for a time when we are not premenstrual, and so on.

Do menstruation and the premenstrual syndrome affect our ability to function effectively and to hold positions of responsibility? It is amazing that we are denied responsibility on the basis of menstrual cycles, and yet men, who are much more prone to seriously incapacitating diseases, such as heart problems—even though these problems are discovered—continue in highly re-

*For an excellent discussion of the menstrual cycle, and especially dysmenorrhea, see *The Menstrual Cycle,* by Dr. Katherina Dalton, which treats the subject far more clearly than any of the gynecological textbooks we consulted. Much of the material on menstruation here is summarized from this book.
†*The Menstrual Cycle,* pp. 60–64.

sponsible positions (the presidency of the country, for example). There also is some evidence that men too have hormonal cycles.* We are still allowed to work where we are "needed": at home, in factories, in offices, with no concessions to schedules or routines that might take account of our cycles.

Sometimes expecting to feel premenstrual tension and depression may increase the severity of the depression. We must not forget that the problems we get depressed about bother us all the time, but we can't handle them as well at this time, or perhaps we have been ignoring them the rest of the time. A lot of us have found that if we are feeling good about ourselves we don't get depressed or as depressed before our period.

Dr. Katherina Dalton theorizes that both types of dysmenorrhea are caused by a hormone imbalance.† She has found that dysmenorrhea can be induced by the wrong hormone. This can be important if you are taking birth-control pills or are having hormone therapy. The spasmodic type is a result of too much progesterone in relation to the estrogen, and the congestive type (also premenstrual syndrome) is a result of too much estrogen for the amount of progesterone. She treats both types with the appropriate hormone therapy.

Another theory about a possible cause of menstrual discomfort is that of Dr. Elizabeth Connell: "We now know that prostaglandins (hormone-like chemical substances) are manufactured by the lining of the uterus—the endometrium—and that shortly before the onset of menstruation there is a sharp increase in the amount of prostaglandins produced. We think, therefore, that per-

haps the pain of menstrual cramps may be a result of the presence of too much of the type of prostaglandin that causes contractions."* Dr. Connell does not suggest a related form of therapy.

Another menstrual problem is amenorrhea (absence of menstrual periods). Primary amenorrhea is the condition of never having had a period by the time menstruation usually starts (age eighteen), and secondary amenorrhea is the cessation of menstruation after at least one period. There are quite a variety of causes. Some are: pregnancy, a congenital defect of the genital tract, hormone imbalance, cysts or tumors, disease, stress, or emotional factors relating to puberty. Amenorrhea is treated extensively in most gynecological textbooks, since it is a frequent symptom of infertility. In fact, considerably more attention has been paid to amenorrhea than to dysmenorrhea, although dysmenorrhea is by far more common. Doctors once again show more concern for and do more research on a dramatic, less common problem than on a less dramatic problem that bothers many more women.

APPENDIX: HORMONES OF THE MENSTRUAL CYCLE

The main glands involved in the normal menstrual cycle (Latin *mensis,* "month") are the ovaries and the pituitary. The ovaries produce eggs (usually one per month), female sex hormones (estrogen and progesterone), and small amounts of male hormones (androgens). The pituitary is called the master gland of the body because its hormones affect almost all other glands and organs in the body. Its interaction with other glands is

*See Estelle Ramey, "Men's Cycles."
† *The Menstrual Cycle,* pp. 44, 46–50, and 64–70.

*Elizabeth Connell, M.D., "Prostaglandins: A New Wonder Drug?" *Redbook* magazine, January 1972, p. 11.

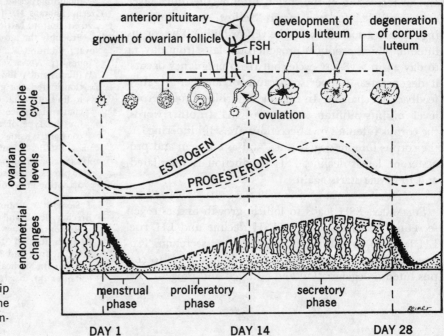

THE MENSTRUAL CYCLE—Relationship between follicle development, hormone cycle, and the endometrial (uterine lining) build-up and disintegration.

controlled by various mechanisms. For instance, by secreting Y, it may stimulate another gland to produce X.
However, if X inhibits Y, as the level of X rises the level
of Y will fall. Thus, eventually less X will be secreted.
This type of control is called "negative feedback mechanism" and is important for our discussion.

The cycle starts with FSH (follicle-stimulating hormone), a pituitary hormone that stimulates an ovarian
follicle to grow. FSH is secreted in greatest amounts during menstruation, is lowest at ovulation, and then rises
again. This is logical, because FSH must be present in
greatest amounts to start each follicle's development; a
follicle begins developing during menstruation. Then,
at the time of ovulation, FSH is needed least; the follicle
is doing what it was "meant" to do. Then it must rise
again, to a level where another resting immature follicle
is stimulated to grow.

What makes the FSH level rise and fall? A rising level
of FSH causes rising amounts of estrogen to be secreted
by the cells in one layer of the follicle. Because of the
negative feedback mechanism, however, increasing estrogen causes a decrease in FSH. A word here about atretic
follicles. We have mentioned that most of the follicles
in the ovary degenerate before completing development.
This degeneration (called atresia) is normal, but before
the follicles die they have secreted small amounts of
estrogen. As follicles are constantly degenerating, there
is a constant low level of estrogen being secreted. This
keeps the FSH level manageable; only one follicle generally grows each month.

Getting back to the cycle, as the estrogen level rises,
not only does it inhibit FSH but it eventually stimulates
the pituitary to release another hormone, LH. LH, or
luteinizing hormone, is a causative factor in ovulation
and in formation of the corpus luteum, the outer layer
of the follicle. (*Luteum* means "yellow," and "luteinizing" is thus associated with the yellow body.) The corpus
luteum, which produces progesterone, lasts from day 14
to day 25 in a 28-day cycle, but if no pregnancy occurs,
it degenerates. It does so because of another negative
feedback mechanism. In this one the rising progesterone
level inhibits pituitary secretion of LH. In other words,
the corpus luteum's own secretions are self-hindering. As
the corpus luteum degenerates, and as estrogen and progesterone levels decline, FSH production is stimulated,
and the cycle starts again.

SUMMARY. FSH leads to follicle growth and estrogen
secretion. Estrogen leads to FSH decline and LH rise.
LH leads to ovulation and progesterone secretion. Progesterone leads to LH decline. LH decline leads to corpus luteum degeneration and estrogen and progesterone

decline. Estrogen decline leads to FSH rise; new cycle
begins. Estrogen and progesterone drops cause menstruation.

This has been the ovarian cycle—from follicle growth
to ovulation to follicle degeneration. The uterine cycle,
covered in this chapter, and the cervical cycle are both
essential for understanding how birth-control pills work.

CERVICAL CYCLE. The cervical mucus, under the influence of estrogen, becomes thinner and wetter. Under the
influence of progesterone, after ovulation, it becomes
thicker and dryer. In addition, the two sex hormones,
estrogen and progesterone, affect the content of the
cervical mucus. There is a sharp peak in calcium (Ca)
and sodium (Na) concentrations at the time of ovulation,
and this is apparently very beneficial to the sperm.
(About 24 hours before ovulation there is a sharp drop
in Ca, and this is the basis of a new test for telling when
a woman ovulates.) The thinness and wetness of the
mucus at ovulation aid the sperm's entrance into the
uterus at that time.

FURTHER READINGS

Anthony, Catherine P. *Textbook of Anatomy and Physiology.* 7th
    ed. St. Louis: C. V. Mosby Co., 1967.
    Basic nursing text. Very readable, well illustrated, and com-
    prehensive, as are many nursing books and magazines.
Dalton, Katherina. *The Menstrual Cycle.* Pantheon, 1969.
    The best book we've seen on menstruation and menstrual prob-
    lems. Her preferred treatment (hormones) may not be for
    everyone, but her analysis makes sense.
Frankfort, Ellen. "Vaginal Politics," *The Village Voice,* November
    25,1971, Health Forum column, pp. 6, 74.
    Article about the activities of the Los Angeles self-help clinic,
    including period extraction.
Green, Thomas H., Jr. *Gynecology Essentials of Clinical Practice.*
    2d ed. Boston: Little, Brown & Co., 1971.
    Probably the most readable of the gynecology texts.
Novak, Edmund R., Georgeanna Seegar Jones, and Howard W.
    Jones, Jr. *Novak's Textbook of Gynecology.* 7th ed. Baltimore:
    Williams and Wilkins Co., 1965.
    Considered *the* gynecological textbook. It's good if you want
    to find out what the recommended doctor's text is. It is pretty
    chauvinistic—see the first part of "Women and Health Care"
    for the type of attitudes expressed. It mystifies medicine by
    constantly using jargon when simpler words are sufficient.
Ramey, Estelle. "Men's Cycles (They Have Them Too, You Know),"
    Ms. (Spring 1972), pp. 8–14.
    Explores evidence of male cycles. Includes some discussion on
    accepting and working with cycles.

See "Sexuality" Bibliography for:
    Brecher, Ruth and Edward, eds., *An Analysis of Human Sexual
    Response.*
    Deutsch, Ronald M. *The Key to Feminine Response in Marriage.*
    Hegeler, Inge and Sten. *An ABZ of Love.*
See "Common Medical Problems and Procedures," Further Readings
    (Chapter 15), for: *Hospital Medicine.*

3
Sexuality

INTRODUCTION

FOR many of us it has been difficult to be open and honest about our sexuality. As we managed to be more trusting with each other we found that talking about ourselves and our sexuality can be very liberating. It was a big step for us to write down our experiences, to expose our feelings and fears. However, with each other's support, we have become more accepting of our sexuality, and we have begun to explore aspects of ourselves that we hadn't thought much about before.

Many of us had been very dependent on men's approval for our self-esteem. This carried over into our sexual life, where we felt that pleasing men was more important than pleasing ourselves. The focus of sex for us was genital. We thought about our sexuality in male terms—intercourse was the goal, and foreplay was almost a dispensable preliminary.

We are learning to define our sexuality in our own terms. In the past three years we have come to see our sexuality in broader ways. First, by getting acquainted with our individual sexual patterns and responses, and not just letting sex happen to us, we are learning to listen to our own rhythms. Second, we are learning to see and to express our own needs as valid. Only by learning to please ourselves can we have more mutual and honest relationships. Third, we have come to be more open to a range of sexual expression. Fourth, we have realized that we don't express our sexuality in a vacuum. Our sexuality is complex because it involves physical, psychological, emotional, and political factors. And it is expressed in the context of a relationship with ourselves and with others.

This chapter is the cumulative work of three years of thinking, and talking, and living by many, many women. We are experts on our sexuality in the sense that we are women sharing our experiences and insights. This proc-

ess has been more helpful and informative to us than all the how-to-do-it, what-is-it-all-about books we have ever read. If you are just beginning to explore your own sexuality, you have to start where you are. Only you know that. Trust your feelings and take from this book what you need. We can't emphasize enough how important it has been for each of us to go at her own speed.

We begin with a general cultural orientation toward sexuality and move on to more specific topics like masturbation, fantasies, and lovemaking. We are not learning more about our sexuality in order to produce bigger and better spasms in orgasm. We are concerned about why women are encouraged to think about sex in such competitive, objectifying ways. We want to unravel the myths that put us down. We want to help ourselves and each other grow to be full people capable of open, loving relationships. And before we can really love another, we must learn to love ourselves. By looking carefully at our needs, by dealing honestly with our sexuality, we free up lots of energy for other satisfying work, activity, and living.

A CULTURAL ORIENTATION

We are all so oppressed by sexual images, formulas, goals, and rules that it is almost impossible even to think about sex outside the context of success and failure. The sexual revolution—liberated orgastic women, groupies, communal lovemaking, homosexuality—has made us feel that we must be able to have sex with impunity, without anxiety, under any conditions and with anyone, or we're uptight freaks. These alienating, inhuman expectations are no less destructive or degrading than the Victorian puritanism we all so proudly rejected. Robin Morgan says (and so do we): "Goodbye to Hip Culture and the so-called Sexual Revolution which has functioned toward woman's freedom as did the Reconstruction toward former slaves—reinstituted oppression by another name."*

We are simultaneously bombarded with two conflicting messages: one from our parents, churches and schools —that sex is dirty and therefore we must keep ourselves pure for the one love of our lives; and the other from *Playboy, Newsweek,* etc., almost all women's magazines, and especially television commercials—that we should be free, groovy chicks.

We're learning to resist this double message and realize that neither set of images fits us. What really has to be confronted is the deep, persistent assumption of sexual inequality between men and women in our society. "Frigidity" or "inadequacy" in bed is not divorced from the social realities we experience all the time. When we feel powerless and inferior in a relationship, it is not surprising that we feel humiliated and unsatisfied in bed. Similarly, a man must feel some contempt for a woman he believes not to be his equal. This male-dominated culture imbues us with a sense of second-best status, and there is no reason to expect this sense of inferiority and inadequacy to go away between the sheets.

*Robin Morgan, "Goodbye to All That," *Rat: Subterranean News* (New York), February 6, 1970, p. 6.

SEXUAL FEELINGS

Part of the reason so many people have problems about sex is that sexual feelings are thought to be separate or different from other kinds of feelings we have. Sex has to do with the body—that alien part of us residing below the neck that has needs and responses we don't understand. But our feelings reside in our bodies. Fears make their presence felt by our pounding heart, our chest caved in, our stomach turning. Joy is tingly—our head feels a little light, our fingers and toes sort of shimmer, and the rest of us feels warm and all in one piece. For some of us anger feels like a pounding in the head, hands tighten and clench, and so on. When you feel these feelings, or any others, try to stop and feel them in your body—below the neck as well as above it. Don't judge, just sense what's happening. It's one way of getting more in touch with you.

* * *

I watch my daughter. From morning to night her body is her home. She lives in it and with it. When she runs around the kitchen she uses all of herself. Every muscle in her body moves when she laughs, when she cries.

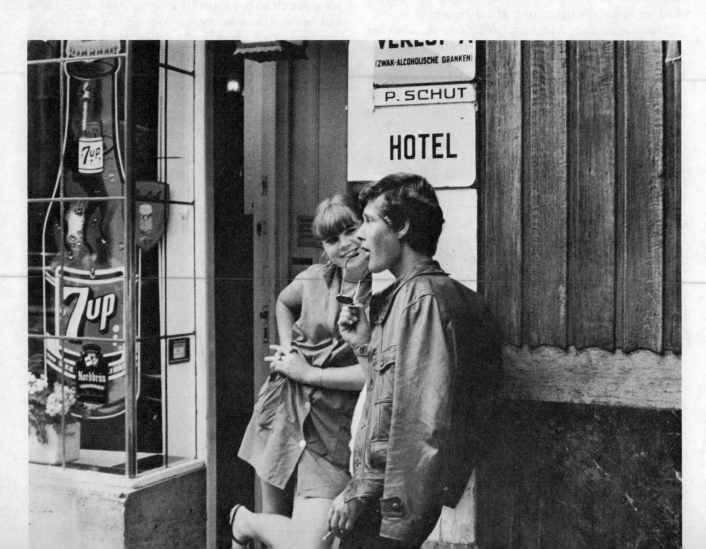

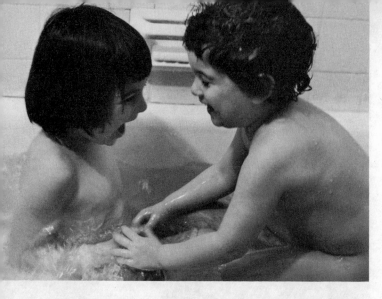

When she rubs her crotch, there is no awkwardness, no feeling that what she is doing is wrong. She feels pleasure and expresses it without hesitation. She knows when she wants to be touched and when she wants to be left alone. She doesn't have to think about it—it's a very direct physical asking or responding to someone else. It's beau-

tiful to be with her. I sometimes feel she is more a model for me than I am for her! Occasionally I feel jealous of the ease with which she lives inside her skin. I want to be a child again! It's so hard to get back that sense of body as home.

* * *

But difficult as it is, there is hope. A lot of current therapy is based on getting back in touch with those physical feelings, integrating our minds and bodies so we can function in a fuller way.

* * *

It has been very hard for me to allow myself to feel good sexual energy in my body. "You mean it's okay, it's not dirty, it's not loose?" I can hear one little voice saying to another little voice inside me. The other voice answers: "Sure, it's fine, that's what you feel." With a lot of support from other women, I have gotten to feel it's fine, and it feels great to feel that energy and know it's mine. What's even harder for me is, when I feel tension in my body to respect it. I keep wanting to shove the

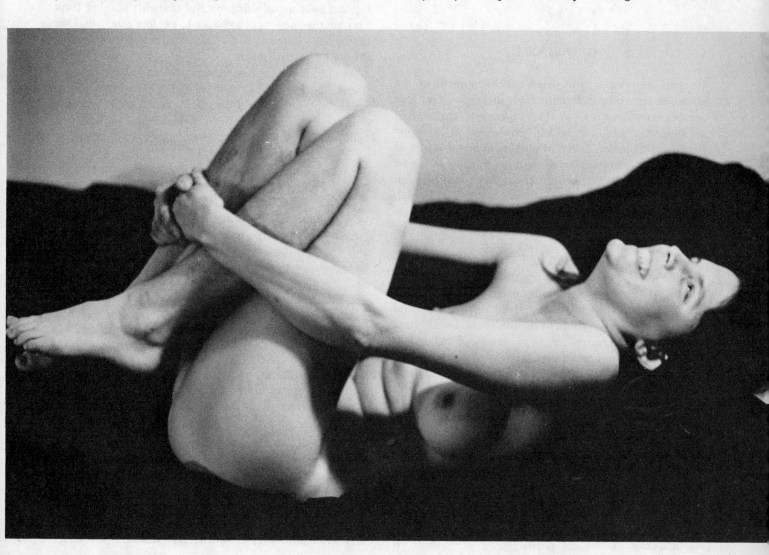

tension under, yell at it to go away. But I realize that sometimes my body responds more in my self-interest than my mind does. I had an experience where my vagina felt tight, closed. I tried to ignore that feeling and force myself to have intercourse. I felt afraid that maybe I was frigid. I think what was happening was that I was scared in that situation. My body knew that and wouldn't let me be vulnerable in certain ways. It didn't let my mind take over. That was a very important experience for me. It's very hard for me to fully respect what my body says—I'm so used to pushing that it's hard to slow down and listen, listen to new and different sounds.

* * *

What we need to do is to get rid of all the standards we have previously used to measure ourselves, not to treat sex as a sexual-achievement exam, and not to make love to "judges" who then pass or fail us. We can help one another do this by talking together and taking support from each other.

GROWING UP

It seems pretty clear to us that from the moment we are born we are treated differently from little boys. Our toys are different: dolls instead of chemistry sets. Our clothes are different: dresses to be kept clean instead of sloppy pants. Pocketbooks instead of pockets—something else to keep us from swinging our arms, using our bodies freely. Over the years the distinctions keep being made between boys and girls. We're emotional; they're intellectual. They're clumsy; we're graceful and dainty. They're athletic; we're domestic. They are going to go on to become doctors and businessmen. We are going to get married.

Some of us had fantasies and dreams of glamorous, exciting careers, yet wound up as wives and mothers, with no other strong interest, playing roles we had fallen into, not chosen. In short, we think of men, and men are socialized to think of themselves, as intellectual, aggressive, and creative, while women are molded as passive, gentle, and emotional. Okay, you say, that's not so bad—separate but equal characteristics. We don't think that's true. We think we have suffered by this characterization as passive creatures, noticeably in relation to our sexuality.

We are not supposed to be interested in sex—that's for men. We are not supposed to admit it if we are— that's dirty. The ideal woman *responds*, she does not initiate.* Men will act sexually aggressive toward us,

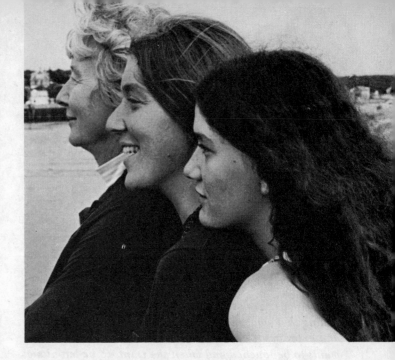

and we must worry about how to set the limits on the sexual encounter. We are always so busy setting the limits, and holding off this powerful sexuality coming from him, that we never get a chance to explore our own. Our bodily functions and our own sexuality are always something of a mystery to us.

As kids, if we are caught masturbating or exploring a friend's body, we are either told to stop immediately or we are questioned carefully about what exactly we were doing. Certain ideas begin to make themselves felt—like young ladies don't do that sort of thing.

* * *

My three-year-old daughter and I were visiting my parents. We all sat in the living room. Lisa sat on the carpet holding a paper-towel tube to her naked vagina. "What would happen if I peed in this?" she asked in her heaviest, gurgling, teasing, curious voice. "Don't do it—the pee will come out on the floor," was what I told her. My father was extremely upset and told me afterward that I had handled it all wrong. I should have scolded her and told her not to talk that way. Not, he assured me, because he cared, but because there are some pretty small-minded people out there who will give her a rude awakening if she's not trained now.

* * *

We also learn that physical affection is acceptable only in some relationships, but not in others:

* * *

When I was about seven or eight, I had this best friend Susan. We loved each other and walked around with our arms around each other. Her older sister told us not to do that anymore because we looked like lesbians. So we held hands instead.

* * *

We also learn that a woman's bodily functions are mysterious and slightly smutty. For instance, an ad for

---

*"By anatomic and physiologic necessity, feminine sexuality is characterized by a receptive readiness for arousal by the male" (N. J. Eastman and E. Hellman, *Williams Obstetrics*, New York: Appleton-Century-Crofts, 1966, p. 341).

sanitary napkins says: "When you have your period, you should be the only one who knows."

* * *

When I first got my period, my mother dragged me into the bathroom and told me to take off my clothes. I stood naked in front of her while she grumbled, "You can have kids now, so you better be careful."

* * *

When I first got my period, I came and told my mother. She slapped me across the face and then congratulated me. Later she told me that the slap was an old custom.

* * *

The books I sent away for explaining menstruation arrived in plain brown wrapping. My father got to them first, and taunted me by holding them over his head so that they were out of my reach.

* * *

The messages go on and on. There is something shameful about our bodies. Our sexuality seems to shock and anger our parents; it scares us, and adds to the growing sense of alienation and mystery we have about our bodies.

By the time we are teen-agers we discover that there is only one norm for beauty, a commercial norm that sells products to us as we agonize over breasts, hair, legs, and skin that will not—no, never—measure up. Again we are left with shame and anxiety. We have body smells and our feet are too big. We lose all respect for our own uniqueness, our own smell and shape and way of doing things. We buy vaginal deodorant and read in a variety of women's magazines articles telling us "Six Ways to Be Sexy."

The shame and anxiety also make it hard for us to raise our own children. We want to be more open about our sexuality than our parents were, but it is very hard. When our kids ask about where they came from, we use different words from those our parents used, but feelings of discomfort remain.

* * *

The other day I was taking a bath with my almost-three-year-old daughter. I was lying down and she was sitting between my legs, which were spread apart. She said, "Mommy, you don't have a penis." I said, "That's right, men have penises and women have clitorises." All calm and fine—then, "Mommy, where is your clitoris?" Okay, now what was I going to do? I took a deep breath (for courage or something), tried not to blush, spread my vagina apart, and showed her my clitoris. It didn't feel so bad. "Do you want to see yours?" I asked. "Yes." That was quite a trick to get her to look over her fat stomach and see hers, especially when she started laughing as I first put my finger and then hers on her clitoris.

At least, I feel that I can have some greater ease and openness about sexuality with my daughter than my

mother had with me. It took us time to develop bad feelings about our sexuality, and we must allow ourselves more time to undo those feelings and develop new and healthier ones.

VIRGINITY

What does virginity mean, anyway? Maybe virginity is a physical state but, much more important, it's a state of mind. Those of us who grew up in religious families feel that to lose our virginity before marriage is to have sinned. We are no longer chaste, unsullied, pure white . . . like the Madonna.

* * *

For a long time after I began to have sexual experience, I, like many women in the early 1960s, knew little about birth control. I was afraid to seek medical help because of the laws of my state and my own guilt-ridden Roman Catholic background. I confined my sexual involvement to heavy petting, since the Catholic Church makes intercourse seem like such a sin. The day I left the Church was the day I had an argument in the confessional with the priest about whether having intercourse with my fiancé was a sin. I maintained it wasn't; he said that I would never be a faithful wife if I had intercourse before marriage. He refused me absolution and I never went back.

* * *

The virgin-whore contrast is not only a religious notion. It runs through a lot of literature and art, and it is part of our everyday growing-up experience as well.

* * *

As I was growing up in the 1950s, the group of kids I went to school with accepted the virgin-whore dichotomy. Those specific words weren't used, but the value judgment was certainly there. There was a clear difference between a "good" girl, who wouldn't sleep with a man until he married her, and a "bad" girl, who was considered "hot," "fast," and "an easy touch" because she would succumb and have intercourse with boys. There was no parallel judgment made on the boys. They had sex with the "bad" girls, but planned to marry a "good" girl; in fact, they were expected to get experience so they could teach the girls they married.

* * *

The sexual revolution of the 1960s and the advent of the pill started to change these feelings about the importance of virginity. Its loss before marriage was less disapproved of if you grew up in the sixties rather than in the fifties. But new problems were created. In the fifties if a guy was pressuring you to sleep with him and

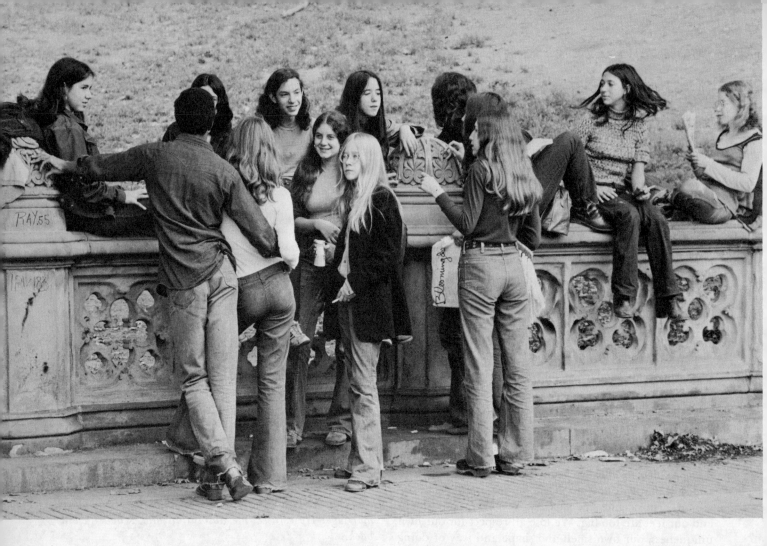

you didn't want to, you could use the virginity bit on him. Or you could use fear of pregnancy as an excuse. In the sixties it became harder to say no; being a virgin was passé, and birth-control methods were more widespread.

The loss of virginity, the loss of the state of purity and innocence, is viewed as a move from childhood to adulthood, a definite breaking away from parents and a move toward more autonomy and independence. Autonomy is surely a good thing, but the cost of sexual exploration should not have to be a sharp, brittle separation if that doesn't seem necessary.

* * *

It's ironic that my mother who had been sexually repressed herself *should in turn protect* my *virginity for the sake of a man she doesn't even know (and surely won't like!).*

* * *

The linking of virginity and marriage often forces us into marriage before we are ready, before we know it's something we want.

Men, traditionally, have made a big production of the bursting of the hymen. Marriage manuals spend chapters on it. Pornographers go wild over it:

At length by my fierce rending and tearing thrusts the first defenses gave way and I got about halfway in . . . as I oiled her torn and bleeding cunt with a perfect flood of virgin sperm. Poor Rose had born it most heroically, keeping the bedclothes between her teeth, in order to repress any cry of pain. . . . I now recommenced my eager shoves, my fierce lunges, and I felt myself gaining at every move, till with one tremendous and cunt-rending thrust I buried myself into her up to the hilt. So great was the pain this last shock caused Rose that she could not suppress a sharp shrill scream, but I heeded it not; it was the note of final victory and only added to the delicious piquancy of my enjoyment. . . . I drew her to a yet closer embrace, and planting numberless kisses on her rosy lips and blushing face, which was wet with tears of suffering which the brave little darling could not prevent from starting from her lovely eyes, I drew out the head and slowly thrust it in again: my fierce desires goaded me to challenge her to a renewal of the combat. A smile of infinite love crossed her lovely countenance, all sighs of past pain seemed to vanish and I could feel the soft and juicy folds of her cunt.*

This episode has all the usual ingredients repeated *ad nauseam* in most pornography: the man's energetic thrusts, the difficulty of penetrating the barrier, the

*"La Rose d'Amour," *The Pearl: A Journal of Facetiae and Voluptuous Reading* (Copyright © 1968 by Grove Press, Inc.), pp. 253–54.

woman's screams, the man's triumph, the woman's bliss-ful acceptance of her new role. In *The Pearl* the scene occurs at least twenty-four times. This, in perhaps a gentler form, is what men have been brought up to ex-pect in their first sexual relation with a virginal woman.

Even sadder, and much more subtle, is the way we have come to accept the inequality between the sexes as the norm, and are disappointed when we do not live up to the mythified scene.

The hymen is a pliable membrane. Hymens often get stretched before first intercourse. General physical activity (i.e., horseback riding or climbing trees) won't stretch your hymen, but petting (digital intercourse) or inser-tion of a tampon will. (For pictures of hymens see draw-ings in the chapter on "Anatomy.") First intercourse often takes place with no physical pain at all. The man need not be a battering ram; the woman need not scream and faint. The mythology* distorts reality to make women seem more helpless and men more aggressive than they are.

Why are we urged and expected to feel this pain? Marriage manuals give hints on how the husband can reduce the pain of penetration, but with the mention of the possibility of there being no pain at all, a note of apology creeps into the text. The books hardly ever sug-gest that a man is not due his quotient of pain, for pain is part of what keeps the two unequal.

It is the easiest thing in the world for a woman to stretch her own hymen by inserting a finger into her vagina and periodically exerting a little pressure on the sides of the entrance. Simple as it is, most of us don't think of it, because we don't have any information, we are uneasy at examining our own bodies, and most im-portant, we are afraid of depriving men of their drop of blood. We are afraid of having our offering questioned as not pure enough.

Virginity and all that surrounds it has had a powerful hold on the lives of many of us. We have been shaped by society's norms about virginity without specifically ask-ing ourselves what we want and need. It is another ex-ample of how we are expected to respond to others—parents, men, friends, the Church, the values of our cul-ture—and not to ourselves.

FANTASIES

We are continually selecting actions and repressing im-pulses in order to conform to what we feel we ought to do. Our discarded or unrealized impulses and desires

---

*Note that myths that go way back in time and span different cultures express many similar and negative attitudes about female sexuality, e.g., the teeth-in-vagina myth, the menstrual uncleanli-ness myth, and so forth.

---

very often stay with us and appear and reappear as fantasies—short flashes or long constructs, stories we tell to ourselves—in which we try out experiences that seem impossible or feelings (desires, sensations) that are for-bidden.

Many kinds of fantasies are outside the scope of this chapter—such as work or success fantasies, or more seri-ously, fantasies that reflect deep emotional disturbances, becoming a world that a person can't get free of. There is also the romantic love (and marriage) fantasy, which tantalizes us, making us hope that our lives will conform to its false promise.

As we talked together about our sexuality we found that most of us have all kinds of sexual fantasies—fanta-sies we have always kept very private. They generally come into our heads when we are making love or mas-turbating, and they often scare and confuse us. They seem abnormal. The part we play in them threatens our self-image. Or they seem disloyal to the people we are involved with. Or we are afraid we may act them out.

* * *

I never felt the freedom to explore parts of me that might come out in fantasy, dreams at night, daydreams, nonverbalized thinking. I was scared they would take me by surprise, tell me things about myself that I didn't know, especially bad things, and I was having enough trouble dealing with what came up without fantasizing. "Let well enough alone" was my attitude.

* * *

I imagined I was sitting in a room. The walls were all white. There was nothing in it, and I was naked. There was a large window at one end, and anyone who wanted to could look in and see me. There was no place to hide. There was something arousing about being so exposed. I masturbated while having this fantasy, and afterward I felt very sad. I thought I must be so sick, so distorted inside if this image of myself could give me such intense sexual pleasure.

* * *

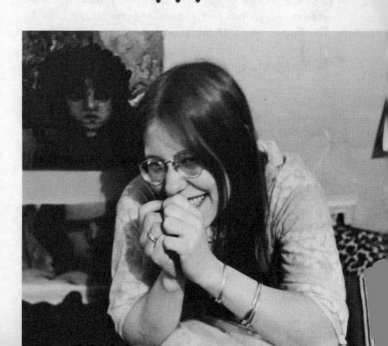

Telling our fantasies, sharing our feelings about them has given us a new freedom to enjoy them and learn from them, to accept ourselves as we are. We realize that these stories and flashes are pieces of us wanting to be known. Some of them we won't ever act on; others show us directions we want to go in.

* * *

Enjoying a fantasy is a new and liberating notion for me. I always felt restrained because I thought I might act on my fantasies—whatever they were. Now that I know I don't have to act—now or ever—I can enjoy them.

* * *

If we are aroused and scared by an image of ourselves that is aggressive, we might first prefer to deny it. Fear of our fantasies, like the fear of leftover myths about destructive femininity, has helped to keep us sexually passive. But learning from our fantasies instead of repressing them can free us to act. To take the initiative in sex. Or, if we fantasize about women, to learn about and accept the sexual feelings we have for women, knowing that we can choose whether or not to act on those feelings. If fantasies of being sexually humiliated are erotic to us, we might examine our sexual expectations. What does this say about how we feel about our bodies or our sexuality, in or out of bed?

Because it has been so exciting for us to learn to accept our fantasies and to enjoy them instead of pushing them down all the time, we want to tell a few of them here. Their range shows us that our sexuality is very complex; we are glad to be starting to explore that complexity.

* * *

A fantasy before I made love to a plumber I know: I was entertaining myself one night by imagining I was dancing with a stillson wrench (the most enormous wrench I ever saw, very businesslike!), and it turned into the plumber. He said, "Well, men are still good for something!" We were fixing the pipe when we were dancing, and the scene changed. We were swimming in a sea of rubber doughnuts (the connector between the tank and the bottom part of the toilet), and the doughnuts got stuck over our arms and legs. The scene changed again, to the beach, where we fell asleep.

* * *

One time, just as I was climaxing with Steve, I suddenly saw and felt someone else. I didn't realize until right then that that other person was on my mind.

* * *

I've had fantasies of having to drink urine from a man's penis while he was peeing.

* * *

When I was a kid every time I masturbated I imagined my parents spanking me as I climaxed. When I got older

it changed to my parents making love, then to my being kissed by someone, then to my making love.

* * *

I used to have a recurring fantasy that I was a gym teacher and had a class full of girls standing in front of me, nude. I went up and down the rows feeling all their breasts and getting a lot of pleasure out of it. When I first had this fantasy at thirteen I was ashamed. I thought something was wrong with me. Now I can enjoy it, because I feel it's okay to enjoy other women's bodies.

* * *

I fantasize about sleeping with my brother, who is nineteen and groovy and looks just like me. I fantasize sleeping with him because he's the person most like me. I acted on it by sleeping with his best friend.

* * *

I had the fantasy of making love with two men at once. I pictured myself sandwiched between them. I acted on this one, with an old friend and a casual friend who both liked the idea. It was fun.

* * *

I fantasize making love with horses, because they are very sensuous animals, more so than cows or pigs. They are also very male animals—horse society is very chauvinist.

* * *

I have been celibate for six months now. The longer the celibacy has continued, the more sexual fantasies I've had.

* * *

At the height of making love with a man I wished he was a woman. I wished he didn't have a penis. I wished he wasn't him, but more like me.

* * *

Sometimes when I'm making love with myself or someone else, I think about the ocean roar and feel the waves swirling about me. Perhaps this means that I'd rather be floating in the sea than be in my bed. But it's also a way of heightening the experience for me. The fantasy makes me feel loose, easy, fluid. It makes me more relaxed. I usually have the fantasy just before orgasm, and it helps me let go.

MASTURBATION

We had a house with old plumbing. The bathtub faucet sprayed a hard stream of water out at an angle. I learned to masturbate with it, had orgasms at seven or eight with it. One day, when I was just under ten years old, my mother surprised me going at it. She said, "What are you doing?" "Just washing myself." "Oh." I was totally freaked out that she didn't know. I figured it must be something pretty weird if she didn't know. I figured I was part boy and part lesbian and certainly a sinner.

When my father went to the hospital with an infection and there was talk of his having a leg amputation and dying if that didn't work, I got real scared and guilty. I figured it was happening to him because I was masturbating, or at least because I hadn't confessed to my mother. I was sure he would die if I didn't.

* * *

We all heard that masturbation was bad, and we felt guilty about doing it. But some of us did do it, which means it must have felt good. Taboos did keep some of us from learning about it until we had sex with men.

* * *

I was fourteen or fifteen years old and a virgin. I was sitting cross-legged on my bed one day, and became aroused by memories of petting with my boyfriend and having orgasms. I was also aroused by the sex smell I was exuding. I suddenly realized that I could do to my clitoris what he had done. I masturbated for the first time, had an orgasm, and wasn't so sure that what I had done was right.

* * *

When we got older, we got sold a myth that masturbating would keep us from enjoying sex with men, it would "fixate" us. So claimed Sigmund Freud. Whereas somewhat more objective observers now suspect that women who masturbate are more likely to have orgasms in intercourse than those who don't.

Masturbating can be a useful part of a person's sexual development. Besides helping you learn to enjoy your body, it can also teach you what techniques are best for arousing yourself, so that you will be able to show your sexual partner how to arouse you. It can be especially important for women: both Kinsey and Masters and Johnson discovered that women who have never had an orgasm before marriage are less likely to have them after. However, don't worry if you never feel a need to masturbate; masturbating and non-masturbating are both in the range of normal human experience.*

* * *

I only put my fingers in "there" or near "there" when I had to—to put in a tampon or my diaphragm. Then I'd run to the sink and wash myself, quick! That's how I felt for many years. So the thought never entered my head that masturbation could be something that was positive or nice. And I had my man for sex, which wasn't so great anyhow. Then the women's movement began. In some early discussions of sexuality I heard some women talk about masturbating. Just the openness of the talk shocked me at first.

They said it was fun, pleasurable! And many of them were women who were married or with men. I was stunned. I had so many questions that I didn't dare ask.

*Marjorie W. Hackmann, *Practical Sex Information*, pp. 16–17.

How do you do it? Do you do it when you're alone? Do you do it in bed with your lover or husband there? Do you let him watch? Do you let your children know? Etcetera, etcetera.

* * *

It is hard to feel good about allowing time and space to give pleasure to ourselves, an affirmation by us of our sexuality. Masturbation is not something to do just when you don't have a partner. It is the first and easiest way to experiment with your body. It's a way to find out what feels good, with how much pressure, at what tempo, and how often. You don't have to worry about someone else's needs or their opinions of you. The more you know about your body, the easier it is to show someone else what gives you pleasure. *It is different from, not inferior to, sex for two.* It is unfortunate that the comparison even has to be made, but that is realistically what we are starting from.

We women have a great number of ways of masturbating. Some women masturbate by moistening their finger (with either saliva or juice from the vagina) and rubbing it around and over the clitoris. You can rub or tweak the clitoris directly; you can rub the hood or a larger area around the clitoris, which stimulates the clitoris indirectly. You can use one finger or many. You can rub up and down or round and round. Pressure and timing also vary. Some women masturbate by crossing their legs and exerting steady and rhythmic pressure on the whole genital area. Some of us have learned to develop muscular tension throughout our bodies resembling the tensions developed in the motions of intercourse. Some women get sexually excited during physical activity—climbing ropes or trees, riding horses. Still other ways of masturbating include using a pillow instead of a hand, a stream of water, or an electric vibrator.

It's nice to make up sexual fantasies while masturbating or to masturbate when you feel those fantasies coming on. Some women like to insert something into the vagina while masturbating—a finger, candle, vibrator—but few women get more satisfaction out of vaginal penetration than they do from clitoral stimulation. Some of us find our breasts or other parts of our bodies erotically sensitive and rub them before or while rubbing the clitoris. Loving ourselves doesn't just mean our clitoris and breasts. We are learning to love all parts of our bodies.

LOVEMAKING

When I was six years old I climbed up on the bathroom sink and looked at myself naked in the mirror. All of a sudden I realized I had three different holes. I was very excited about my discovery and ran down to the dinner table and announced it to everyone. "I have three holes!" Silence. "What are they for?" I asked. Silence, even heavier than before. I sensed how uncomfortable everyone was and answered for myself. "I guess one is for pee-pee, the other for doo-doo and the third for ca-ca." A sigh of relief; no one had to answer my question. But I got the message—I wasn't supposed to ask "such" questions, though I didn't fully realize what "such" was about at that time.

* * *

I had been doing heavy petting for years when I was out on dates. One night I realized I felt something strange inside me. It was his penis. I didn't realize this was what intercourse was, but I said, "Hey, this is going too far!"

* * *

I always had a lot of trouble with intercourse. I thought it had to be very romantic. It never quite happened the way I imagined it should happen. In a woman's group I was in, one woman said you had to work at having intercourse. A very strange idea to me. She described what she did, what her husband did. And she added that the most important thing she had learned from her mother was to use saliva. That evening changed my life. I worked at it, I made Mark work at it.

It was a threat to Mark that we would share equally in lovemaking. He just saw it as another DEMAND—"I do half the housework, half the child care, and now half of this—this is going too far!" I was so furious. . . . It took us a long time to work this out.

* * *

All of these stories indicate that we grow up with a lack of basic information about "the sex act," and are made to feel uncomfortable when we ask for it. We grow up ignorant because people don't talk about intercourse or orgasm in real and helpful ways. In this section we want to break down that ignorance.*

Intercourse is an incredibly personal thing. You know for yourself just when you have reached a stage in a relationship where you want to make love. Maybe you are being pressured into it, maybe not; only you alone can feel inside yourself just what you want. Your body is yours; what someone else wants or thinks or what parents or friends might say should not be what makes you decide whether or not to have intercourse. Intercourse is not some ultimate sexual goal. Our culture puts a tremendous emphasis on genital sex, but what is much more important is feeling good about the totality of your own body. We have been put down for feeling erotically sensitive in other areas but our genitals (our

*We are talking for the most part in this section about heterosexual lovemaking. However, most of the information about the sexual response cycle is applicable in relationships between women.

breasts, necks, whatever, are only "secondary" erotic zones). Men, out of their own repression, often don't want to touch us all over as much as we want to be touched. We shouldn't be afraid to ask for what feels good. If intercourse does make us feel good, we'll want to have it; if it doesn't, we won't.

What Happens in Intercourse?

What is it like to have intercourse and to experience an orgasm, and what happens? Here is a rough sketch to give some idea of the main events.

Maybe you have just had a bath and are warm and relaxed, or maybe you have been flirting and teasing each other and are excited and aroused. One way or another you end up on the bed (sofa, floor, lawn) with some or all of your clothes off, and begin making love. You stroke each other all over, maybe give each other a back rub. You take turns concentrating on *giving* and *receiving* pleasure. Before long you become aware of your genitals: the penis and clitoris begin to get hard, the woman may feel a faint tingling or swelling in the labia, and a wetness inside the vagina. (This wetness is an early sign of arousal and doesn't mean that the woman is ready to accept the penis.)

You begin to concentrate more on the genitals. The man may enjoy having his penis stroked, or maybe licked, and perhaps having his testicles pulled gently or fondled. The woman may like her clitoris and labia stroked, or massaged or maybe licked. You can tell each other what feels good. (Women have a myth that men automatically know how to make love. This is not true. Not only do they have to learn, but since every woman's nerves are a little different, you have to tell them what *you* find stimulating.)

If there were an observer, he would notice that your heart was beating faster and you were breathing harder. These manifestations will continue up to orgasm, and then slowly subside.

In a little while you are feeling much aroused; you may be moaning from the excitement. Maybe one of you feels inside the vagina with your finger to see if it has loosened up. If you are using foam or a condom, it's time to put it in or on. Then one of you holds the penis in your hand, and you gently guide it into the vagina.* Maybe you just lie together for a minute, letting the vagina get comfortable around the penis and enjoying each other. Gently at first, by rolling your hips or moving in and out, you begin to move the penis inside the vagina. For some women these motions can stimulate the clitoris enough to reach orgasm.

Exactly when orgasm occurs depends on the person,

*This may be what you feel like doing. However, since a woman's orgasm originates in the clitoris, you may want to stimulate it more directly before intercourse. See "The Myth of the Vaginal Orgasm" by Anne Koedt. This is the paper that taught many of us about the source of our orgasm. It first appeared in *Notes from the First Year,* published in 1968 by New York City women active in women's liberation. Copies can be gotten from the New England Free Press, 791 Tremont St., Boston, Mass., 10¢ a copy.

and it's unusual for both people to reach orgasm at the same time. At some point the penis or clitoris has received enough stimulation, and it triggers off. First there is a feeling of expectation, as if your genitals were about to sneeze; the clitoris or penis may tingle. Then your whole body, especially the penis or clitoris-plus-vagina-plus-uterus goes into a glorious spasm (actually a series of rhythmic contractions), followed by a sense of relief.

Sometimes the woman, with continued stimulation, can have several or more orgasms. The man will have a "refractory period," during which he can't come to orgasm again. This can last from a few minutes to several days, depending on his age and physical condition.*

What Is an Orgasm?

What is an orgasm? An orgasm is not a mystical experience. It is a physical experience, and here is a description of the whole human response cycle:

What happens during the response cycle can be divided into four parts. First, there is the *excitement* phase. It begins as the body reacts to some kind of sexual stimulation. Blood rushes into the clitoris (also the penis) engorging it and causing erection. The rate of breathing increases, nipples become erect, body muscles (some voluntary, some involuntary) tighten, and you may notice a sexual flush or rash. The woman's vagina becomes moist, lubricated by fluid which passes through the vaginal walls from the body cavity in a kind of "sweating" reaction. As it lubricates and becomes more sensitive, the vagina begins a process of lengthening and expansion. The compacted folds and ridges smooth out and the whole cylinder straightens, enlarging and tenting at the upper end to make room for the fully erect penis and the ejaculated semen. This causes the uterus to balloon upward.

Excitement is followed by the *plateau* phase, although it would be hard to say exactly when one phase stops and the next begins. During the plateau phase the changes increase. The rate of breathing increases. Most dramatic is the swelling of the tissues around the outer part of the vagina, which makes the width of the vagina half its normal size, and able to grip the penis. The clitoris elevates like a male erection, and the inner lips change in color from pink to bright red. Both sexes feel increased involuntary muscular tension. The testes in the male move closer to his body. If stimulation continues (about a minute from the time of color changes in the vagina), the changes in your body build up to a climax of heightened feeling and body tension, which suddenly spills over into *orgasm,* a series of genital muscular contractions that release the built-up tension.

Orgasm itself is the third phase. There is a feeling of intense pleasure as the vagina goes into rhythmic muscu-

*Hackmann, pp. 14–16.

lar contractions which have come down from the top of the uterus; then the intensity tapers off.* The number of contractions vary with the intensity of the orgasm. The uterus also contracts rhythmically but the contractions are rarely felt. All the body's muscles respond in some way (even hands and feet, and facial muscles often contract into a grimace).

After the orgasm a kind of final *resolution* (fourth stage) occurs. The swelling of the nipples subsides, the sex flush disappears, and the clitoris returns to its normal position.† It may be as long as a half hour after orgasm before a woman's entire body returns to the state it was in before she was stimulated. If she has reached the plateau stage but has not reached orgasm, it will take much longer. Orgasm can be a very mild experience, almost as mild as a peaceful sigh, or it can be an extreme state of ecstasy with much thrashing about and momentary loss of awareness. It can last a few seconds or half a minute or longer. There is, in brief, no right or wrong way to have one.‡

The physical source of our orgasm is based in the clitoris, not in the vagina. Our sexual response to having a penis inside us depends very much on how much stimulation our clitoris receives either before or during actual intercourse. In intercourse the man's penis moves in and out of the vagina, alternately stretching and relaxing the inner lips (*labia minora*), which are swollen and partially erect as a result of sexual arousal. Since the minor lips form a hood over the clitoris, they move back and forth over the sensitive *glans* or tip of the clitoris, stimulating it so that sometimes orgasm occurs even though the penis has not directly contacted the clitoris. Often a couple will arrange their bodies so that there is more direct pressure on the clitoris.

This is not to say that the clitoris is the only sexually responsive part of our genitals. As we become increasingly aroused, the whole genital area including the swollen inner lips and the outer third of the vagina can become so sensitive that every movement of the penis feels good. This generalized sensitivity, however, does not come until the clitoris has had enough stimulation. The tissues are so connected that it is appropriate to say as Masters and Johnson do that we have not just vaginal orgasms and not just clitoral orgasms but sexual orgasms.

*"During a woman's orgasm many muscles are in function—including muscles in the walls of the vagina. Many women are unaware of these muscular contractions.

"The muscle consciousness can become greater. Most women can report discovering more and more things about their own orgasm with the years. Many women thus discover that their vagina contracts rhythmically during orgasm—something they had not realized before" (Inge and Sten Hegeler, *An ABZ of Love,* p. 193).

†A woman can have another orgasm right away; a man cannot. (See Hackmann quote above.)

‡Wardell Pomeroy's *Girls and Sex* is helpful on this.

Sex Without Intercourse

There are other ways of coming to orgasm besides intercourse. Sometimes people discover them in the course of heavy petting. Many people use them for variety after the first thrill of intercourse has worn off, or as an addition that makes lovemaking more enjoyable.

The first technique is masturbation. Most people in our generation were brought up with the idea that masturbation is bad, or that it will cause all sorts of problems and disease. This is *not true*. In fact, it is becoming clear that children brought up this way are likely to be uncomfortable with their own bodies and out of touch with their sexuality.

(For more on masturbation refer to the "Masturbation" section of this chapter.)

Masturbating your partner, aside from the variety, can sometimes be useful when one wants sex and the other is too tired to be aroused. The one being masturbated should show the other what motions work best and guide the other's hand until he/she catches on.

Oral stimulation is a very effective technique; the mouth and tongue are very sensitive and can give much finer variations of feeling than even the fingers. In cunnilingus, the man licks and sucks the woman's genitals, and in fellatio, the woman licks and sucks the man's. Some people have a strong, involuntary gag-reflex which interferes with making love this way, but that doesn't mean they don't love their partner.

Some people . . . find that anal stimulation is a great addition in making love. Some enjoy anal intercourse; be gentle about this, the anus is not as elastic as the vagina. Some enjoy a finger or candle in the anus during regular intercourse. Some enjoy having the anus licked. You will want to use a lubricant when inserting anything in the anus. It is very important to wash the penis, finger or candle after anal stimulation, before inserting any of these into the vagina; if you don't you're asking for an infection.

For some women, manual or oral stimulation, or the use of a vibrator, works better than intercourse; many couples use a combination of intercourse for the man and other stimulation for the woman. The French have a saying: "Anything that works, we do it!"

All of these techniques have advantages in addition to their variety. You can use them for physical relief if you don't want to have intercourse yet, and if you're caught without a contraceptive you can use them without getting pregnant.*

More Thoughts About Lovemaking

Some of us like to wash our genitals before making love, some of us don't. What counts is that you feel good about yourself and come to value your body's tastes and smells.

*Hackmann, pp. 18, 19.

If a woman washes her genitals regularly, she shouldn't need either douches or vaginal deodorants. The vagina cleans itself by shedding everything down to the entrance, where your washcloth takes over. Douching (except for a specific medical reason) interferes with the vagina's natural cleansing process and makes infections more likely. The natural smell of your genital area is designed to be attractive . . . so it's silly to cover it up. Also, the ingredients of deodorant suppositories and douches can be irritating to the vaginal tissues of some women. If you start to get a very strong and unpleasant odor, in spite of washing, you probably have an infection, and you should go to the doctor.

. . . .

If you have trouble touching each other in a sensual way, Masters and Johnson* have discovered a simple trick that should help. They tell couples to take turns rubbing hand lotion all over each other's body, finally coming to the genitals. Using the lotion, being told to cover the person's whole body with it, seems to give people "permission" to touch their partner in a way expressing love and enjoyment and to touch places they might not have dared to otherwise.

. . . .

You should generally count on one of you coming to orgasm before the other (the "ideal" that both people should reach orgasms at the same moment is unrealistic). Also, remember that people have different amounts of sex drive, and one person may not need or want orgasms as often as another.

. . . .

It is important never to begin making love with the idea that you are *definitely* going to have intercourse (though you should always have a contraceptive ready). This puts a lot of pressure on both of you to "perform." If it turns out that you are too tired, or have had too much alcohol or other drugs, it can be a real blow to your ego; you begin to worry, and a worried person can't relax and enjoy himself. If making love leads to intercourse and orgasm, fine; if not, that's fine too, we have both enjoyed ourselves.

. . . .

Try different positions for intercourse. The missionary position (man-on-top: so-called because some sophisticated natives had never used it until a missionary told them to) isn't necessarily the most arousing. Various ways with the woman above give her room to roll her hips freely, resulting in better stimulation for both. When the man enters the vagina from behind, there is the advantage that he can reach around and stimulate the clitoris with his fingers. Try not to be hung-up about the man being "dominant" or the woman "submissive"; you'll only miss out on a lot of human enjoyment. Sometimes you may want to try a really way-out position, even if it turns out not to work very well, just because the idea of it turns you both on. At any rate, experiment. Different people are different shapes and even the hardness of the bed you're on can make one position better than another.

. . . .

There is nothing wrong with having intercourse dur-

Human Sexual Response.

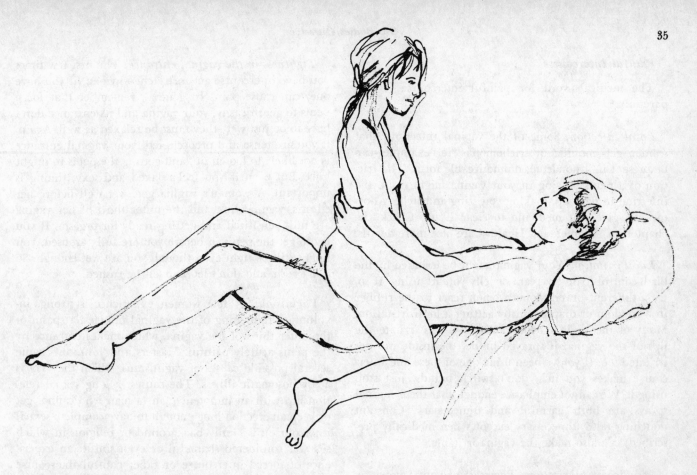

ing the woman's menstrual period, unless it is personally distasteful to one of you.

. . . .

There can be a real benefit to having intercourse (or masturbating) during menstruation; Masters and Johnson discovered that if a woman has cramps, coming to an orgasm will make them go away for a while.

It's also all right to have intercourse during pregnancy. Masters and Johnson studied some pregnant women and decided that, except for people with unusual medical difficulties, intercourse is OK as far into pregnancy as both partners are interested. After birth you can start again as soon as the woman's vagina is healed and she begins to be interested.*

Problems of Lovemaking

People have a lot of problems in lovemaking. When we finally started talking with each other about sex, we realized we had been putting up with a lot of the same ones. Also, we were putting up with these problems without doing much about them. Some of the reasons why:

Because we're dependent on the man and/or he'll go someplace else for sex, we don't complain.

Unconscious guilt—we grew up feeling that sex was bad or dirty in some way, which keeps us from actively finding out why our sex isn't better. While most of us

*Hackmann, pp. 20–24.

can sleep with a man without *consciously* feeling guilty, it has been difficult to assert our right to pleasure during lovemaking. First we have to realize that lovemaking can be pleasurable, then to work at getting what we need and want.

Even when we are aware that men have problems with sexuality, we often don't make a connection between their problems and our problems. We have not dealt with problems men have with sex here. Yet we realize that premature ejaculation, ejaculatory incompetence and impotence are very real problems.* Not only for the man but for us women who care about those men and also get frustrated by their problems. They thus become our problems too. In this area we must examine how our expectations of men contribute to their sexual problems. Mutuality in lovemaking hasn't been stressed enough; we need to take more shared responsibility in lovemaking than we have in the past.

If we don't have a gynecologist with whom we feel like talking about our sex lives, we don't have many good places to get information.

We haven't gotten information from each other.

Some of the problems of lovemaking are problems around intercourse that is physically painful, and around orgasm.

*See *Understanding Human Sexual Inadequacy* by Fred Belliveau and Lin Richter, Chapters 9–11, for more details.

Painful Intercourse

The medical word for painful intercourse is dyspareunia.*

Local infection. Some of the vaginal infections that women get—monilia or trichomonas, for example—can be present in a nonacute, nonnoticeable form. The friction of a penis moving in your vagina might cause the infection to flare up, making you sting and itch. A doctor can give you medicine to clear it up. Check the chapter on "Women and Health Care" for more details.

Local irritation. Your vagina might be irritated by the birth-control foam or cream or jelly you are using. If so, try a different brand. Some women react to the rubber in a condom or diaphragm by getting a local irritation. Many of the vaginal deodorant sprays can irritate the lips of the vagina; if sprayed inside, the inside can get irritated too. If you've been using one of these and intercourse makes you itch, don't switch brands, just stop using it. We cannot emphasize enough that these vaginal sprays are both harmful and unnecessary. Constant douching (also unnecessary except when medically prescribed) can also make the vagina irritable.

Insufficient lubrication. The wall of your vagina responds to sexy feelings by "sweating," giving off a liquid that wets your vagina and the entrance to it, to make the entry of the penis easier. Sometimes there isn't enough of this liquid. Some reasons: (a) You may be trying to let the penis in (or the man might be putting/ forcing it in) too soon, before there has been enough foreplay to excite you and set the sweating action going. (b) You may be nervous or tense about making love (maybe it's the first time, or maybe you're worried about getting pregnant), so there isn't enough liquid. (c) If the guy is using a rubber (condom) you are missing the lubrication supplied by the drops of liquid that come from his penis when he gets aroused.† Be sure to give your vagina time to get wet. If you still feel dry, try using saliva, K-Y jelly, or a birth-control foam, cream, or jelly. Occasionally, insufficient lubrication is caused by a hormone deficiency. After childbirth (particularly if the woman is nursing her baby) and during menopause are the two times when a lack of estrogen can affect the vaginal walls in such a way that less liquid is produced. A doctor can give you vaginal suppositories or some kind of hormone therapy. Meanwhile try the lubricants suggested above.

*See the section on dyspareunia in Belliveau and Richter, *Understanding Human Sexual Inadequacy* (pp. 195–206, paperback edition).

†This is just as well, as these drops can contain enough sperm to make you pregnant.

Tightness in the vaginal entrance. The first few times you have intercourse an unstretched hymen (if you have one) can cause pain. In general, remember that for a penis to get in easily, your vagina and its entrance don't have to be just wet—they must be relaxed as well. Again, if you are tense and preoccupied, your vaginal entrance is not likely to loosen up, and getting the penis in might hurt. But even if you feel relaxed and sexy, timing is important. A woman's vagina gets wet well before her clitoris, vaginal lips, and the outer third of her vagina are fully sensitized and getting ready for orgasm. If you try to get the penis in before you are fully aroused, you might still be tight even though you are wet enough. So don't rush, and don't let yourself be rushed.

Vaginismus. A few women experience a strong, involuntary tightening of the vaginal muscles, a spasm of the outer third of the vagina, which makes entrance by the penis acutely painful. Masters and Johnson* name several possible causes of vaginismus, which they say is a psychosomatic illness. The causes: a long sexual relationship with an impotent man (a man who cannot get or keep an erection long enough to have complete sexual intercourse); a family background or religion in which sex was considered shameful or even sinful; an experience of forced intercourse or rape; painful intercourse tolerated over a long period of time. If you think you are suffering from vaginismus, read about it in *Understanding Human Sexual Inadequacy* or in the detailed Masters and Johnson report, *Human Sexual Inadequacy*, and take the book to your gynecologist. There is an effective and simple physical treatment for vaginismus. You may want or need some psychotherapy to help you deal with the cause of your vaginismus.

Pain deep in the pelvis. Sometimes the thrust of the man's penis hurts way inside. Masters and Johnson say this pain can be caused by: (a) tears in the ligaments that support the uterus (caused by childbirth, a botched-up abortion, gang rape); (b) infections of the cervix, uterus, and tubes (such as pelvic inflammatory disease—the end result of untreated gonorrhea in many women); (c) endometriosis; (d) cysts or tumors on the ovaries. These can all be treated successfully. Also, if the penis hits the cervix during intercourse, it can be painful. That pain can be relieved by having the man not go in so deeply.

Clitoral pain. It may hurt if the man tries to touch your clitoris directly, as it is very sensitive. Also, a collection of material under the hood that covers the clitoris can cause irritation and make penetration painful. When you wash, be sure to pull back the hood of your clitoris and clean it gently.

*Human Sexual Inadequacy, pp. 184–194.

Not wanting to have intercourse in the first place. Sometimes a woman will feel pain in intercourse just because she doesn't want to have it. Another woman may hurt because she feels she *shouldn't* be doing it. As we begin to understand and be proud of our sexuality, we will increasingly feel good about having intercourse when we want to and saying no when we don't.

Several women we know have talked about intercourse as a kind of ritual rape for them. As we take more control of the situation for ourselves, and society changes its notions about sex, we hope these feelings about intercourse will cease.

So, if intercourse is at all painful to you, don't put up with the pain! Find out what is causing it and do something about it. And until the problem is solved, figure out other ways to make love. Use your hands, your mouths, your bellies, your thighs. An extra benefit—your clitoris can get more direct stimulation in other ways of lovemaking than penis-in-vagina intercourse, anyway.

Problems Around Orgasm

There are many reasons why we have problems with orgasm. Despite all the scientific evidence, male psychologists persist in treating the orgasm as a subject to which they can apply their own personal theories. The damaging and degrading images of women that these theories project can best be shown by quoting from one of them. Alexander Lowen, a well-respected psychotherapist, wrote his *Love and Orgasm* (see Bibliography) after Masters and Johnson published their results. Here's what he has to say about our sexuality. The italics are ours.

> The *problem* of orgastic potency in a woman is complicated by the fact that *some* women are capable of experiencing a sexual climax through clitoral stimulation. Is a clitoral orgasm satisfying? Why are some women capable of having *only* a clitoral orgasm? These questions should be answered if we are to understand the *problem* of orgastic impotence in the female.
>
> Most men feel that the *need* to bring a woman to climax through clitoral stimulation is a *burden*. If it is done before intercourse but after the man is excited and ready to penetrate, it *imposes* a *restraint* upon his natural desire for closeness and intimacy. Not only does he lose some of his excitation through this *delay,* but the subsequent act of coitus is *deprived* of its *mutual* quality. Clitoral stimulation during the act of intercourse may help the woman to reach a climax, but it *distracts* the man from the percepion of his genital sensations, and greatly interferes with the pelvic movements upon which his own feeling of satisfaction depends. The *need to bring a woman to climax* through clitoral stimulation after the act of intercourse has been completed and the man has reached climax is *burdensome* since it *prevents him from enjoying* the relaxation and peace which are the rewards of sexuality. Most men to whom I have spoken who engaged in this process *resented* it.

I do not mean to condemn the practice of clitoral stimulation if a woman finds that this is the way she can obtain sexual release. Above all *she should not feel guilty* about using this procedure. *However I advise my patients against this practice since it focuses feelings on the clitoris and prevents the vaginal response. It is not a fully satisfactory experience and cannot be considered the equivalent of a vaginal orgasm.*

It is astonishing to us to find ourselves so totally disregarded by Lowen. In a paragraph about women's orgasms he talks exclusively about male burden, male pride, male pleasure, male resentment, and then has the audacity to tell us not to feel guilty for seeking our own pleasure. How outrageous that he can use his moral authority as a therapist to tell women *not* to go after clitoral stimulation and to write a book whose only effect is to make us deny everything natural about what we need and to make us feel we're frigid or neurotic.

Here is a fantasy that indicates a lot about the reality many of us have experienced:

* * *

I have a fantasy about making love to David. We are having intercourse. I have an orgasm before him. I pull off of his penis and lie beside him, enjoying myself fully. He's very hurt. I say: "I should, but I don't want to continue." (His words to me on former occasions.) He insists. I scream at him: "Selfish pig! Can't you take what you dish out? Now you know what it feels like most of the time for a woman having sex. You're supposed to say: "It's okay. Just lie back and enjoy yourself. I'll wait until next time."

* * *

Even when we're aware of the facts of orgasm, even when we know that Lowen is wrong, and even when we know that the men we're sleeping with should be as interested in our orgasms as theirs, many of us still have trouble with orgasm. Here are some of the reasons:

We don't notice or else we misunderstand what's happening in our bodies as we get aroused. We're too busy thinking about abstractions—how to do it right, why it doesn't go well for us, what he thinks of us, whether he's impatient, whether he can last—when we might better be concentrating on sensations, not thought.* (Many of us grew up with the notion that a man just had to "come" or he was going to explode. His erection felt hard to us, and we were sure it hurt him. He is not going to explode, and his not climaxing hurts no more than our not climaxing.)

We know what we want at a particular moment, but we're too embarrassed to indicate what it is.

We are afraid of asking too much, asking for more than he can give.

*We refer to the sexual partner as "he," here, although we know that there are bad times in relationships between women. Most of us have had much less or no experience with women.

We are afraid the man will take requests and suggestions as an attack on his manhood.

We rush into it—or let our partners rush us into it. We end up fucking with great intensity, swept off our feet just like in the movies, and swept under the rug when it comes to climaxes. If you are getting passed by, it makes sense to slow everything down drastically, and never to escalate the situation without a clear and pressing physical impulse that tells you to. At this point we tend to get afraid that something is wrong with us—the impulse will never come. Sometimes it feels better just to hold each other for a while, or if being in bed feels bad, to get up, to take a walk, for instance, alone or together.

We feel ourselves becoming aroused, but we are afraid we won't have an orgasm, and we don't want to get into the hassle of trying, so we just repress sexual response.

We get interrupted.

> . . . a woman as a rule prefers a calm, constant, regular form of titillation without interruptions. The intensity of the titillation may vary during the period concerned and the woman may wish to have the rhythm changed a little, but as a rule she is less able to tolerate direct interruptions than a man. She is more easily distracted and then has to start all over again from the beginning in order to build up the tension that is to culminate in orgasm. Her orgasm would appear to build up more slowly, remain at peak longer and ease off more slowly.[*]

We are trying to have a simultaneous orgasm.

> . . . simultaneous orgasm is something that takes place very, very seldom and . . . it is by no means the normal, natural thing so many have tried to make of it. As a rule both first concentrate on the woman's orgasm, after which the man has his. Or one of the partners may peacefully go without once in a while if the sexual urge doesn't happen to be so great.[†]

We get on the right track, but we expect instant results, so we get tense and don't give ourselves enough time.

We have been making it with the same man for a long time and never or practically never have been satisfied. We feel angry (naturally), but find it difficult to break the pattern and assert our needs (ourselves). If a situation like this goes on long enough we can develop a real aversion to sex.

We expect to be instantly free and at ease with men we don't know very well or feel very close to. Maybe some people can do that. If you can't, you can't.

We don't want to be making love in the first place.

We feel guilty about having intercourse and so cannot let our body really enjoy it.

[*]I. and S. Hegeler, p. 193.
[†]Ibid.

Some Experiences

NAOMI. I have trouble asking that Jonathan continue to stimulate me after he has had an orgasm. It's hard for me to stay excited. I can't explain why because I haven't figured it out yet. Maybe I'm too self-conscious and not able to lose myself in my feelings. Also, part of what I find exciting is Jonathan's excitement and that is gone at that point.

The times when I make love with Jonathan and I'm only a little turned on I enjoy hugging him. It feels good to be close with him. Do I feel maternal, sisterly, a friend? Maybe a need to be mothered? It's not sorted out, but I know I do feel good. It satisfies one of my needs—for joyous physical contact with another person—but it isn't really the intense sexual one.

I don't worry as much as I did several months ago about whether I am going to have an orgasm. I am trying more and more to enjoy this physical relationship with Jonathan as it is. I hope this can continue—it's a lot less pressured than it used to be. I don't expect to have an orgasm when I make love with him now. I don't think I will very often, unless he can control his orgasm more or we start to make love differently. Sometimes we make love so that I have an orgasm before he enters my vagina. That's not bad, though I wish I could have one more with his penis inside me. The other way is a lot like masturbation and I feel I can do it better myself.

MAUREEN. The first time I had an orgasm which I was conscious of, was in the middle of my freshman year in college, in the middle of a heavy petting session with my regular date. I felt a mild, rhythmic and pleasurable sensation inside my vagina. I had not even known where my vagina was a few weeks earlier, since I had never used a tampon. I was not sure what had happened and had no knowledge that I had a clitoris or that it was my main organ of sexual pleasure.

I began to have orgasms more frequently during petting sessions by rubbing against the man and having him touch my genitals. The intensity of the pleasure feeling increased and I learned to feel more, become unanesthetized. In my second year in college I learned to masturbate with the bedclothes, rubbing against my genital area. It was often very hard for me to achieve orgasm this way. I think my guilt was enormous and blocked my ability to stimulate myself. My fantasies were not particularly vivid. I remember agonizing over whether I could confess masturbation—I was beginning to leave Catholicism. I think a lot of my trouble learning how to have orgasms with men is connected to the same wall of guilt about genital pleasure that I found preventing me from masturbating.

I frequently didn't have orgasms, because the man I was with didn't care to caress me in a way I found pleasurable. Because I sensed that he didn't want to pay attention to my needs, I didn't care to tell him about them.

MELISSA. I fell into a pattern of frigidity and experienced sexuality in marriage as a disguised ritual rape, which I now call "the Victorian syndrome." One of the things which characterized my sexual deadness was the emphasis on intercourse I had experienced in my marriage. Sex was something that was "done to me." I felt an incredible lack of mutuality and lack of control. I became, over a time, a passive instrument for my husband's pleasure. I felt very distanced from him during intercourse. I had the sense that he was relating to his own fantasies while he was having contact with me. He later told me this was often the case. It was not just my husband's fault. Neither of us was conscious of the emotional dynamic of our marriage, or the effect of our monogamy on our sexuality. Neither of us had people close enough to talk to about the problem, nor a sense of other people going through similar things. I felt sexually destroyed. I could not seem to make headway in improving the sexual expression in my marriage.

Three years ago I began to change my life. I stopped playing a "wifely" role and began to establish a life of my own, still within the context of marriage. As I began to feel stronger as a person and a woman, I became aware of and began to identify with the women's movement. I decided to open up the possibility of having sexual relations with other men than my husband, since that aspect of our relationship seemed at an impasse.

I have had some positive experiences and some very painful ones in exploring sexuality with other men. My ability to express myself sensually and to have joy in sexual relationships has increased.

FURTHER READINGS

Historical Books on Women and Sexuality

de Beauvoir, Simone. *The Second Sex.* New York: Bantam Books, 1961 (paper).
    This is a classic book about us—women, the second sex. It is divided into two books, "Facts and Myths" and "Woman's Life Today." The approach is philosophical, historical, literary, experimental—in other words, very broad. Some parts are easier to read and more relevant to our lives than others; some of her experiences are peculiarly French. The book (originally published in France in 1949 and in America in 1953) predates the current women's movement, and was the first book that many of us read that made us aware that we were oppressed as females.

Freud, Sigmund. *Three Essays on the Theory of Sexuality.* Translated by James Strachey. New York: Basic Books, 1962.
    No bibliography would be complete without an annotation on Freud. This work outlines his basic theories on female sexuality, part of a larger psychoanalytic view that we are not whole human beings because we lack a penis. Lot of nonsense, we say. But we should give him some credit. By the end of his life he recognized that he didn't know everything about women. He suggested that until there were further scientific studies we would have to look to our own experiences or to the poets. Quoting from "The Politics of Orgasm" by Susan Lydon from *Sisterhood Is Powerful*: ". . . he also expressed the hope that female psychoanalysts who followed him would be able to find out more. But the post-Freudians adhered rigidly to the doctrine of the master, and, as in most of his work, what Freud hoped would be taken as a thesis for future study, became instead a kind of canon law" (p. 199).

Friedan, Betty. *The Feminine Mystique.* New York: Dell Pub. Co., 1963 (paper).
    One of the first current and popular books about our condition as women in America. It gave impetus to the women's movement and to us. Recommended highly.

Herschberger, Ruth. *Adam's Rib.* New York: Harper Row Books, 1970 (paper; original, New York: Pellegrini & Cudahy, 1948).
    This book was written before the first Kinsey *et al.* study. It remained unread history until it was discovered by the women's movement. Filled with sexual theories, analysis, and general discussion of women's oppression. Her quote from Dr. R. L. Dickinson is especially relevant here: "Indeed Kobelt states that the glans of the clitoris is demonstrably richer in nerves than the male glans, for the two stems of the dorsalis clitoridis are relatively three or four times as large as the equivalent nerves of the penis" (p. 32).

Kinsey, Alfred C., Wardell B. Pomeroy, Clyde E. Martin, and Paul H. Gebhard. *Sexual Behavior in the Human Female.* Philadelphia: W. B. Saunders Co., 1953 (also paper).
—— *Sexual Behavior in the Human Male,* Philadelphia: W. B. Saunders Co., 1949 (also paper).
    Long studies of human sexual behavior that give lots of information and many experiences of women in the first book and of men in the second. They are historical books in that they opened up a new era of actual sex research. Masters and Johnson follow them.

Reich, Wilhelm. *The Function of the Orgasm.* New York: Noonday Press, 1961.
—— *The Sexual Revolution.* New York: Noonday Press, 1963 (both paper).
    Very important and original works on human sexuality.

Sexual Histories

Brecher, Edward. *The Sex Researchers.* New York: Signet Books, 1969 (paper).
    A very lively history of discoveries in the field of sex, with information about the people who made those discoveries. Enjoyable to read, conscious of female sexuality.

Lewinsohn, Richard. *A History of Sexual Customs.* New York: Harper & Row, 1971 (paper).
    The title describes the book. It is full of lots of interesting information. Lewinsohn is very sensitive to women as he writes the history. You can see the development of our oppression through time.

Current and Popular

Firestone, Shulamith. *The Dialectic of Sex: The Case for Feminist Revolution.* New York: Bantam Books, 1971 (paper).
    This book is considered a heavy, theoretical book. It is inter-

esting that it has been reviewed by journalists but not discussed very widely by the women's movement. The book is uneven: certain parts are fascinating and brilliant; others seem simplistic and boring.

Greer, Germaine. *The Female Eunuch*. New York: McGraw-Hill, 1970.
As with *Sexual Politics* this book and its author have been well advertised. *The Female Eunuch* has good sections on how we feel about our bodies and sexuality. In these areas the book is very useful to us. On the question of life style it is not as helpful to most women. Germaine Greer is a very talented, witty woman who perhaps generalizes too much from her own strengths. We certainly believe that we should be autonomous people, lead independent lives, and not be subjected to oppressive marriages. Yet for many of us her model of motherhood, for instance, is a little too extreme to relate to.

"J." *Sensuous Woman*. New York: Lyle Stuart, 1970.
A highly publicized but very sexist book; emphasis is on how women can be more sexy to please men. His needs are most important in the book. On the positive side, it does encourage masturbation, and it stresses that in lovemaking a woman should use her body and the man's body for her sexual pleasure in the same way that the man does.

Millet, Kate. *Sexual Politics*. New York: Doubleday, 1970, and Equinox Books (Avon), 1970 (paper).
The book and its author have gotten a lot of publicity for themselves and the women's movement. It is a basic book about the politics of sex—particularly sex and literature. It was designed for the college-educated person who has read a a lot of the literature she refers to.

Morgan, Robin, ed. *Sisterhood Is Powerful: An Anthology of Writings from the Women's Liberation Movement*. New York: Vintage Books, 1970 (paper).
This book is a collection of writings from the women's movement. It includes an enormous range of material, and has an excellent bibliography. Several pieces in the section "The Invisible Woman: Psychological and Sexual Repression" are especially applicable to the sexuality chapter of this book.

Solanas, Valerie. *S.C.U.M. Manifesto*. New York: Olympia Press, 1968.
A strong treatise on female superiority.

Other Current but More General Material

Cade, Toni, *Black Woman*. New York: Signet Books, 1970.
Anthology of writings by black women. Excellent.

Cooper, David. *The Death of the Family*. New York: Vintage Books, 1970.
Written by a young British radical who has had contact with the American situation. It's much more difficult to read than necessary—male philosophic obtuseness at its worst. Yet, if you can plow your way through, there is a good discussion of the oppression of the nuclear family and the limitations of monogamous relationships. The author has a good grasp of the importance of loving ourselves—feeling joy, having the ability to grow and change and not stagnate because we place security and happiness over love of ourselves.

Laing, R. D., and A. Esterson. *Sanity, Madness and the Family*. London: Pelican Books, 1970.
An excellent study of schizophrenic women and their families. It talks a lot about the oppression of the family. Very readable.

Roszak, Betty and Theodore. *Masculine/Feminine: Readings in Sexual Mythology and the Liberation of Women*. New York: Harper Colophon Books, 1969.
Diverse collection of readings on topic.

Slater, Philip. *The Pursuit of Loneliness*. Boston: Beacon Press, 1970 (paper).
This book is about American culture in general. It has very interesting things to say about the relationships of women and children. Most relevant for this chapter is the author's economic analysis of sex and romantic love.

Stevens, Barry. *Don't Push the River (It Flows by Itself)*. Real People Press, P.O. Box 542, Lafayette, Cal. 94549 (paper, $3.50).
Experiences of an older woman. She worked with Fritz Perls to become a Gestalt therapist. This book is a journal of sorts. Very helpful and supportive in understanding yourself, your own rhythms.

Pamphlets and Journals

Much of the most current material is published in this form and in newspapers of the movement. Here is some material that we used or are aware of. There are many more sources in your area.

Allen, Pamela. *Free Space: The Small Group in Women's Liberation*. Times Change Press, 1023 Sixth Avenue, New York, N. Y. 10018 ($1.25).
Pam Allen writes about the women and history of her small group. She also discusses the basis and process of such groups. Many of us have grown more aware of ourselves by being in small consciousness-raising groups. This pamphlet can help you understand the process of our growth—about sexuality as well as in all other areas of our lives as women.

The Female State: We Choose Personhood—A Journal of Female Liberation, Issue Four (April 1970). Copies of these journals are available from New England Free Press, 791 Tremont Street, Boston, Mass. 02118 ($1.25 plus postage).
Articles relating to dress and sexuality, motherhood, and so on.

No More Fun and Games: A Journal of Female Liberation.
One of the first women's journals. Put out by a Boston group. Some of the first current writings on the liberation of women.
Issue One (Spring 1967): Articles on celibacy, sexuality, asexuality, and "dress to go human in" first began to raise our consciousness about these topics.
Issue Two (February 1969): Articles relating to sexuality and other topics—being a beautiful object, sex and the single girl.
Issue Three (Fall, 1969): " 'Sexual Liberation': More of the Same Thing" was the source for some of the ideas in this chapter.

Unbecoming Men: A Men's Consciousness-Raising Group Writes on Oppression and Themselves. Times Change Press, 1023 Sixth Avenue, New York, N. Y. 10018 ($1.25).
Many men are trying to change in response to the women's movement, but for themselves. Here is an account of that process for men.

Fiction

Angelou, Maya. *I Know Why the Caged Bird Sings*. New York: Bantam Books, 1971 (paper).

Arnow, Harriette. *The Dollmaker*. New York: Collier Books, 1961 (paper).

Chopin, Kate. *The Awakening*. New York: Capricorn Books, 1964 (paper).

Drabble, Margaret. *The Waterfall*. New York: Alfred A. Knopf, Inc., 1969.

——— *The Garrick Year*. New York: William Morrow & Co., Inc., 1964.

Holiday, Billie, and William Dufty. *Lady Sings the Blues*. New York: Doubleday & Co., Inc., 1956.

Lessing, Doris. *The Golden Notebook*. New York: Ballantine Books, 1970.

——— *A Proper Marriage*. New York: New American Library, 1964.

——— *A Man and Two Women*. New York: Simon and Schuster, 1963.

Moody, Anne. *Coming of Age in Mississippi*. New York: Dell Pub. Co., 1970.

Stead, Christina. *The Man Who Loved Children.* New York: Bard Books (Avon) 1969.

Tolstoy, Leo. *Anna Karenina.* New York: Signet Books, 1961.

Walker, Alice. *The Third Life of Grange Copeland.* New York: Harcourt Brace Jovanovich, 1970.

There are growing numbers of women's fiction writings that give lots of insight into our sexuality. These are just a few.

Specific Information About Sex and Sexuality

Belliveau, Fred, and Lin Richter. *Understanding Human Sexual Inadequacy.* New York: Bantam Books, 1970.

Shortened and more readable version of the Masters and Johnson second study, *Human Sexual Inadequacy,* for someone who doesn't want to have all the clinical details. It can be used as a handbook also for those who can't get to a sex counselor and need some help. For instance, it has specific therapeutic exercises for premature ejaculation.

Brecher, Ruth and Edward, eds. *An Analysis of Human Sexual Response.* New York: Signet Books, 1966.

This book is just what the title says it is, an analysis of the Masters and Johnson study. The analysis was done by the editors and is very readable. It also contains sections on other sex research, practical applications of sex research, and sex research and our culture—a wide range of articles by people who have been involved in the study of sex. The book has lots of bibliographical references scattered throughout the book.

Deutsch, Ronald M. *The Key to Feminine Response in Marriage.* New York: Random House, 1968.

A popularized account of how women can have better orgasms (and incidentally prevent many "female troubles") by strengthening their pelvic-floor muscles. A how-to book. The last third of the book explores some reasons why women have trouble enjoying lovemaking. The author makes many perceptive comments, but doesn't consider working to change society in order to change conditions.

Ejlersen, Mette. *"I Accuse."* New York: Award Books, 1969 (paper).

A book by a woman about female sexuality. She talks a lot about clitoral orgasm. The book is brief and supportive to women. There is an Afterword to the book by Sten and Inge Hegeler.

Hackmann, Marjorie W. *Practical Sex Information.* Waking Woman Press, c/o Hackmann, 1637 N.W. Kings Boulevard, Corvallis, Ore. 97330 (50 cents plus postage).

Excellent pamphlet filled with practical sex information. Written simply and clearly. Good for all ages.

Hegeler, Inge and Sten. *An ABZ of Love.* New York: Alexicon Corp., 1967 (paper).

A superb book about sex. It's written as a dictionary of sex terms, but don't let that put you off. The authors, a doctor and a psychologist, have a very open, honest, human view of sexuality; they take us as women very seriously. The book can be used as a marriage manual of sorts, but one that deals with feelings, not techniques. They make you feel that it's natural and normal to want to know more about sex and explore your own sexuality. Get a copy! They have a second book, *An XYZ of Love.* New York: Crown, 1970. If it's anything like the first book, I'm sure it's good.

Masters, William H., and Virginia Johnson. *Human Sexual Response.* Boston: Little, Brown & Co., 1966.

The authors' research into real human sexual behavior in the 1960s was at first shocking. It is truly a revolutionary book because it considers sex a legitimate topic for scientific inquiry. We as women will always be thankful to Masters and Johnson. Their research began to destroy many myths that have kept us down sexually—most notable among them the myth of the vaginal orgasm or that the source of sexual pleasure in women is in our vagina, not in our clitoris.

Pomeroy, Wardell B. *Boys and Sex.* New York: Delacorte Press (Dell), 1968.

——— *Girls and Sex.* New York: Delacorte Press (Dell), 1969.

These two books are simply and clearly written. They have information and good attitudes about accepting ourselves, our bodies, our sexuality. He is a man who has essentially the same politics about sexuality as we have. Good books for adolescents. Pomeroy worked with Kinsey.

Yale Student Committee on Human Sexuality. *The Student Guide to Sex on Campus.* New York: Signet Books, March, 1971 (first edition).

Complete and up-to-date information.

Lesbianism

Writings are sparse at this point. Look to current gay newspapers, journals, and any other publications.

Caprio, Frank S. *Female Homosexuality: A Modern Study of Lesbianism.* New York: Grove Press, 1954.

Has some good historical facts—for instance, just how common lesbianism is all over the world. But the author's basic attitude toward homosexuality is bad: you can be "cured" if you want to.

Grahn, Judy. *Edward the Dyke and Other Poems.* Graphics by Wendy Cadden, Brenda Cridler, and Gail Hodgins.

Write to Women's Press Collective, 1018 Valencia Street, San Francisco, Cal. ($1.25 plus postage).

Hall, Radclyffe. *The Well of Loneliness.* New York: Pocket Books, 1959.

A classic novel about lesbians. Sympathetic, not pornographic. Life was depressing for the two lesbians about whom the book is written.

Love Songs of Sappho. Translated by Paul Roche. New York: Mentor Books, 1963.

Information about Sappho and other lesbians of the past is included in Lewinsohn, *A History of Sexual Customs* (see page 39).

Miller, Isabel. *A Place for Us.* Bleecker Street Press, Box 625, Old Chelsea Station, New York, N. Y. 10011 ($2.25 plus postage).

Reissued in 1972 by Macmillan as *Patience and Sarah* ($5.95).

An excellent book. Isabel Miller (a pseudonym) received the first annual gay book award from an affiliate of the American Library Association for this book. It is supposedly the true story of two women who lived and loved each other during the early part of the nineteenth century in upstate New York. The book is positive about lesbianism and also has a feminist consciousness.

4
Living with Ourselves and Others: Our Relationships

INTRODUCTION

WE LEARN from our culture that the relationship of a married woman with her husband is the most intimate and lasting relationship a woman has. A woman is always expected to put this relationship before everyone and everything else in her life. What we want to do in this chapter is counteract this misleading and confining message. We want to open the definition of marriage and we want to explore intimate relationships in addition to marriage, intimate relationships instead of marriage, and intimate relationships with ourselves. For those of us who decide that marriage *is* a very deep and important relationship for us, our marriage will be far better if we feel that it is our clear choice rather than our only alternative or our life-defining duty.

We have found for ourselves that broadening the scope of our close relationships has been very difficult and has taken a lot of time and energy. The support of other women has allowed us the space to grow in many directions. In this chapter we present the experiences of a lot of different women. They are not meant to be models. We don't want any woman reading this chapter to feel that these are goals she has to get to someday. We want to share our experiences, our confusions, and the choices we've made so that every woman can be more aware of what her own choices are. We're still growing and changing. A year from now we would probably tell our stories differently.

Good relationships are difficult, if not impossible, if we don't understand ourselves and our own needs. Asking and being given, telling a need and having it fulfilled, free us to be able to give. This is very difficult when people come together not as equals but as teacher and taught, the admired and the admiring, the assertive and the acquiescent. Good relationships are mutual. They are built on each partner feeling as competent and in control of her or his life as the other.

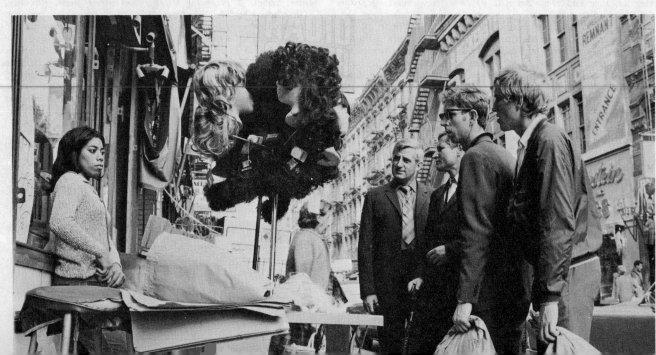

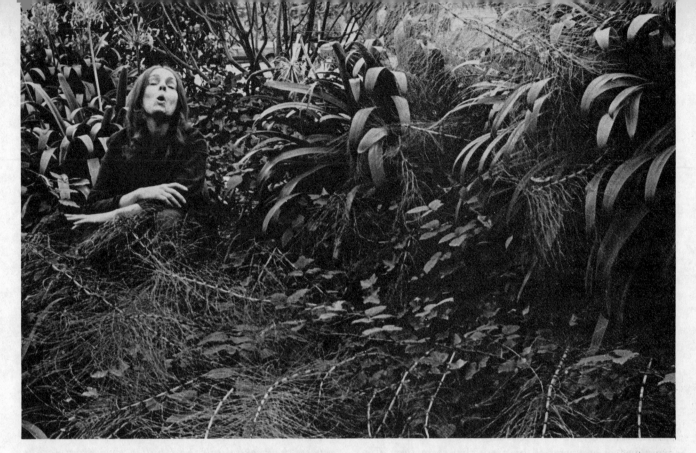

In this chapter we present a range of experiences and feelings about our relationships with ourselves, with men, and with women. Two aspects of our relationships that we have neglected in the past have been the possibility of periods of celibacy—that is, having no sexual relations with others—and the possibility of accepting and coming to terms with our sexual feelings for women.

FEELINGS ABOUT CELIBACY

Sexual relationships often create anxieties and distractions that keep us from getting in closer touch with ourselves. We wonder why we didn't come, or if the other person liked it, or if he or she wouldn't rather be in bed with so-and-so, and so on. This takes up lots of psychic energy that could be used for other thoughts and activities.

Celibacy, for different periods of time—two weeks, a month, a year—allows us to explore ourselves without the problems and power struggles of a sexual relationship. We can begin to define ourselves not just in terms of another person.

Many of us have entered periods of celibacy with apprehension—we have feared the insecurity of being without a partner. Yet often this anxiety diminishes because being alone is a very positive experience. It has given back to us our integrity, our privacy, our pride.

* * *

At this point I realized that I had been initially frustrated by not having a man, because I felt incomplete without one: a man meant completion. After several months of celibacy I saw that I could feel whole by myself.

* * *

My first reaction to being without a man was frustration and anger. I thought, Well, here I am feeling pretty liberated sexually, and there's no one to sleep with. Over time, I thought less and less about being with a man. I had very relaxed times with my friends, and never had to think twice about making plans with them for dinner. I was not asexual during this time. I was masturbating with much pleasure, having different kinds of orgasms— some long and slow and ripply, others short and jerky and tenser. I explored my sexuality in a way I had not with men. It was also easier to work at what I wanted to, because I was my only obligation.

* * *

I have been celibate for over a year, since the beginning of my involvement with the women's movement, which gave me a lot of support. I work very hard and feel good about working. I have created my own physical environment building a house and provided my own psychological space—a good combination. I masturbate a lot and enjoy it. I feel happy, independent, and free to figure out my own expectations of me.

* * *

Some of us come out of celibacy deliberately, feeling that we need a primary relationship. Some of us, feeling isolated and outside the norms of society, give up and flee into the arms of the first person to come along. Some of us may find we feel better being more autonomous.

The luxury of this kind of solitude has been very liberating. But for most of us being celibate has not provided a long-term solution to the problems posed by sexual relationships. There are also some very real drawbacks to long periods of celibacy.

Most of us crave physical contact and physical affection. To be alone, or to receive physical affection only from our animals and children, doesn't quite work. We can have fantasies about sleeping with them, but it doesn't feel right to act on them. We need other adult human beings to meet our deeper sexual/sensual needs.

Going without physical affection for long periods can be a kind of starvation. We won't die as we would without food or air, but the effects may still show in our bodies. We may get stiffer and out of touch with our sensuality. Though we can masturbate a lot and enjoy it, masturbation doesn't fill the same need as sex with someone else. When celibacy no longer feels good we should get out of it—but that's easier said than done. And it feels harder the longer we have been celibate. Coming out of celibacy, we may feel awkward or defensive, or we may feel embarrassed by needs that seem insatiable. Sometimes it's easier to start a new relationship with someone else who is also coming out of celibacy.

One unresolved thought: Do we ever choose celibacy out of fear of any kind of physical intimacy? What does this mean?

It's hard to take on the loneliness, the bad parts of being alone as well as the good parts of getting in touch with ourselves. It's also difficult to explore fully what being celibate can mean to us, since society does not generally accept the idea of choosing to refrain from sexual activity.

FEELINGS ABOUT HOMOSEXUALITY

We do each other a lot of harm by being scared about homosexuality. Our fears are understandable: parents who joked about fags and dykes, teachers who carefully avoided the subject, doctors who pronounced that homosexuals were maybe not sinful but indeed very sick—all left us with no clear information and a lot of prejudice and fear in our attitudes toward people who were sexually and emotionally attracted to other people of their own sex.

Here is a friendship that suffered because these fears had been so well taught:

* * *

When I was a junior and senior in high school I had an intense friendship with Jan, a girl in my school. We wrote notes and went on walks and climbed trees, shar-

ing dreams, reciting poems that we liked, and talking about coming back to the school in later years to teach together. We vowed lifelong love and friendship, but physically we could express the energy that was between us only by clowning around, bumping into each other— and once when she was asleep I kissed her hair. The intensity of my friendship with Jan made my family uneasy—I remember comments about seeing too much of one person. Their uneasiness got to me a little, because I was a bit uncomfortable with my strong pit-of-the-stomach feelings about her anyway. I remember being shy about undressing with her in the room, although I undressed with other friends without thinking about it. Then during the summer after we graduated, having not seen Jan for several weeks, I was leafing through a psychology book and found a section that talked about the intense, bordering-on-homosexual friendships of young girls.

Before long I had labeled it as a silly, childishly intense friendship. I made no efforts to see her when we both went to college, for I figured we had nothing in common.

I think our feelings grew more intense as we tried to repress their sexual side. So I pulled away from Jan because I couldn't handle the natural sexual part of my feelings of affection for her.

* * *

We're not saying that we all want to sleep with each other, but that we don't want to pull out of friendships or repress whole areas within friendships because of fears of homosexuality. We can be conscious of sexual feelings between us and choose not to act on them.

Some of our feelings revolve around thinking that having homosexual feelings and acting on them is very abnormal and unusual. Quite the contrary. Fewer people act on homosexual feelings than experience them, but in both cases the number of people, women and men, is surprisingly greater than most of us know. The Institute for Sex Research of Indiana University found that "between their adolescence and old age, about 37% of all males have some overt homosexual experience to the point of orgasm . . . for females the estimated incidence of homosexual behavior is about half that for males."* The actual incidence, particularly for women, is surely higher. (See Bibliography for historical references and references to other cultures.)

For some of us there will be times in our lives when we will feel sexual rapport only or mainly with women. The fact that the women's movement has opened up that option for some of us is very exciting:

* * *

*Isadore Rubin, *Homosexuality*, SIECUS Study Guide No. 2 (October 1967), p. 7.

I have felt as strong, if not stronger feelings for a certain woman as I felt for my husband. She was a good friend I had known as long as I'd known my husband. We loved each other very much, and with support from the women's movement, became more comfortable being openly physically affectionate, and this grew into our sleeping with each other. It wasn't just sexual, but deeply emotional too. When I touched her breasts I knew what she was feeling because I had breasts too.

But just because we were women, it did not mean that we could avoid all the problems of power, control and competitiveness we had experienced in relationships with men. That frightened me. I still have a lot of sexual feelings toward women and feel good about being physically affectionate, but I have chosen for now not to sleep with women.

At the time, one year ago, when the Gay Liberation Movement was beginning to blossom, it felt easier to me than it does now. The fear of being different, to the extent that I would call myself lesbian, is too scary for me.

* * *

The women's movement has made me feel both good about women and also hesitant about intense sexual involvements with women. After the high times of the first year of the women's movement, when we discovered how wonderful women were, believed everything was possible, we came down to earth. Women did not always act in the most friendly and supportive ways to one another. The gap between the ideology of sisterhood and the reality became very apparent to me in the second and third years of the women's movement. In fact I even found that in some instances I got more support and understanding from men friends than from women.

It took me a long time to accept this as true. (I wanted very much to believe in the ultimate power of sisterhood, when in fact people are people, and just because someone is a woman, doesn't necessarily mean we're going to be close friends.) I realize now that it makes sense. It is very hard to change the deep patterns of competition between women for men. At least the pattern has begun to change—we've begun to be open, honest, and able to cooperate, be supportive to each other. During these changes I've felt a new commitment to women. I also am able to accept men as friends and lovers again. Perhaps this is part of my and other women's greater mellowness and openness to men this year than in the last two years.

* * *

My first homosexual experience felt very natural and right. Afterward I wasn't guilty or confused, and I wished it had happened sooner. I blamed this delay on our culture and my upbringing—I grew up without ever having seen a woman expressing sexual feelings for another woman.

I've slept with several women. Although sex with one of them was incredibly intense and ecstatic, much like my best experiences with men, on the whole I've felt less "electricity" in my relationships with women. Instead, I've felt more sensual and affectionate and more of a back-to-the-womb comfort. It's been a different experience, though—not better or worse.

I've recently been celibate (except for an occasional night spent with a dear friend living several hours away), and for the first time have noticed the extraordinary amount of energy I've put into men and trying to change them. Much typically masculine behavior really bothers me, so when I've spent lots of time with a man who's learned to be "properly virile" I've struggled a lot. Now, since almost all my important relationships are with women, and these relationships are much less draining, I see this all much more clearly.

I'm not gay, but I see now it's a real possibility for me, at least for a while. I've come a long way from childhood expectations of marrying a "special" man and having four kids.

OUR EXPERIENCES

Although in this society marriage is considered the model arrangement for adults, and the monogamous, nuclear family is seen as the ideal living situation, there are, in fact, other choices we can make about how and with whom we live. Instead of systematically separating the different options for discussion one by one, we have chosen to use narratives from the lives of several of us who have passed in and out of one or a number of these options on our way to finding what's best for us.

We have no one opinion about monogamous or non-monogamous relationships. We want to express both our good and bad experiences. We want to begin to separate the good reasons for staying in monogamous relationships from the good reasons for leaving. (And remember, monogamy is not limited to just heterosexual relationships.) We want to explore the possibilities of getting love and support from several people, rather than having one primary intimate relationship that is supposed to satisfy all needs.

Laura: Family, Marriage, and Separation

I grew up in a progressive, middle-class family: mother, father, sister, brother. I learned by watching, listening, asking my parents what was important to them. Their relationship to one another was special, different from their relationships to other people. Before their marriage they slept with other people, but after marriage they only slept with each other, as far as I knew.

They never put in words that the marriage relationship was sacred, but I knew it; when friends of theirs got divorced there were sounds of "How terrible!" Even when they were feeling miserable and unhappy, it was clear they would "stick it out." I was never afraid my parents would separate, but I had to hold inside me any tensions and negative feelings that they pushed under. For instance, instead of each of them visiting different friends because that's what they felt like doing, they would fight until one won and one lost. And they both went off together—but angry and resentful.

My parents have functioned as a unit for almost thirty-five years. Their marriage has a sense of continuity, a sense of love, caring, and security, which is not easy to come by in this crazy world. I have a very real respect, even admiration, for much of what grew out of their commitment to one another. But the lack of questioning in their relationship, their failure to meet problems head on, and their idealization of the nuclear family and monogamy—all this I felt was destructive to both of them and to me.

Okay. So I am twenty-nine years old now. Following the only model I knew, I lived with and then was married to my husband for ten years. We had two children together. I separated from him six months ago.

I got married at nineteen. We were both in college, both young, scared, and alone. We got together. It was a way to break ties with our parents, to be on our own in a comforting, secure way. For many years we grew alongside each other as friends and as lovers.

As we grew up we felt our differences more, too. But we found it hard to see those differences as legitimate, since all our expectations told us that we were a special "unit." If I wanted to spend time with him and he wanted to read, I felt hurt. If I wanted to visit my friends and he needed to be with me at that time, he felt hurt. If one of us didn't want to make love and the other did, the hurt was worse. At times the hurt turned to anger and resentment.

Being intimate with only one other person did not seem to be enough to meet our needs. But it was hard to go outside the marriage for intimacy, since that would break the "contract." Friendships with others was okay, but sexual intimacy was another matter.

At the point that we both reached out for other intimate relationships we were reaching out for ourselves. Friends still referred to us as the Greenways rather than as Laura and Joe. But the need for each of us to feel whole, distinct, separate, and centered in ourselves was pressing; it took priority over the marriage.

How do you know when you reach the point when you no longer can change together? When is separation a copout? When is it a positive moving forward? These are crucial questions with no easy answers. Many, many couples get to this point, sometimes over and over again. There are different ways of dealing with the impasse—keeping up a marriage of convenience, splitting up angry, splitting up when the kids are less dependent. For me it was very difficult and painful to think about separation and finally separating. Breaking up doesn't have to mean the whole relationship was bad, but deep down the myth is that marriage should be "for always" and we are failures if our marriages come to an end. I still feel the pain of losing the closeness and intimacy that we had built up over ten years. It was hard to give up even when the marriage lacked joy, and things between us were clearly sour.

Ungluing our marriage took at least two years. It began with the women's movement, which gave me support to move out on my own, to develop new skills and

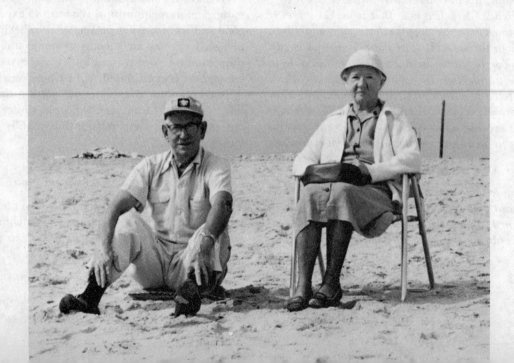

new relationships. I still felt in contact with my husband on some levels. I was involved in two different relationships during that time—one with a woman, one with a man. They were each long-term friendships that grew more intimate—emotionally and sexually.

During this time my husband and kids and I were living with a group of people. With other people around, we thought we could perhaps be more independent and still live together. It didn't work. For us, more people meant more conflict and tension as well as more resources.

I split for a while. I left the house to sort out my feelings, though I still wanted to live with my husband and kids. I wound up staying away for several months, and finally left for good. The decision to leave was especially painful because I was breaking up a family as well as a marriage.

So where am I now? I feel in many ways I've exchanged one set of problems for another. I live by myself half time, and with my kids half time. (Relative to other women, I'm fortunate that my husband and the people he lives with are willing and able to care for the children half time.) I feel much more centered in me than when I was married. Sometimes my center feels warm and strong, other times cold and lonely. My kids are very important to me, especially now. They are a stable, loving element in my life.

And my friends—I couldn't be living alone without support from them. Some of them have lived or do live alone. They tell me, "Keep going, it's good for a time." It's the first time in my life I've had space to focus on me, to love myself more, so that I can deeply love others, whether men or women.

So what about my husband, ex-husband? Our relationship continues. Tentative. Slow. Tense at times, happy at others. I feel much more love for him than the last couple of years together. We are clearly separate now; I don't waste energy resenting him for not meeting my needs, or making demands he can't meet.

Because of the kids and child-care arrangements we have regular contact. Beyond that, our relationship is far from ended. I like to think it's just beginning in other ways. Sometimes I think I'd like to be married to him again, and then the other side comes pouring out. . . . I am where I am now. Where I'm going tomorrow I don't know, and part of me likes the excitement of not knowing.

Mathilde: A Deepening Relationship

Julien and I met when we were very young, eighteen and nineteen years old. We had a fiery, emotional, storybook love affair. Read poetry to each other, took long

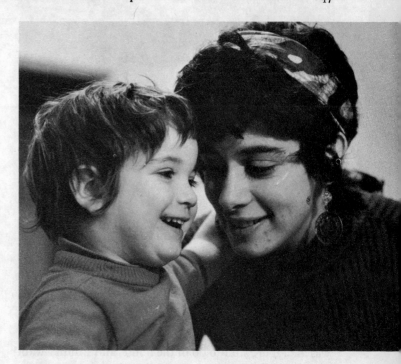

walks in the country, went skiing. We spent whole afternoons, days, weekends in bed, holding and touching each other, bringing each other to orgasm many times, even though we didn't actually have intercourse with each other for over a year. After a couple of years we got married.

The years before we had kids we spent a lot of time together studying, working, traveling, and making friends, building up a reservoir of experiences we shared and talked about. They have become a part of us both, have somehow made us part of each other.

Over the past ten years we've had plenty of fights and disagreements, but I've had only one huge trauma. In our third or fourth year of marriage we had a fight over something—I don't remember what—and he wouldn't talk to me for over a week no matter how much I cried. I hated that coldness more than anything else in my life.

When we were first married and had gotten over the first high excitement of early lovemaking, we started talking about how we would handle it if either of us wanted to have an affair. Well, we blissfully thought, that would be easy! We would simply bring the third person into our relationship and all make love together! It actually almost happened once.

We also talked about having sexual relationships with other couples. Both of us had had very little sexual experience before we met each other and wanted to "broaden our love relationships" (though we didn't want to betray each other). I realize now that those things could not possibly have happened the rational way we planned.

The women's movement coincided with my very little

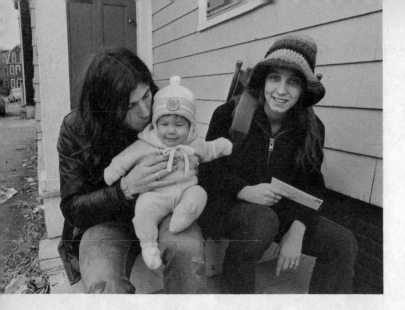

babies and with Julien's getting a job for the first time. Before the movement we played traditional roles—I worked from nine to five and did all the things in the house too. It never occurred to me to ask him to cook, clean, or do the marketing. When the kids came, there was a lot more stuff to do in the house, and I didn't want to do it all. There were lots of fights around those things, but he really changed a lot. Now we share much of the child care. But, still, he has a full-time job, while I stay home with the kids and work part time.

Julien has always been a good lover, has always wanted to do what I liked. It was a couple of years before I had orgasms during intercourse, but I was never left unsatisfied. Our love affair remained a love affair for a long time after we were married. Then, inevitably, it became more tranquil. But our relationship never lost the closeness, the basic understanding we have of each other: we love each other very much and we tell each other so, often.

That wild sexual excitement of our early lives has been gone for a long time, along with all those wild positions, antics, lotions, honeys. But, then, we're now much more proficient at lovemaking, and when we do it, we do it very well.

We have both made compromises in our lives for each other, for our kids. We have both changed a good deal over the years we have been together. I often think that it was just luck that our individual changes did not make us grow apart, but allowed us to draw together. I'm very glad they did.

Sarah: Thoughts and Feelings About Monogamy

After many years of struggle we have reached a plateau of trust together, and these trustful feelings allow us to take risks with each other and ourselves. I also feel less hung up about the traditional roles of male and female, because through our openness and the resulting intimacy I have learned that my husband has many of the same weak feelings, fragile feelings, that previously I thought were female—just as he has learned that I have certain kinds of strengths he doesn't have. This kind of relationship provides a unique opportunity, I feel, for self-exploration and deep understanding about oneself and one's mate. I think the crucial thing here is time, to build up feelings of confidence and trust and comfort and kindness, and time also to foster a special atmosphere that seems to be a combination of closeness and openness which teaches one the confidence to begin to explore, search, and grow.

I want to stress that at this point in my life, knowing all the things now I didn't know when I got married, I would again choose monogamy, not for the sake of the children or the family, but for myself, and my husband. I don't prescribe my choice for everyone. I just feel—I have tasted love and it is good.

The Experience of Being Single: Many Voices

Excerpts from taped conversations among a group of single women in Boston

It is an old belief that heterosexual couples are the only natural and necessary form of existence. Think of Noah's ark. Everything leads up to finding a mate—for love, for intimacy, for economic security, for survival of self, and for the survival of the species. Any other form of adult life is an exception to be pitied (old maid, widow), maligned (homosexual), or possibly tolerated (playboy bachelor, eccentric artist).

We all grew up with these assumptions. People outside our families were defined as "outsiders." We expected to be inside a couple and inside our own families when we grew up. We might be single women and do exciting things for a while, but that would be just a breathing space before marriage.

It didn't work out that way for us. We are a group of

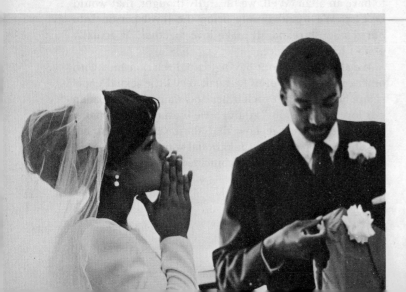

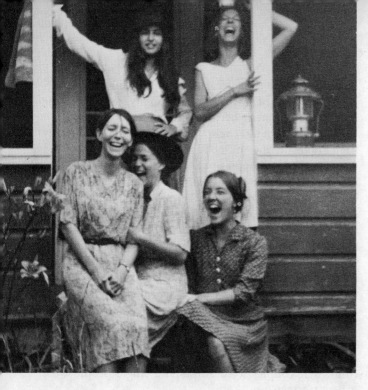

single women in our twenties. We have all had relationships with men that have been important to us, but none of us has ever been married. For the past few years we have all been deeply, personally involved in the women's liberation movement, and our lives have changed drastically. All of us have varying degrees of intimacy with people now, primarily with women. None of us has a primary relationship that defines who we are. Together we are trying to explore our independence and find positive identities for ourselves—not in isolation from other people, but outside of relationships that feel limiting or defining.

We have different fantasies for the future. Some of us want more intimate relationships. But in our lives outside of couples we've felt a lot of strength and joy—alone and as part of a group. What we've learned from being single is much more than the skills of survival in a "transitional" state. And we look forward to new options for women in the future. Here are some of our experiences and thoughts.

ELAINE. As a child I was often told it was impossible for a woman to take care of herself alone in the world, that she needed a man to manage things for her. No one took a woman seriously. I knew a repairman would come immediately if my father called, but it would take my mother many phone calls before he'd finally come around.

JUDITH. I was brought up with the idea that not getting married was the worst thing that could happen to you. If you didn't get married, your life was doomed to loneliness.

My mother had one single friend named Janice. She was the only adult I called by her first name. I remember my mother always trying to fix Janice up with the few eligible men around. There was always the problem of how to include Janice in social situations where there were all married couples. As a result, Janice came to our house alone, usually in the daytime. She was the only adult I had a real independent friendship with.

From junior high school through high school my close friends were mainly women. But after junior high school I stopped having one best special girl friend to whom I could reveal everything. In fact, around fourteen or fifteen I stopped confessing all my innermost feelings to anyone. I remember, in spite of all my girl friends, feeling lonely and thinking that no one understood me.

At this time I started to dream about Prince Charming, though I had few dates and knew very little about sex. Sometimes I would share my fantasies about meeting Prince Charming with a few friends who shared similar dreams, but our actual experiences with boys became more and more private.

I remember when I first started going to parties. Now everyone says they had similar experiences—feeling awkward, ugly and unpopular, no one asking me to dance, not knowing how to start conversations. I kept wondering what was expected of me, what did guys like. I could never talk to anyone about those feelings, and I was always mystified about what did happen between men and women.

DEBORAH. I'll always remember the day I was supposed to go to the movies with my friend Darlene. She called me at the last minute and told me that a boy she knew from camp had called her up and they were going to go somewhere instead. I got really upset. I hung up the phone and said I didn't understand why she had canceled her date with me. I really didn't understand it—I hadn't learned yet. My older sister and my mother said that I shouldn't get upset, because that's what girls do. It's more important for them to be with boys, and I just had to start getting used to it.

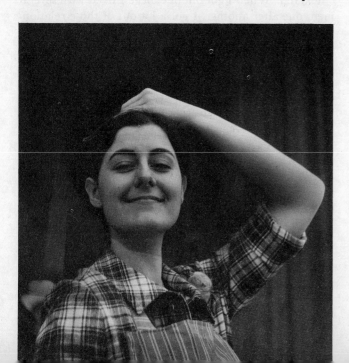

In high school I decided it was silly that boys should pay for girls. So I remember saying to my family that I should pay for myself, and my father started ranting and screaming at me, "If you have that attitude, Deborah, boys will never like you and no one will ever take you out and you'll never get married!"

SUSANNE. In high school I found it harder to be without a boyfriend than it is now at twenty-three. All of us were expected to have a rocky time in adolescence, but those of us who didn't go on to get boyfriends and husbands still have a rocky time.

DEBORAH. In college, groups were usually made up of couples. Any activity for couples excluded me, so I felt bad. It seemed like you had to have a boyfriend to go places. It also affected my relationships with women in the couples, since they shared and talked about their relationships with their boyfriends.

ELAINE. Sometimes I accepted dates to get out of the dorm.

JUDITH. I found that it was hard to just date. Also, women with serious boyfriends often implied that if you weren't with one man consistently you were promiscuous.

I would talk with many of my women friends about careers, but by the time of my senior year I was the only one in my group who wasn't getting married. When I thought about going to graduate school, a male professor told me not to go—that I would become too much like a man and never get married.

Like many other single women, I went to New York after college. I spent months looking for an "exciting" job to meet "exciting" people. Of course I didn't get the ideal job, but finally settled for enough to live on.

I came home after the battle in rush hour to eat dinner with my roommates and talk about meeting men. The evening was spent waiting for someone to call for a date or trying to find someone to do something with. There was one guy I remember who had listings of open parties in all the boroughs.

I went to those parties dressed in my new and most sophisticated attire. I tried to learn the art of cocktail chatter, taking subtle initiatives, looking confident and above it all. Going out on dates was another ordeal. Coolness and dishonesty seemed like the only qualities of the early parts of relationships. Informal socializing over real interests was almost impossible. Then, of course, there were the sex hassles—will you or won't you? What you learn quickly is that New York is filled with lonely people—women petrified that they will never get married, men on the make. I know that I wasn't ready to get married. There were still so many things I wanted to do—travel, meet people, find exciting work. But I didn't know how long I could last; marriage seemed the only

way out. For me the horror of being single was the loneliness, the lack of intimacy and honesty, as well as the lack of commitment between women.

As a single woman I felt a lot of anger and pain in my life. There was no outlet for the feelings, no focus for my anger and disappointment. I wanted freedom and independence, but I also wanted to be loved. Getting both seemed impossible. In retrospect I realize that I chose to be single. I wanted independence and excitement more than marriage. But at that time I couldn't see it as a choice. It seemed impossible to share my feelings with other women. Everything made me feel ashamed. It must be my fault, there must be something wrong with me if I didn't have a permanent and lasting relationship with a man.

ELAINE. One of the things I hated most was to be around married friends. Seeing their closeness reminded me of my aloneness. Around couples I often felt like a child, that couples were adults and single people were still not grown up.

KATHY. As a single woman I was constantly worried about my image to the outside world. A lot of my married women friends used to romanticize my position and tell me that I should stay single since it was a better and freer life. A lot of times I wanted them to think I was happier than they were.

CAROLYN. When I tried to "make it," become successful in my own right, I became aware of the incredible social stigma put on independent women. It became clear that one could not be seen as womanly and at the same time be successful in the "active work world of men."

DEBORAH. I gained a lot of respect for being politically and intellectually aggressive. But I always felt that men wouldn't see me in a romantic way, although I knew they liked me. My girl friends told me it was great I was direct and honest, but they acted differently around men.

RACHEL. When I got out of college I lived with several men, one after another. I got a lot out of those relationships—love and security and understanding and support. I thought I had what I'd always wanted. But underneath I was terrified. I was very dependent on my sexual relationships and that frightened me. Instead of feeling nurtured by the sense of "losing myself" in sexuality, I began to feel I was shutting out the world and dying when I made love.

Being out of a couple for several years has let me grow up and learn to function independently in the world. I really feel as if I can rely on myself now. And I feel I want more intimacy and am ready for it, but I don't know if I'll ever want to be part of a couple that develops a lot of dependency.

As a group of women we felt free to talk about our

problems, and begin to act on our feelings; we began to look at each other differently. We rediscovered a common bond that allowed us to stop judging ourselves and other women by men's standards. We tried to stop competing with one another. We worked to respect our emotions and to support each other's strengths. We learned to take each other seriously.

We joined women's consciousness-raising collectives and worked on various women's projects and organizations. We moved into houses with other women and began to acknowledge our feelings of love toward women. We changed our lives—our expectations, our environments, our definitions of meeting our needs.

Within the women's movement we found that our interests and our needs sometimes differed from those of married women. At times we felt excited that single women seemed freest to change their lives. At other times we felt burdened and saddened by the insecurity of being single. We want to find new ways of relating to men, but we have no models. The possibility of gayness has opened new options for us, but gayness does not resolve the conflicts we feel about couple relationships.

When we tried to summarize the differences that the women's movement has made in our lives, we ended up with a lot of confusion. There is still fear, but also joy and relief about the roles we have grown out of and the possibilities we see ahead of us.

DEBORAH. Basically the difference is that you no longer feel alone. When you're with someone you have the whole women's movement behind you. Last summer I was dancing with a man at a party and he started making a pass at me. I remember thinking at the time that a few years before, I would have sidled away or clung to someone else. Instead I just told him I didn't want to have anything to do with him. It felt so good, and it was so easy.

Now it seems if I wanted a relationship with a man I could get in touch with him, or we'd just decide on a good way to get together and spend time together. Probably what would determine who picked up whom would be who had a car.

ELAINE. Now at most parties I go to, people function independently whether they're in couples or not. There's some sense of community. Your goal at a party is not necessarily to meet someone.

JUDITH. When I felt there was a clear community of women that was autonomous, I think I stopped thinking about myself primarily as a "single" woman and started to think of myself more as a woman.

DEBORAH. Now I don't have to feel second best to a friend's husband or boyfriend. When Susan and I started becoming friends I was able to say that I had fears about becoming friends with her because I knew she had a commitment to her husband. She said she didn't see that as an issue between us.

I realized a year ago that more and more women really wanted to hear what I had to say and considered it legitimate when I chose not to have a boyfriend.

KATHY. I think there has been a growing respect for women who are more aggressive. A woman who is single is now given a certain amount of respect for having the strength to go out on her own. I always liked doing things that were thought of as boys' things, and in the women's movement these have become acceptable for women for the first time. Learning auto mechanics and feeling that people respected me for it has been very important to me.

SUSANNE. Now I really count on other women as being prominent in my life. I no longer feel that I just happen to be there with other women who happen to be there because they aren't married or aren't with men.

KATHY. I still look toward the future with a lot of dread. I'm really scared that it's all going to collapse and I'll still be left alone. I have an absolute fear of what it means to be forty—I mean for me. The fact that many women are going back into couples—some with men and others with women—is what brought that fear back, since I've never related primarily as part of a couple.

DEBORAH. The women's movement opened up to me for the first time the option of not getting married. That's frightening, because it means that I have to create something new; there aren't the old forms of security. On the other hand, I feel better, since those old forms never really seemed quite so secure or didn't really give me the kind of happiness they were supposed to.

In giving up the idea of getting married I gave up one sense of the future. Now it feels as though I'll be making certain decisions for a few years at a time, but I don't have any sense of where my future is headed. Some of that's really good. It allows me to live from day to day and to express my needs for the present. On the other hand, I do need a greater sense of continuity.

I still want some kind of permanent relationship, to feel security and love. I want to have children of my own or share ongoing responsibility for friends' children. Now both those possibilities seem so hard to achieve I have no models for what I want.

RACHEL. I've been a single woman for a long time and my heterosexual identity is very unclear to me. I feel like I'm in limbo about my sexuality. If you're a single woman who's not gay, then what are you?

I don't like to think that I would necessarily have to be in a sexual relationship with either a man or a woman to experience that trust and commitment I've felt with men. I still feel confused about what a couple is, what needs it meets, and how much it's possible to meet those needs without becoming part of a couple. A woman friend said to me two years ago that she felt there was a part of myself that I really held back because I was waiting for a man. I don't see my life in the last three years as "waiting for a man," but I do feel like I'm waiting for something.

I get scared when I think about the future. The greatest fear I have is of stagnation. I need to believe that my life won't be static and I won't stop working for what I want, whatever that is.

Abigail: Search for New Forms (Excerpts from the Diary of an Eleven-Year Marriage)

Looking back on my first five years of marriage, I realize how unformed I was then. I acted and talked mystical and poetic. In reality I had very little imagination about myself; I couldn't project myself into the future with a vision of whom I wanted to be, and I was so often lonely and unhappy in the present. But that first year was a good one, for I did recognize that I lived in an unreal world and Gene, my husband, was a form of reality for me. But sometimes I felt I hardly knew Gene. Sometimes I hated him and felt like I was in hell. I was going to leave him, but decided to stay (I was too afraid to leave him, afraid of what people would say). The summer after we'd been married a year I went home to my mother's house and literally slept for a whole month (in a single bed).

Sexually Gene and I gave each other pleasure. I was always able to have orgasms, even though they didn't seem to me to be much. We made love very conventionally, usually without much passion. I rarely if ever masturbated. I wasn't a very sensual person it seems. I was fairly passive. Also, I would use sex to punish him by refusing to make love, by holding back, without ever going into why I felt so negative all the time.

One night we had a very deep talk about ourselves and what we were expecting from each other. We wondered together: why did we stay sexually monogamous? I said, I was afraid of my own jealousy of other women. I told Gene jealousy arose because I wanted to be a complete woman for him. He said, wasn't I betraying myself when I wanted to be everyone and satisfy his needs completely? I realized I had been leaning on him too long.

Well, two months later I became pregnant and fell in love with Peter. I think a lot of my sensual opening-out and heightened existence (including my feeling of being in love) was due to my pregnancy (Gene's child). I passionately loved Peter, and he me for two months. I felt torn between him and Gene and stopped seeing Peter.

During the past four years Gene and I have grown together, talked a lot more. We had a second child in April 1969 (first child was born in 1965). We spent a fine summer together. Then came fall 1969. We moved to a new house and again I felt that Gene was very distant from me. When he told me that he was ending an affair, he expressed a lot of commitment to me and our marriage. He said he had been feeling very guilty. I told him I was in love with someone, with Lou. Then somehow our whole marriage opened up. We talked and talked together, clashed, reconciled, clashed again. We really opened up to each other. We agreed to deal with the problems that loving people outside our marriage brought to us. We agreed to try and understand our anger and jealousy and resentment and fear of being deserted.

We are still working on that! I find it terribly hard to understand the roots of my strong anger and jealousy now that he loves another woman. We have chosen an unusual form of marriage. We know why we've chosen it, we know the problems that will come up.

Because we are dependent on each other in many ways, if only one of us has an outside relationship, there's an unbalance that takes place. If he's loving another woman, he is out of my life in a sense, because of her. I certainly am busy enough. I love the work I'm doing. I need all the space away from him and the children that I can get. Yet still he's depending on or communicating emotionally with a woman who's not me. That's hard.

I don't know if I will fall in love as I have before. I feel I have been brainwashed in part, because though married so long, part of me still waits for the shining prince to come. Yup, I'm still waiting, still longing. At the same time I am highly critical of most men I meet and critical of myself. I feel stuck and bounded by structures of thinking and feeling about other men and women. I want to be much more open to everyone, not only sexually but in all ways. It's extremely difficult to break down all our fears and barriers, to invent new structures, to find a new language. . . .

Lesbian Relationships: A Few Words

Some of us choose to relate solely to women—an option for more of us since the women's movement.

Since there are many myths surrounding lesbians, we feel it's important to read the entire chapter "In Amerika They Call Us Dykes." It will present a better and fuller understanding of lesbian relationships than one or two experiences we could have included in this chapter.

Elena: Marriage and Multiple Relationships

In the seventh year of our marriage I got involved in the women's movement and began to sort out a lot of issues in my life. I had been at home for several years with two small children, and although I had chosen to become a mother, I found myself overwhelmed by the total responsibility, and became deeply depressed. With the support of other women, I began to question the traditional roles we had drifted into since becoming parents. Because I had been so much into myself when I was depressed, for a whole year my husband had been feeling a lot of unmet emotional needs. He began to talk about wanting to have other relationships.

I felt hurt and rejected because our exclusive sexual bond was somehow the price of certain household duties. Some of my women friends, too, had begun to question the validity of monogamy, emotionally as well as sexually. But I had grown used to depending on one person, and was fearful of exchanging the security of marriage for the rat race of adolescence, which was my only other model.

At that time there were other areas of my life that I was more concerned with changing; I wanted to put my energy into work, personal development, and friendships with women. I was learning that I liked women after all, and was liking myself better too.

I didn't think I wanted other relationships, and feared I would drift into having them if my sexual needs were not met by my husband, Jim. I wanted my sexuality to be determined by my own choice and not by fiat. I was feeling very turned off to men at the time, and didn't want to be intimate with men I didn't feel emotionally close to just to prove some obscure point about women's rights and equal sexual capacity. Yet who would meet my emotional needs if my husband was intimate with others?

Because I was seeing myself more as a separate person, I began to see my husband that way too. I didn't think we should possess each another, so I told him to do what he thought was best for him, but not to put pressure on me. During that time Jim and I became friendly with a couple who turned out to be living with another couple. Both women were in the women's movement. All household chores were shared equally by the four adults. One of the men assumed a large, possibly major role in his young son's care. After we became friends they told us they had a group marriage, exchanging marital partners when all four agreed to do so. They proposed that we might be interested in this arrangement. My husband was quite interested. I was frightened and opted out. I was turned off by the "contracting" (to safeguard the basic marital relationship), which meant that if he joined, I did too. It seemed to me even more oppressive than conventional marriage.

The next fall we started a couples group. After many weeks of rehashing old hurts—how Lucy always had to cook after both she and John came home from their jobs, etc., etc.—we came to the realization that the nuclear family was somehow tied to the economics of one adult going out to earn money while the other kept the life systems operating at home. Because women earn less for the same work, and because part-time work pays less per hour, the option of each partner working half time is economically not feasible for most families. The majority of us were interested in starting a commune, or cooperative household, in which child care and housekeeping duties would rotate, and all adults would work part time (about three days) outside the home—an arrangement impossible to achieve within the restriction of the nuclear family.

My husband and Anne were the major proponents of sexual openness. We resolved to be monogamous within the group, keeping open the option of discussing changes of feeling in group meetings as they developed. I was still threatened by Jim's wanting to have a sexual relationship with another woman and thereby rejecting me.

After several months in the house I found myself growing closer to Michael, Anne's husband. We both enjoyed child care and going to community meetings, and so began to spend a lot of time together. We became more and more aware of being attracted to each other and began to touch and kiss more (which was generally accepted.) Since both my husband and Anne wanted to break out of monogamy, we felt open to developing our relationship, but realized that there could be problems. One evening when I came home from my job, both my husband and Michael kissed me as I came in the house. This seemed really strange to me.

One afternoon while visiting Jim at his office, I made a chance discovery that led to his telling me that he had slept with a woman about a month before while out of town on business. I was hurt and upset and went about with a lump in my throat for days. I was especially upset that he had not told me, and felt it as a breach of trust.

Jim had been having a lot of trouble living with a group. I enjoyed having people around the house during the day. I had more free time than ever and my life seemed more integrated than before. I could be a "good mother" and still have time for myself. Most important, I was getting a lot of positive feedback from the group and getting and giving a lot of emotional support.

One evening when I was talking with Michael, an electric current or something almost tangible passed between us; I knew at that moment that I could not continue living in the same house if we did not have a sexual relationship.

We discussed it first with our spouses and then in the women's caucus of the house, and got supportive responses from our spouses and the women in the house.

When we first slept together it was Christmas Eve. Half the group were away (the pro-monogamy faction). It turned out to be a really fine sexual experience and the beginning of a strong emotional bond. Both our spouses were upset. After we had made love we could hear Jim pacing the halls and taking a shower. Anne was upset because we hadn't told her clearly that we were going to make love that night and perhaps because it was Christmas Eve.

Anne, who had had other relationships before, quickly got over being upset and was supportive of our relationship, as were the other women in the house. The other men were rather noncommittal and just didn't speak of it. Jim continued to be upset and insisted that he had to be out of the house or sleeping with his lover when I slept with Michael.

My preference was to be spontaneous about sexuality and to move in the direction of breaking out of our "coupleness," only sleeping together when we felt like it, and sleeping with others when we were feeling close to them. (The group considered separate bedrooms at several points, but it was never acted upon. The group norm was for spouses to share bedrooms, although occasionally one or another of the women would spend the night in a study or on the living room couch.) Since we lived in an essentially monogamous group, where Michael and I had the only intragroup relationship, I could see the basis for my husband's feelings of isolation, and tried to reassure him as much as I could. The new relationship was of greater intensity, but my marriage had a lot of strong ties and was satisfying and comfortable in an entirely different way.

The group broke up for a whole range of reasons, and half the people left for the country.

With the four of us left, Jim became progressively more distrustful of Michael, whom he had considered his closest friend throughout the year in the house. Anne and Jim had never gotten along too well, and there was some friction, which expressed itself as "Well, I'm not attracted to you, either!" Anne had mentioned once the possibility of she and I having a sexual relationship, and although this was not followed up much by either one of us, I think Jim felt doubly rejected (excluded) by the idea of the three of us being close sexually.

The four of us who remained were an untenable group because of the emotional dynamics.

My husband and I and our children are living together. We still have an important relationship with the other couple. Michael and I are very close and continue to have a sexual relationship. We would like to live together again in a group, but it is not yet clear how Jim feels about going back to any group-living situation, let alone one with Michael in the group. I may have to choose between my commitment to my husband and my feeling that I can grow more in a group-living situation. I must also sort out the issues of group living and my attachment to Michael. It seems important not to confuse the two.

Anger and Relationships

We realize that a lot of the anger we feel in our personal relationships hasn't come through in our stories. One reason is that many of us have held back from expressing those negative and angry feelings, which might have exposed our true identities. We realize now how important it is to let our anger out, rather than keeping it inside where it poisons us and our relationships.

A second reason is that anger, and the irrational rage and fury that often go with it, are powerful emotions and ones that all of us have difficulty expressing at the time we feel them directly to the person we're angry at. Even when we have expressed that anger it is difficult to convey those feelings in our stories. So instead of concluding this chapter with an incomplete sense of relationships, we want to quote some poems that illustrate the angry feelings all of us have felt in our relationships.

DECLARATION

For years I charted my independence
in miles traveled away from you.
You were New York and I a car
fleeing in every artery.
That I made you the center, there is no question.
No question I could rule on
without your opposition. No adventure unless
it wasn't yours. Today I think of Concord grapes,
those little pyramids, depending;
of the bay's water angrily repeating
its leap up the beach. One man's
violent need becomes a woman's service job.
But I don't work for you.
I'm crazy now.

MIRIAM GOODMAN

THE EDGE

Time and again, time and again I tie
My heart to that headboard
While my quilted cries
Harden against his hand. He's bored—
I see it. Don't I lick his bribes, set his bouquets
In water? Over Mother's lace I watch him drive into the
     gored
Roasts, deal slivers in his mercy . . . I can feel his thighs
Against me for the children's sakes. Reward?
Mornings, crippled with this house,
I see him toast his toast and test
His coffee, hedgingly. The waste's my breakfast.

LOUISE GLÜCK

5

In Amerika They Call Us Dykes*

INTRODUCTION

THIS chapter is a beginning, the beginning of our efforts to define for ourselves what it means to be a lesbian in this society. It is part of a larger beginning, as more and more gay women throughout the country have started to write, argue, sing, and shout their message to the straight world.

A lot of people worked on this chapter. The continuity was provided by a group of about nine women in Gay Women's Liberation who had been meeting together for a number of weeks before they decided to write this chapter, most of whom had been friends for some time before that. We had no connection with the group that was writing the rest of the book—except individual friendships between some of us—and in fact we disagreed, and still do, with many of their opinions. However, we took on the project because we thought that it was very important for any book dealing with women and sexuality to have a good section on lesbianism, and because we thought that writing it would help us sort out some of our own ideas, feelings, and politics around being lesbians in this society.

In addition to the nine of us, another half dozen women contributed pieces they had written, took part in tape-recording sessions, and helped edit and put material together. We write from many different points of view. But we all have in common that we dig being gay; we think it's one of the most positive aspects of our lives.

We want to break down the myths, misrepresentations, and outright lies that make possible our oppression and exploitation as lesbians, and that control not only our lives but the lives of straight women as well. The horror and fear with which others view us have served to ghettoize us, to isolate us not only from the straight world but from each other, since we must stay hidden to sur-

*Since the gay collective insisted on complete control over the style and content of this chapter, the Health Book Collective has not edited it. Because of length limitations, however, the gay collective has had to leave out much material that they feel is important.

vive. The problems of our lives—from medical questions to the difficulties of living in a society that condemns our very existence—are not viewed as legitimate by straight society, which insists that our only problem is that we are queer. The fact that we are lesbians is used to discredit everything that we say, and to make us into scapegoats for everyone else's problems. The fear of lesbianism is used not only to divide us from other women but also to keep all women isolated from each other, to keep women from becoming close friends. It also serves to keep women "in their place": any woman who acts assertive or holds a "man's" job may be labeled a dyke.

This chapter is a beginning—that means there is much more to come. There are many things we had to leave out, because of space limitations or because we do not have the experience to write about them. We have included nothing about lesbianism in prisons or in the armed forces, about the problems of black lesbians or older gay women. We do not deal adequately with questions of class, role playing, legal problems, and many other subjects. We hope eventually to expand this chapter and use it as the beginning of an anthology by and about gay women. We welcome your criticisms and ideas. Write to us c/o Lesbian Liberation, The Women's Educational Center, 46 Pleasant Street, Cambridge, Massachusetts 02139.

We have included four of our lives so that you may see us as we see ourselves—as real people. We weren't born lesbians. Coming to think of ourselves as gay was part of a process. We went through social conditioning, had experiences with men and women, and made choices, conscious or not. We have always loved some women—friends, mothers, sisters—but that did not make us gay. At some point our love for our women friends found expression in sexual feelings, and we acted on those feelings. For Clyde this happened when she was nine; for Nell, not until she was thirty-seven, married, and the mother of three children.

From this point on, we continued to turn to women

56

for love and friendship. Bisexuality might be possible in a healthy society, but it's not possible in this one. Relationships with men in this society have a built-in power imbalance, and few of us who have explored the possibilities of relationships between women would choose again to start with that handicap.

SARAH. I'm twenty-five, and I "came out" when I slept with a friend a year ago. We have been lovers ever since. But it took me about six months to actively assert my gay identity and feel bound to figuring out what gay politics was or could be. I understood my reluctance to being labeled "lesbian" after listening to a couple of gay women at a gay bar react violently to the word. They saw themselves as human beings, not as labels. But, I thought, that's just not the way people deal with each other in this society. They give you labels whether you take them or not. They reminded me too much of myself ten or fifteen years ago when I responded similarly to being called a Jew.

From the sixth grade on, I was the only Jew in my school. Everyone informed me of that; and it was no compliment coming from their mouths. I thought of myself as smart, capable, good at science and math. I was going to be another Marie Curie. But I was also intimidated by other peoples' judgments; I had to figure out how to fit in. "No, we don't bury our dead standing up," I would say. I really wanted to have friends, and I did get close to girls and boys. But I was always on the

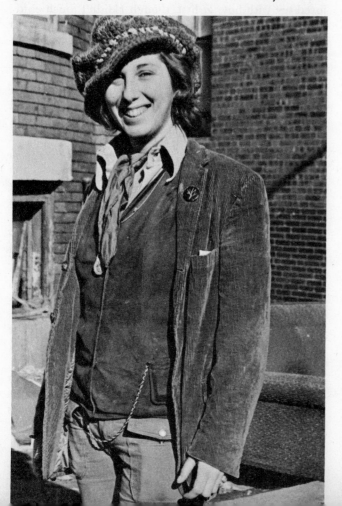

fence; they might always turn around and say "You're a Jew." This explains a lot of my reluctance to identify myself as gay and say "I'm a lesbian."

I thought I could have what people would call a gay relationship with my friend and not have to get into gay women's liberation or see myself as a lesbian. I had the choice not to do that. I knew by calling myself a lesbian I was asking for disapproval, distance, and perhaps violence, from most people. And since I had gone through it once, why ask for it again? So for a long time I did not identify. Then I realized that while ideally no one wants to be labeled, I do live in a society where people react to each other that way, and I don't have any control over that. I can't deny how people relate to me. Yes, I'm Jewish and I'm a lesbian.

I'm one of those women who "came out" with the women's movement. Women's Liberation made me think about my past, about when I was a kid and liked to play football and baseball. To me the accusation "You throw like a girl" was a terrible put-down—I didn't want to be lumped in with the "girl" category. I realized when thinking about my family that my parents had similar expectations for me and my brother—except that it was impressed on me to be nice, considerate, concerned for others in ways my brother was rarely pressed to show.

I thought about how, in junior high, the boys looked at the girls as developing bodies. They would yell, "Pearl Harbor, surprise attack!" as they grabbed our breasts and forced us down on the ground to get the "big feel." I know it scared me then, but how could I deal with my anger and fear when what was so important among girls was to be accepted by the boys? And having a boyfriend was often a protection from those other boys.

In ninth grade a group of girls got close. We used to hug and kiss each other a lot and have slumber parties. Most of us had boyfriends, but we seemed very important to each other. Once in a while someone would say, "What are you, a homo?" and we'd laugh. It didn't mean anything and it didn't change our behavior in any way.

That's the only reference to homosexuality before college that I can remember. In college I got hit with Freud and latent homosexual tendencies. What did this mean for me, who had always been more emotionally attached to women than to men? In freshman year my roommate and I became very close and dependent on each other, but neither of us could handle the intensity; that happened to me a lot with female friends. In psychotherapy I asked (indirectly of course) if I had "those tendencies." After about fifteen minutes the therapist figured out the question and asked, "Are you wondering if you're a lesbian?" Me: "Not really—ahh, I'm just wondering what you think about those tendencies." "You've given no indications of that," he said. Phew! was my reaction, not knowing what those "indications" were! (That's a story of how expertise has power over people's lives.) So I didn't worry about being a lesbian, but continued to build close friendships with women; and the problems those emotional attachments brought weren't lessened.

After college I felt the sadness of women friends going in different directions without the question of sharing our lives, like there would be with boyfriends. I went with a guy for three years, but he was never more important to me than two of my female friends. That was to my liking, not his. He wanted to get married, but since marriage wasn't part of any world I could imagine for myself, he married another woman two months after we split up. Sometimes my friendships with women were threatened by their jealous boyfriends. With these feelings, I could no longer ignore the women's movement. I read something another woman had written about her—and my—experiences. Fantastic! I wasn't alone. I began thinking that men didn't understand friendship, that they were sexual prowlers wanting all the attention focused on them; whereas my relationships with women seemed natural, exciting, and intense.

Working with Women's Liberation in Boston meant being with women all the time. A group of us who weren't really close but were friends would hang out together, circle-danced at a bar, played basketball. Diana was one of them. She and I found we could tune into each other's survival tactics: her piercing, allusive quips weren't offensive to me. What a relief. We could accept each other without many hurt feelings, we shared a lot of interests and criticisms of the women's movement. Eventually we slept together. That was over a year ago.

DIANA. When I was a kid, I was always a tomboy. In seventh grade the situation changed—I went to a private school where I didn't know anyone and all my friends were girls. I never got to know any of the boys and couldn't see why anyone would want to—they were picking on younger kids, harassing women teachers, and so on. It seemed as though you couldn't get to know them as friends, but only flirt with them. I didn't want to flirt, so I didn't go to parties everyone else was going to. I knew of course that when boys and girls grew up they were supposed to mysteriously start being attracted to each other. I thought that would happen to me, too, later. But the kids in my class just seemed to be playing at being grown up.

In junior high I started identifying more strongly as a girl. Boys were becoming more and more of an alien group. I still hated stockings and frills, but I certainly didn't want to be a boy anymore.

We had dancing classes in junior high. One night between dances a cold breeze started blowing through the open window. I reached over and touched Margaret's knee and asked her if she was getting cold too. She shrank back in mock horror and said, "What's the matter, Diana, are you a lesbian?" Everyone nearby started snickering. I didn't know what a lesbian was, but I knew I didn't want to be one. Later I found out; there was a lot of joking and taunting among girls in my class about lesbianism, which they viewed as sick and disgusting.

I went to an all-girls boarding school for high school. I was happy to be in an all-girls school, because I thought of boys as people you couldn't act naturally with, people who would make the classroom atmosphere tense and uptight. I began to worry consciously about being a lesbian. I knew that wherever I went, women attracted my attention, never men. If I rode on a bus or subway I would watch the faces of all the women. My emotional attachments were all to women and I had crushes on women friends. But I thought that if my attachments weren't sexual I was okay. I tried imagining sex with one of the seniors and was repelled by the thought. That was a relief. I said to myself that I was attracted to girls' *faces,* not their bodies. I told myself, "I just think Kitty's body is beautiful from an *esthetic* point of view, not a sexual one."

I was a tactophobe—a word we invented to mean someone who was afraid of touching people. I was afraid that if I touched other girls I would like it and keep on touching them. So I became repulsed at the idea, to save myself from perversion.

I went to college, and as I began sleeping with boys I began to lose some of my fear of being a lesbian. I enjoyed sex with boys at first, though I didn't much enjoy being with them otherwise, and was always trying to think up reasons not to see my boyfriend. I thought men were boring, and I still felt I had to act very artificially with them.

I began to go on a campaign to become more boy-oriented. I tried consciously to watch more men and fewer women in the subway. I wanted to feel turned on to men, not because it would be enjoyable, but because I was afraid I would not be a complete woman otherwise.

One summer I went to Latin America. There the women are much more physical with each other, walking arm in arm, dancing close together, and touching each other more. I liked this freedom and thought that it showed how culture-bound our definitions of homosexuality are. I got close to one woman, a nurse named Edna. Before I left I spent a day at her house. We were sitting on her bed and she started sucking my finger. I was totally turned on. As I left I thought, Oh no, there's no denying it anymore. I'm a lesbian. Bisexuality did not occur to me as a possibility, although I knew the term. I thought if I was turned on to women, I must accept the fact of being a total queer.

I got into the women's movement, and felt an enormous relief that I would no longer have to play roles with men and act feminine and sweet, dress in skirts and heels, and do all the things I'd done on dates. Then I began to feel hatred for men for having forced me into these roles. During this time I would buy women's papers as soon as they came out and look immediately for articles by gay women. I began to hang out with gay women, who turned out to be regular people, not the stereotypes I had imagined. On a gut level I was beginning to realize that gayness was not a sickness. One night I went out for a long walk, and when I got home I had decided I was a lesbian. For me it was not a decision to become a lesbian. It was a question of accepting and becoming comfortable with feelings that I had always had.

I don't know if I would ever have "come out" if it hadn't been for the women's movement. The women's movement first led me to question the "naturalness" of the male-female roles that I had always largely accepted. Because I thought that role-playing heterosexuality was "the way it's supposed to be," whenever I rebelled against these roles I was afraid that this meant I was not a complete woman, that there was something wrong with me— not enough sex hormones, no doubt. The women's movement helped me to reject these roles, and with them every reason for struggling to be heterosexual. I realized femaleness was something I was born with, it was not something others could reward me with when I acted "feminine," or take away from me as a punishment.

RONNIE. When I was a little girl I was very pretty and very good. My mother made me frilly dresses and set my hair into blond ringlets. She had had a hard time in a male-oriented immigrant family, and was determined that her daughters should be as good as her sons. She dreamed about sending us to college.

My parents loved each other, and my family seemed different from those of my friends because of all the affection. My sister and I have always been close. We slept in the same bed for fifteen years and usually snuggled, and she and I and girl cousins, drawing on our European background, would walk around arm in arm or holding hands and gossip about our periods.

As a teen-ager I hung out with a group of girls. We got crushes on boys and gossiped about them. In high school I didn't date much, but I wasn't unhappy about it. Instead I read books, learned to smoke, cut classes, and hid a bottle of Scotch in my locker that it took me two years to drink. I had fantasies of a career as a politician and said I didn't want to be a housewife, but as I talked big and tough I was shortening my skirts, dieting, and putting a rinse on my hair.

I went away to college, not knowing I was strikingly pretty, and faced with the wealthy girls in my dorm, I felt like I would always be an onlooker in other people's lives. I felt angry that I had to iron other girls' clothes to buy little Villager outfits, while other girls got money from home. I began to date fraternity boys,

though I thought they were snobs, and to look for someone with whom to lose my virginity. After several boyfriends I settled down with one man, and we spent five years living together, part of that time married.

My marriage was a good marriage, as marriages go. But it was hard for me to integrate my job, my friends, and my politics into a full-time relationship with my husband, and after enthusiastic starts I would usually quit what I started out to do. He didn't help me with the housework, and I, who had always wanted kids, began to think that if we had them, I would have to do all the work—and that scared me. After five years of living what got to be progressively more his life I began to feel cheated, and looked for something of my own to do. We tried a group marriage with friends, and it helped for a while, but it ended because it scared all of us. I tried professional school but didn't go to classes much. I thought about Women's Liberation, and a woman friend at school suggested that we start a women's group. I had new life in me. One night I suggested separation for a while, but when I left I knew it was for good. About this time a married woman friend at school, Susan, fell in love with me. This was not the first time I had to deal with my sexual and emotional feelings for women. At college my roommate Alice had been lovers with Sylvia. But Sylvia freaked out, married someone who was studying to be a psychiatrist, and told Alice never to talk to her again. Consoling Alice and getting closer to her, I felt drawn to her sexually, but was too shy to tell her for fear she would think that I felt that way because she was a lesbian.

One night we both got drunk and made love, but she fell asleep. After that we could drink wine by candlelight, reach out for each other's hands, and have bad fights just before I would go out to spend the night with my boyfriend. We loved each other, but I in my shyness and she, trying to draw back from lesbianism, did not know how to make it deeper.

My love for Alice had opened me to women sexually, but did not make me gay. I had more respect for my women friends though. But I never sought out gay women. I was aware of the sexual attraction that existed between me and my friends, like if we slept in the same bed together, but I never acted on it, because living with my husband took up all my energies.

After my marriage was over I responded to Susan, although I still needed men. We would often sleep in each other's arms, but it was becoming clear that she was married and that our love was a secondary secret garden. Once, when she and her husband had been fighting and were separated, I surprised myself by suggesting that she stay with me and sleep with me. She said no, and pulled back into her marriage.

All this was two years ago. Soon I got into the women's movement with all my energy. I let my relationships with men slip and became celibate. I wondered if I was gay. I was changing; I cared for women, and I could not lead the kind of life I wanted to with men. My commitment to women was making me stronger in every way.

The first woman I slept with after I decided I was a lesbian was someone I did not know well. She and I had dinner and we talked until it was too late and cold to go home. I slept on her bed, and because she had been a lesbian a long time, it never occurred to me that I could sleep with her and not make love. The sex was good, and I never told her she was my first gay lover. But when I woke up I felt sick, repulsed at having made love to someone I did not want to love, and frightened at being a lesbian. I never got past dealing with her as an obligation. I went through a period of self-consciousness, thinking there were rules to learn, not realizing it takes time to get used to a new identity. Fortunately, many people I knew were going through the same crisis too, and we talked often about our new experiences.

I never expected to be so much on my own, without a man, and sometimes I worry about being dependent on only myself for money. I am a hard worker, and whatever skills I have will be used for women. I like my life to be busy, and I guard my freedom. I feel really good about the relationships I can have with women. I never feel smothered and without power, the way I did with men. I feel that I will make mistakes, but no matter what I'm creating, it will be my life.

MIKI. I am a twenty-four-year-old gay woman who has been into the women's movement for approximately one year. Although I "came out" many years ago, the movement has helped me accept myself as a woman and accept my gayness in a new way.

I was the older of two girls. I always knew my mother wanted a son, and consequently I have always had a high value on achievement (something that is usually more important for sons than daughters). As a young child I played mostly with one boy, because he was the only other Jew around and the other kids were Catholic and didn't want to play with us. From age seven to ten I was a tomboy but lived near more kids and I had several girl friends and one special friend. I always felt pretty normal—just a little smarter than the others in school. When I was in the sixth grade we moved again (still in Queens, New York City), and it was then that I began to feel different. I got crushes on girls, while everyone else had them on boys. My tomboy interests were no longer acceptable, especially to my mother, for I had gotten my period and was now "a woman."

I felt different from girls around me in many ways—they had money and clothes, and their fathers were professionals. They could dance and flirt with boys. I was segregated into special classes in junior high, and thus my social life was confined to bar mitzvahs of the boys in my class, at which we petted and made out. I was increasingly aware of my attraction to other girls. In high school I was placed in a special science class designed to make us all into nuclear physicists. There were forty boys and four girls in this class. I was friends with the girls, but developed a really close and important relationship with a boy, M. We talked about many things, and he accepted my feelings toward women as natural. Our relationship was based mostly on intellectual stimulation, since I didn't feel turned on to M. sexually. In a lot of ways I thought of girls as silly and didn't want to compete with them for boys; but I did compete with boys for achievement in school. I wanted to be a boy so that I could have the career that I wanted and also in order to have a girl friend, for I thought that girls only liked boys.

I had my first gay relationship at about age seventeen in college with an older woman, who looked like a dyke —short greased-back hair, pants, jacket, etc. It made me even more sure that I was gay, but I fought hard to be bisexual.

My years in college were spent with a small group of "druggies" at the beginning of hippie culture. There was a certain level of acceptance of my gayness; I slept with my girl friends, but they were still looking for boyfriends, and thought that all I needed was to meet the "right man."

In college there was a woman whom I spent a lot of time with—who taught me to trust, whom I loved very much. When I told her that I loved her and wanted to

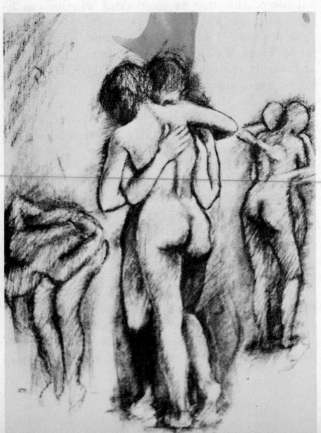

sleep with her she said I was sick and she was going to help me with my problem. There was always a certain amount of sexual tension and rejection that I felt from the women that I related to, because they were straight.

Then I went to work for the Welfare Department in the South Bronx. I had my first real affair with a woman and my first taste of reality outside of academia. At the end of that relationship I couldn't deal with my feelings and started shooting heroin. This went on for two years. I didn't get very involved with the people or the realities around me, because it was too depressing. I had one close friend and lover, who fucked me over in a way cause when she got involved with a boy, that was clearly more important to her than our relationship. I got busted twice for dope, and kicked my habit. I stayed in Manhattan for a while and was part of the bar scene there and got into cruising and one-night stands.

At that time the women's movement to me meant child care and abortion demands, which had no relevance to my life as a gay woman. I went to a Radicalesbians meeting because I liked the title, and met a woman from Gay Women's Liberation in Cambridge who invited me to Cambridge in February 1971. I was really turned on to the feeling of community, and saw so many "freak" gay women that I didn't feel so much alone. Then women from Cambridge and Boston seized a building at Harvard for a women's center. After being at the women's center I went through a lot of changes and started to accept being a woman, identifying with the women's movement, and getting really angry. Only now I had women to help me figure out how to channel that anger. They helped me change the ways in which I was hurting myself and the women I was involved with, because of my former identification with and acceptance of male values.

Now I live my life nearly totally with gay women, and the possibilities for real friendship with women have become a reality. I am totally open with everyone—my family and the people at my job—about being gay, because I feel good about it. I don't feel bad about not being able to get close to men, and I am learning how to make relationships with women work. I don't feel sick and alone anymore, and I have more optimism about the future.

OUT OF THE CLOSET AND INTO THE FRYING PAN

Lesbianism is not a physical characteristic—unlike the quality of being black or being a woman. So most of us have the choice either to be invisible by passing as straight or to be open. If we decide to be openly gay, we become vulnerable to physical and psychological harass-

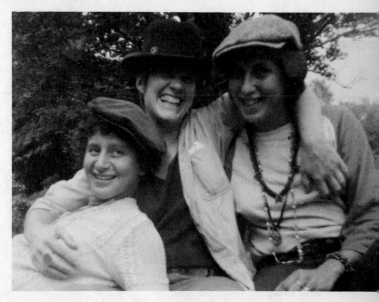

ment. We're labeled sick, kept away from the kids, maybe fired from our jobs. If we keep our gayness hidden, we are constantly subjected to the insult and embarrassment of being assumed to be heterosexual: gynecologists want us to use birth control, friends want to "get us up" with boys, men make passes at us. More important, our lives become controlled by the fear that others will find out. We may be blackmailed (though this mostly happens to gay men)—for money if we have it, for favors and information if we don't.

One of the first decisions confronting gay women after they "come out" is whether to tell their family and friends that they are gay.

HEDY. Sexuality is a very heavy thing with my parents. When my mother found out that I wasn't a virgin any longer she started sobbing hysterically. I think she would rather have heard that I was a mad bomber than *that*. Since I've been more into the women's movement and have "come out" I've felt much more loving and sympathetic toward my parents, especially my mother. She's noticed that I've been happier when I see her and less hostile. She's also relieved that I'm innocently living with girl roommates instead of with degenerate male lovers. It's scary to think of shattering this—the first real affection between us since I was a kid—by telling her I'm now a pervert. I'm sure she'll accuse me of turning into a lesbian on purpose, in order to torture her. I have to tell them soon, though, because it's getting harder and harder to see my family and feel close to them while I'm still withholding this big secret.

SARAH. The mystique of the family really hits me when I think about telling my parents. I look at my parents as being totally isolated. Who can they talk to about their daughter being gay? (I have my gay friends to talk to.) In this society people make very harsh judgments about gay people, and making a judgment about a kid is also making a judgment about the parents. At least my parents feel that they are responsible for the person I am, and they can get into guilt trips about what they did wrong.

After I "came out" I really didn't want to be preoccupied with being gay. That was a drag; I'm a regular person too, who has other interests, other things to talk about. Except that when I left this protected gay colony to venture into home-town, family affairs, I was constantly reminded: I'm gay, I'm gay.

For example, at a wedding an aunt let me know that I was expected to be next in line.

"Sarah, come here. I want to talk business."

"Yeah? What are you selling?"

"I'm old, I don't have many years left. Tell me, when can I expect your wedding?"

"I'm too young. I have too much to do."

"Too young? How old are you?"

"I'm twenty-four."

"Twenty-four! I was married for four years when I was your age."

"So you were too young."

She laughed, thank God—and I went to say hello to a cousin.

RITA. Telling my sister was not so difficult and felt good. We have been pretty close most of our lives. She is divorced and has a child, and she has been broadening her ideas about ideal sexuality. I felt that if she could see my girl friend and me interacting—being friends, doing things together—it would break down the idea that we belonged to a secret, erotic, violent underworld, totally removed from other women. Her reaction was a mixture of acceptance because she loves me and confusion because of all her preconceived ideas. I felt that she accepted my gayness too much on the level of sexual preference, rather than understanding the difference in relationships or what it means for me to be gay in a world that is mostly hostile to homosexuality.

It's not just our family and friends whom we have to worry about telling that we're gay. The problem goes beyond that to all the institutions of our society, to our doctors, our psychiatrists, our employers, our teachers, our friendly neighborhood cops—all of whom have the power to make our lives very difficult if they know we're gay, and many of whom don't hesitate to use that power.

Homosexuality is illegal in every state but Illinois. Though the statutes prohibiting homosexual acts are almost never enforced against women, they may be used selectively, like drug laws, to punish political undesirables or others whom the Establishment wants out of the way. They may be used as an excuse for discrimina-

tion elsewhere, such as on the job. There are also laws in most states against "sex psychopaths," which allow homosexuals to be committed for indeterminate periods from one day to life.

However, most of the discrimination that we face whenever we come into contact with the legal system is based, not on the laws against homosexuality but on societal attitudes toward "queers." The police harass us, especially around gay bars. Since it is difficult to prove that anyone has committed a homosexual act, they arrest us for drunkenness or disorderly conduct, charges for which their testimony is usually enough to convict us. In court, lesbians convicted of crimes often get stiffer sentences than straight women. Gay mothers lose custody of their children. A study of divorce and child-custody cases showed that in every case in which lesbianism was an issue the mother lost her kids. The courts want to "protect" our children from us. One of the women working on this chapter lost custody to her husband without even being present in court to defend herself. Later, out of court, her husband gave her custody, but their separation agreement says that her children may not be "exposed" to her lesbian friends.

Doctors, lawyers, clergy, and counselors are others who because of their position of power over us can cause us much trouble if they know we are gay. Gynecologists pose a special problem. Often we are forced to tell them we are gay, because it affects their diagnosis or the treatment they prescribe for us. However, when we tell them, not only may we be subjected to lectures, snide comments, and voyeuristic questions but we may find that after all that, they are totally ignorant about our problems. Very little research is done on the medical problems of lesbians, and gynecologists often don't bother to acquaint themselves with what is known. One of us went to see a gynecologist because she was hemorrhaging badly. The doctor insisted that she was having a miscarriage although he knew she was gay. A friend of ours was hastily—and wrongly—diagnosed as having gonorrhea by a gynecologist who did not realize that VD is not easily spread from one woman to another.

JODY. I have pelvic endometriosis, a noncontagious disease that women can get from a bad abortion or low progesterone production. The disease isn't very common and doctors know very little about it. After I found out what I had, I knew I should ask my doctor about making love. He said, "Abstain from sexual intercourse for a while." I didn't have the nerve to tell him I was a lesbian. Besides, I figured that if I told him he still wouldn't have an answer, because homosexuality is something people don't even talk about, let alone do medical research about.

About two months later I figured I'd better find out more, so I asked a gynecologist who I'd heard was fairly sympathetic to women. I was scared to death and felt like I had rocks in my stomach. Instead of answering my question, his face got very stiff and "professional," and he said, "Perhaps you should explain what you do sexually, so I'll have a better idea how it affects you." I just sat there flabbergasted. Here was this medical dude who wanted to know how we "do it." Finally I said, "I don't think that's any of your business. What I need to know is if any form of sex is harmful, or if it's just harmful when there's penetration." He kept pushing me to describe how I made love with women, what it felt like, whether I had been a lesbian my whole life, the whole trip. I got really mad, started yelling at him that we did it with bananas, what did he think—after all, everyone knows that the only reason you're a lesbian is that you want a penis or you're afraid of men. He said, "Your disease is psychological, not medical. I know a very good psychiatrist whom I would recommend that you see. He has cured many homosexuals." I said, "Do you mean that I spent five years in pain, spent months in and out of doctors' offices, and finally had surgery for a psychological disease? Are you telling me that I didn't get endometriosis from a rotten abortion six years ago, that it's all in my head?" He quickly retreated and admitted that he knew I had endometriosis and that that wasn't psychological, then rapidly changed the subject to my abortion with questions like "Do you think that having that experience was the reason you began to feel hostile toward men?"

By this time it was crystal clear that I wasn't going to get any information out of him that would do me any good. I was crying as I left, and the last thing he said to me was, "I strongly recommend that you see a psychiatrist. You're clearly very emotionally upset because you're a lesbian, and I think it would help you to deal with your disease if you began to work out your feelings about men. You're young, you can change." By that time I wanted to kill him, but I just told him that only a violent feminist revolution would deal with my feelings about men and that he'd definitely be on the top of my list.

Job discrimination is a big problem for lesbians. We gay women are very dependent on our jobs, since we cannot fall back on husbands for support if we are out of work. Yet in addition to the disadvantages we face as women, lesbians are subject to further job discrimination for being gay. If we are openly gay, we are the last hired and the first fired. Gay people are not protected by any civil rights act. Employers usually need no excuse to justify firing us. If we hide our gayness in order to find a job, we may live in constant fear of being found out.

MIKI. I was involved with my supervisor. She would meet me a block away from the office after work and drop me off a few blocks away in the morning, because she was afraid to be seen with me in public. We would not even go to a bar together, because she was afraid that there would be a raid and she would lose her job.

Despite the risk it entails, many women choose to be open about their gayness on the job, because they don't want to playact all the time, because they don't want to be discovered and fired later, or because they are sick of always being assumed to be heterosexual.

CLYDE. I have worked in many places, mostly factories and plants. When you start a new job it's hard to get to know the people there. The first question I'm always asked is, "Are you married, and how many children do you have?" I just answer, "I have no husband, I have a girl friend." Most of the people in the places I've worked don't have much to say about me being gay. I mean, they're in no position to be worried about my sexuality when they're working in a place like that, because we are both being fucked over by the same people.

THE-RAPISTS: LESBIANS AND PSYCHIATRY

The theories of Sigmund Freud and his successors form an important part of the ideology of twentieth-century middle-class America. They permeate our thought and languages. We use terms like "inferiority complex" and "sibling rivalry" to explain people's behavior, the way the Puritans used witchcraft or pacts with the devil to explain people's behavior three hundred years ago.

The psychoanalysts say homosexuality is a sickness. Middle-class America believes and repeats, "Homosexuality is a sickness." (People seem to think that to call

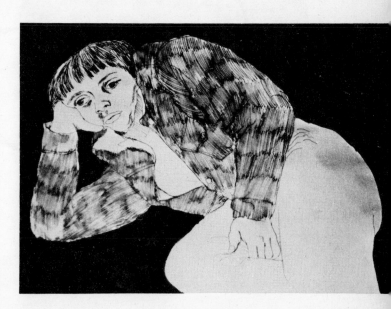

homosexuality a sickness is somehow more humane than to call it a crime. But at least people accused of crimes have a right to due process. Once you've been labeled a deviant, you're convicted without a trial.) After hearing over and over that homosexuals are sick, we may come to believe it ourselves and think that we need a cure. Or we may actually break down under the pressure of constantly being told that we're perverted, being shunned, being harassed. So we get carted off to the hospital, and our problem is diagnosed as (you guessed it) homosexuality. But that's not our problem. Our problem is the doctors and other upstanding members of society who make life difficult for us.

There is always a problem between psychiatric professionals and members of a minority group if the professionals assume that the source of a person's problems lies in the patient's mind and not in the racist, sexist world. For a lesbian this is extremely heavy—every school of psychiatry explains lesbianism as a maladjustment to life. All the theories regarding psychological development are based on male experience and male sexuality— as well as on bourgeois values and the nuclear family. Their "theories" of personality development are all based on a sexist view of women's role in society—as passive, submissive, wife, mother. Lesbians are seen as infantile, perverted, promiscuous, socially malfunctioning creatures. Lesbianism is never seen as a positive life choice for women who refuse to bow to society's demand

that we live our lives subordinate to men. Instead, regardless of what we consider our problems to be, they will always see our homosexuality as the root of all our problems.

MOLLY. I began to seek psychiatric help when the woman I'd lived with for years committed suicide. I was drinking heavily, couldn't accept her death, and had no idea how to continue my life. When the anxiety became unbearable I checked into a hospital. The interviewing doctor told me they would be able to help me. Oblivious to the fact that I managed to get drunk every day for fifteen months in the hospital, they began to assault my lesbianism: sometimes they assigned me an aide to follow me around the ward; they threw me into "preventative" seclusion; they investigated all my relationships with the other women patients, and on occasion threatened to interrupt friendships with massive doses of tranquilizers.

Doctors have told me I was utterly dependent (love women), had anxiety neuroses (alcohol withdrawal), was borderline schizophrenic (failed to conform to their idea of what a woman's life should be), and had a poor prognosis (I believed in myself more than in their theories about me).

In the few years following, things got worse: the drinking that threatened my life wasn't interesting to them. When I was close to dying, a clinic slip read "Patient

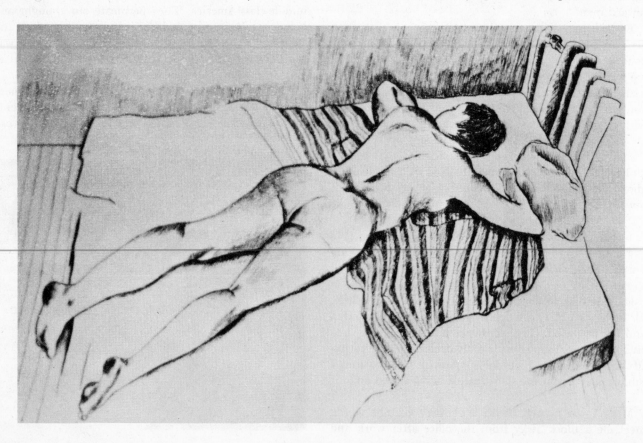

says she is alcoholic." But all the doctors were willing to ship me away permanently to the back wards of state hospitals, not because I was harming myself (drinking is just a symptom, they said), but because I lived wrongly. I could feel their need to punish me for not giving in to their opinions of what was wrong with my life—that is, I defended lesbianism as one of the more positive and beautiful aspects of my life. Yet they were so into forcing my life to conform to their theories that while I was literally dying of alcoholism they wanted to know what my lover and I did in bed.

My experience may seem extreme at first, but if we think about it, we can see that their treatment of me was just the logical extension of their theories. The same attitude is always there about lesbians (if they don't have you locked up in a hospital, it doesn't go that far, but it will be simply a milder dose of the same medicine): medicine seeks to undermine, mutilate, and ridicule the lesbian way of life.

Often doctors tell their patients that they accept their homosexuality and will assure the lesbian that they are able to treat her as a nondeformed being. However, in practice this is rarely the case, since it would mean that the doctor would have to put aside all of his (her) theories of how women develop in order to truly accept the validity of lesbianism. After all, doctors are people who often go through training that lasts up to fourteen years, and training fills their heads with false conceptions about the correct role of women in life. The student can't possibly come out of such intensive training with an open mind about lesbianism.

A therapist can't provide support in other areas if he or she disagrees with the basic tenets of a lesbian's life. And it would certainly be rare to run into a doctor who had had a lesbian experience and who could begin to understand what one was talking about.

I had one resident psychiatrist who assured me that my lesbianism was acceptable to him. However, he told me he was constantly criticized by his supervisors and forced to present a defense of himself for not treating me for my homosexuality, since they insisted that that was at the root of my problems. That therapist subsequently threw me out of a hospital when I wasn't in any shape to leave after I'd discovered that he was a homosexual.

Where does all this leave the lesbian who is deeply troubled and feels in need of help? Obviously, the ideal would be to find group therapy where the members of the group and the leaders were avowedly lesbians. This is rare, although not unknown, as, for example, the Homophile Clinic in Boston. Second, a number of female clinical psychologists have become part of the movement for women's liberation and are very supportive to women including lesbians.

A rule of thumb would be to avoid psychiatrists and analysts—that is, therapists with medical training—as that branch of the psych field is the most reactionary, most grounded in doctrine harmful to women, and its practitioners freely give out tranquilizers under the guise of treatment. Psychology is not always better, but the training is shorter—and more flexible—and it is in this realm that radical therapists and young women and men seeking radical relevant approaches to emotional troubles can be found.

When choosing a group, a lesbian should request that she be put in one with at least some other gay people. She should look for a group in which the leader is also required to participate, not as an inhuman, arrogant authority figure, but as another human being who happens to have a little more information about how people work than the rest of us and would like to share that knowledge.

And last, one should try to find out whether the orientation of the group is totally in terms of adjusting to society as it is or whether radical life alternatives are sought and valued.

THE BARS

We need places where we can go to be with other gay women—to meet, talk, dance, relax, be sexual—to be totally ourselves. We need to be able to meet others like ourselves who will understand us when we talk about our lives. We exist secretly where we work and where we live. And each time we are made to feel invisible, insulted, or freakish, we add more anger and hatred to our stored-up frustrations.

Society, knowing that we need some place to vent our feelings, gives us our bars. Mafia-controlled, they are usually crowded and expensive. If we are lucky, we may have a gay women's bar in our town. Recently one opened up outside Boston; it's run by gay women, sometimes has an all-women band, and there are no men. The atmosphere is relatively pleasant and relaxed, but the Mafia connections are still there, and it's still a profit-making enterprise, with high prices and cover charges.

Often, however, gay women, gay men, and all of society's outcasts are lumped together in one dingy, crowded little bar—such as the Bottom Rock in Boston. The bar becomes a hustling scene, full of pimps and drug dealers, as well as straight men, often with straight women, who come to get their voyeuristic rocks off on watching us. Booze flows, alcoholism is encouraged, and sometimes fights break out. Then the cops, always hovering nearby, start beating and arresting. Some evening's relaxation that is! And the anger that should be directed toward society is directed toward one another, as it always is when people are ghettoized. We get uptight, jealous, and strung-out on the destructive bar atmosphere.

Why do we keep going there? Because there is no other place to be with lots of other gay women, open and unashamed, to dance, hold each other close, and try to forget the straight world for a while.

CLYDE. I go to the bar because it's the only place to go, because my friends are there—friends I've been with since I was fifteen—you know, people who taught me to live with myself being gay. Because I was having a hard time putting up with it. At one point I was just totally gay, then I was bisexual—I went with this kid for two years, but I never had sex with him. But yet I still felt as though I was bisexual. And then I met this girl when I was sixteen. Bobby was my first lover, and I just went on from there.

SARAH. When I started going to the Bottom Rock I just sat there and watched the drag queens. I knew I was objectifying them, but then how could you deal with them in any other way? They were just caricatures of *femmes fatales*. They were like a joke.

I kept going to the bar. I was sleeping with Diana and starting to get to know gay women, and a lot of them went to the Bottom Rock. That was a problem for me, because I never used to go to bars, since I don't drink. But I thought I had to learn to dig it, because all these other people did. And some of my friends from back home would say, "Wow, what do you keep going to a bar for? I never knew you to go to a bar." And I'd ask myself, "Yeah, why *do* I go if I think the bar is totally exploiting all of us?" It was very expensive, and on weekends you couldn't move in there—and the smoke was so bad you choked—so it seemed silly to go.

And there'd be these boy-girl couples sitting at tables, sometimes just making out all night, and straight men standing around gawking. You just knew that the Bottom Rock was for everyone who is rejected from most other places. And I hear the bar is Mafia-controlled. I really don't want to support them much. But, then, it *is* a place where I can act gay and not be intimidated by the judgments I get outside.

But somehow the whole atmosphere seemed sick. I had been feeling good about being gay and being with women, yet at the bar I started feeling like there's something wrong with me. I didn't know why.

CLYDE. Well, like you said before, every type of deviant comes in. I can honestly say I feel as though the people who come in to see the freaks (who are us) just come in to get off for the sake of getting off. I mean, we have love and feeling toward one another, where they don't. These dingaling executive guys, who have six kids and a wife, come over and pick up a drag queen on the corner. There's no love, there's no affection, there's no emotional feeling. It's all sexual when they come in. Like among us there're feelings, but like these freaks come into the bar—I mean, *they're* the freaks and come in to see us!

A hopeful alternative to the bars is beginning to appear. Weekly lesbian liberation meetings, more and more frequent women's dances and gay dances, a large room and an office for gay women at the Boston Women's Center, all provide a chance for gay women to get together, rap, dance, vent our anger and frustration, and celebrate our joy at being together, outside the dreary and sick atmosphere of a bar. We control the atmosphere; we set the terms. Nobody gawks at us, insults us, makes money off us.

LOVING

DIANA. One night I gave Sarah a ride home from somewhere, and I went inside to have a cup of coffee and chat for a few minutes. We ended up talking all night long. During the whole time Sarah was jabbing, punching, tugging, wrestling with me. We felt a physical tension, but were too uptight to be physically affectionate. Finally, at around five in the morning, we began to nod out, and I asked if I could sleep there. She said "Sure. There're two beds in the living room."

We lay down completely dressed, she on one bed, I on the other. Then she started telling me that hers was much softer than mine. So I got up to try it, lying with my feet to her head. We decided that we'd both sleep on that bed (just because it was the more comfortable, of course).

But suddenly Sarah was afraid that my car might have been ticketed. So she jumped up and ran to look out the window. After she had been standing there for what seemed like fifteen minutes, I said, "Hey, Sarah, what're you doing?"

"Oh, I was just watching to see if the cops would come by to ticket your car."

Finally she came back to the bed and started to lie down again, head to foot and foot to head. I made a sour face, and she turned around. At last we were lying together in the same direction. Timidly I put my arm around her. "Hey, Sarah, is this okay with you?" She said "Yeah" and snuggled up to me, putting her leg over mine. Pretty soon we were hugging each other. I tried to get up my nerve to kiss her—I'd bring my face up close to hers, then chicken out and turn away. After about ten false starts I got up the courage to do it—and she seemed to dig it.

That's as far as things went that first night, but soon we were sleeping together every night.

NANCY. (From a letter in July 1967 written to my woman lover after a stolen month alone together—I was then ceasing to be one man's wife and another man's mistress—overwhelmingly attracted by a deep and almost bewitching sense of the endless possibilities that could flow between women.)

"I am asking more than we ever spoke of—offering more than I ever whispered to myself. Let's go through, Judith, let's not stand here quaking, terrified to enter and too numb to turn aside—let's lock eyes and risk that unmapped place where we cannot hide. And soaring, to touch ground with you—to wander, seek, run toward—our lifelines blended and smashed together.

"Hot breath, moans of thirty days and nights—goddesses on a single army cot. Listen, do we both truly long to travel as far as I now suggest—which is more than smiling, daily moving, almost richly touching togetherness, and much less insured, secured, guaranteed and warranted? I mean, on the line with our innards, all parts and pieces exposed.

"I falteringly now say to you that I will at least inventory what I ought to pack for such a journey if you are willing."

Five years ago. The first three together were lived in unwanted social exile from all former acquaintances and circles of friends—in and out of mental hospitals and

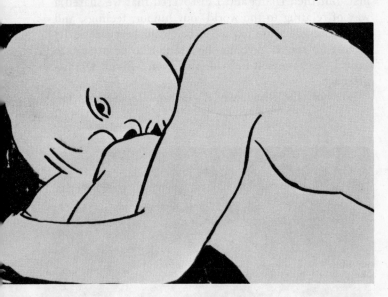

alcoholism. Six months of running in opposite directions, fleeing the pain of love turned mad when severed from the rest of life. Two years of slow building together again, inspired and ignited by the shared vision of a worldwide revolution while living in the wings of the women's community.

MIKI. My relationship with Daphne started when she was doing my astrology chart. We met and talked for hours, getting to know each other, walking and sitting by the river in the springtime. There is something very earthy, very sensitive, and very warm, kind, and understanding about her. She was married and is a mother—that too, and her kids, turned me on. Perhaps being a mother makes a woman more sensitive to feelings in others.

Daphne has had sexual feelings for women all her life, but has always fought them because she was trying to be a good wife and mother. The women's movement gave her the space and support to finally accept her gayness and "come out."

That first night by the river we kissed and touched one another hesitantly. For me there's something very exciting about first times, and I, too, was intoxicated by the freedom and pleasure she felt at finally being able to make love with a woman. For the first time in a sexual relationship with a woman, for me, things were equal. I trusted her, I could relax and enjoy her making love to me, for it was obvious that she got pleasure out of it.

We spent a lot of time together that summer up in Maine living outdoors—making love under the stars, in open fields at midday, in the woods. We had a very beautiful, very private, special and romantic first few months together. I was happy, secure in loving and being loved by a woman so beautiful, precious, and special to me. I was no longer feeling the confusion of having several relationships at once. I was planning that we could live together, that I would have a family with kids to be a part of my life. I didn't feel lonely, and aside from a few areas in my life that I felt Daphne didn't understand or take seriously enough (my past drug problems), I felt that we understood each other and were able to share the pleasures of our love for each other by a passionate, flowing lovemaking and in just being in nature together.

Then the bubble burst—her husband freaked and got custody of the kids just because she was gay. All communication between us was cut off. I've cried a lot.

RONNIE. I've slept with a lot of women. Some people would call this casual sex, but it has involved me in a lot of pain. I took chances sleeping with women I liked, and I have been hurt.

I slept with Lynn long after I first wanted to sleep with

her. I had buried my attraction for her because she was in love with June and living with her. One night she was lonely and we had done something together. We kissed goodnight for five minutes. I remember sleeping with her and being afraid to open my eyes when we were done. I felt like the pauper sleeping with the queen, afraid of her position, her banter. After making love we talked and laughed until morning, and she became a person like me. I liked her for her energy, her love of herself and life. That day we smiled when we met but did separate things.

The next night we went to the bar, the first time in months I had gone with a lover. We talked to many other women, extending ourselves because we were high on each other. That night I made love with her in a way you only can with someone whose pleasure you love.

Then I went back to the country. When I saw her next she was torn apart by the ending of her relationship with June. I knew she would feel different about me. She did, worried about what she had gotten herself into. I was angry that she didn't trust my friendship. Didn't she know that I understood her pain with June, that I hadn't intended sleeping with her to change our friendship? We talked and pretty much worked it out. For the rest of the summer there was some closeness between us.

She moved away, and in the fall I went to visit her. I wanted to see Lynn, but again I felt scared. I walked instead of driving the last five miles to her house. I spent hours with the other people in her house, seemingly chatting about old times, but really being tense. Finally only she and I sat in the kitchen. It wasn't easy. She invited me to sleep in her bed.

Being in bed broke our nervousness. We talked freely, laughed, spoke of our fears and feelings for each other honestly. Secure, we made love. Again I felt a welling up of passion for this incredible she-creature who, with luck, was my lover. Our bodies spoke their own language, but I felt that as I made love to her, I did so with a little less trust than before. Lynn said, "We have something nice. We can talk honestly about sex, and it seems as if we have a relationship with no expectations." I did not feel good with that summary.

When I left, she was still sleeping. I was upset. For many months I never contacted her, feeling that each attempt would only create more distance. I saw her again, and again she did not know how to relate to me; she was distant at first, warmer after a while. I resented her caution as well as her warmth. I closed myself to her, saw those things about her which I had never liked, forgot her beauty and my wonder.

Sometimes there is no way you can sleep with someone and come away feeling good about yourself and her. You have to forget something to survive. Casual is not my word. Every time I open myself to someone, I feel love, anger, ripped off, stupid, dulled, released.

JUNE

It just happened one afternoon
As we were walking home
posters in hand
on our way to day care
for Jesse and Raphael

"Do you think you'll ever have children?"
she asked me

My mind swelled with memories of my mother
asking when I wanted to settle down and have a family
memories of teaching retarded children
memories of wanting a baby so he'd stay with me
memories of needing a child to keep the loneliness away
Thinking of my sister alone with her son
Thinking of now
Thinking of who I have become
of whom I live with and whom I love
Thinking of loving women
of loving her (June)

"Do you think you'll ever have children?" she asked me
I felt the dam breaking
flooding my body and mind with warm liquid energy
alive and real

RITA

SARAH AND DIANA. We're buddies. We live together. We work on the newspaper together. We do the crossword puzzle together. We sleep together. When someone gives one of us a joint, we wait till the other is around to smoke it. When one of us buys chewing gum, we buy another pack for the other. It's not that we have to do all these things with each other—we like to.

SARAH. When I first met Diana I didn't feel capable of expressing my thoughts unless someone else said it first. But then Diana and I discovered that we shared a way of relating to the world—our humor, feelings, and analyses made sense to each other. And that was really freeing for me. It gave me the strength to be myself, to actively assert myself individually, even without Diana's presence.

Lots of the time we do things separately. On

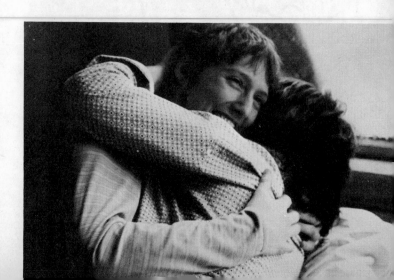

Wednesday nights one of us teaches a French class, the other goes to Lesbian Liberation meetings. We have different schedules at the newspaper.

We spend a lot of time with each other, but we are with other people too. We live with two other women, and there are always lots of people in and out of the apartment. All the things we work on, we do as part of a group. So whenever we get a chance we skip out and snatch a few minutes alone together somewhere beyond reach of visitors and phone calls.

All this is not to say everything's wonderful. We have some basic differences, and we often get into fights:

D. Sometimes I feel like knocking the shit out of her. So I go off into another room and play solitaire for a few hours to cool off. Or I take a walk outside, hoping some man will be foolish enough to try to rape me, so that I can vent my anger in beating the shit out of *him.*

S. Sometimes I feel like I'd like to get a good punch in. But then I don't really want to. So we scream and swear and take swings at each other, and then laugh and hug, all within twenty minutes.

Being buddies gives us the freedom to blow up at each other. We know that underneath our anger we both feel a long-term commitment to each other. So we know we can yell and scream at each other without worrying "Maybe she'll get so mad she'll walk out and never come back," as we would with other people. We can show our weaknesses and our bad points to each other as well as our good points. We can be ourselves with each other.

NELL. I've become very afraid of getting closed into any relationship that looks like it might develop into a monogamy. Maybe it's because I was married for thirteen years and I need a lot of private space around me. It's not that I don't have the same needs as any other woman. Sometimes I feel very lonely and really want to be intensely in love again, or to be able to just relax and depend on someone else to help me make decisions and share my life intimately. I'm thirty-seven and have three children, and I get tired and scared. But then I look at the lives of my monogamous friends, and I become more and more convinced that there has to be a different way for me to live with and love women. I know that a marriage of two women is better than a marriage between a woman and a man, because a woman will take better care of you than a man will. A couple starts off okay, but after a period of time the two people build up a frightening dependency on each other. I don't want to be responsible for someone else's happiness, not even my children's, or feel that she is responsible for mine. I don't want to feel that someone has to know what I'm doing every hour of the day and night. I'd end up lying to her. Even when a monogamous relationship is working well, friends of the couple become secondary.

It is often hard to relate to a tight couple if you are an unattached woman, especially if you're closer to one than the other, and it's not always possible to care for both equally. The other woman will probably resent your friendship with her partner if you're really close, even if it's not sexual. I'm not saying that that's always true, but I think it's common. And then what happens when one partner becomes a little bored with the other or begins to feel trapped? The feelings become unequal, and the pain really starts. If they break up, the process is long and awful. If they decide to loosen up the relationship and start being with other women, they find they can't control their jealousy even if they want to. Or else they agree to keep their thing the primary one and have casual side affairs that don't threaten it. Then these other women may feel second-rate and used. When I talk to my coupled-off friends about this stuff they say, "Maybe so, but no other kind of relationship looks any better." They're right, the way things are now, but I have a vision of what I think could work for me. I want to be very close to several women—live with some of them, sleep with some of them, and love all of them like family. I want the same amount of security and warmth that a couple can give each other, but I want it spread out to more than one woman. If one friendship is having trouble, the other ones can support and help it. If one woman goes away, I won't be totally freaked out and lonely. If I'm sleeping with more than one woman, maybe I can control my jealousy and my desire to own my sexual partners. I know it will be very hard to build free but long-term love relationships among a group of women, but the possibility of that kind of community keeps me going. If it doesn't work, I'll find a nice woman when I'm fifty and settle down.

Women I Love

JUNE. To Nancy: Oldest friend, curious and wondering in your words over so many years, our canoes travel in different streams yet still meet in the forks of the clear mountain water of our minds. I think of your body, liquid strength, rhythmic energy in peace in the bow of the boat, and wonder why we cover our fears in metaphor, and never take a real canoe trip together. Visions of myself as the fearful freak and of the razor-edged distance which may always be between us because my longings are not yours. Who snuffed out those flames in you, my friend whom I can touch with my eyes, my words, but not my skin, nor my soul?

To Lynn: You were the flamboyant Southern writer, I was the daring independent radical woman, our mystifications of each other crashed, sometimes in painful explosions, sometimes in joy. Backing off from the intensity: months of a painful triangle, months of silent healing—for to accept such love would take a self-love hard for a woman to maintain, so maimed are we so often in this country. (Oh sisters, remember where the blame belongs.) Now, with relief and wonder, as a friend/lover, I travel to the place you now call home and enjoy a more slowgrowing love, with glimpses of that first destructive awe and fear which has been so time-subdued and I feel we still will touch when older in years.

To Rita: We are not two jigsaw pieces under the label "couple," you are not my other half, for you are a whole with changing faces, sometimes a distant rainbowed fish I watch in fascination, sometimes octopuslike with arms which scare and entice me. I think, there is no other way to love women than to know that total vulnerability may descend at any moment. Tears on top of toughness, I sit here now with bittersweet memories of our women's skins, women's minds touching.

To Mother: Mistress of a psychoanalyst, wife of a formula constructed by men, you who warned me of the barren jealous homosexual existence, have you never let loose in the depths of women's communication and felt the small spark of the flames which now enrich me? I protest my unwholeness, only partly your doing, and know it is not the right time for you to hear the final blow of lesbian truth. Yet you call on me in your wife/protector role and I will be more real with you. Someday. Soon.

To Gail: It is 3,000 miles to you, my married sister, it is the second summer of my gayness and more steady hues have crept into my lesbian opal. Rita is with me, there is a fierceness of wary commitment singing in our blood. I kiss her on the back of the neck, unaware of your eyes, and so the words I have been groping for must begin—words of history and fantasy and new ways, ways which have filled out my awkward body to a sensuous peace and gathered up my energy for all the storms which will try to quench my desires. Not entirely free of sadness and anger at the men who put you here, still you show your love, and I feel gayness stretch her strands between us, spider webs growing to huge nets catching witches and myths and revolution in strong rope arms as we talk for what seems like, yes, the first time.

"BLESSED ARE THE POOR"

As Lesbian Liberation has grown to include more and more women, and more different women, we have come to understand that many of our differences have a class origin. Here one woman describes how her lower-class background has affected her relationships with other women and with the movement.

JESSE. I've always felt anxious when movement women started talking about role playing. I suppose it's because I'm a pretty "butchy"-looking dyke, supposedly very much into roles. Anyway, the idea of being confronted by a group of middle-class movement women on my "macho" behavior was very intimidating.

In the past I haven't involved myself in the movement to any great extent because I felt intimidated and bitter about that. I have, though, thought a lot about why the movement has isolated me and whether or not it's fucked up, because I want to see the movement grow.

I gradually started to realize I didn't like the way this society set up identities. I didn't like the kind of roles my mother and father played. I liked doing the things my father was free to do, like having the freedom to develop his body. At five or six I was very physically oriented and played basketball and softball. How was I supposed to enjoy wearing skirts when I couldn't climb trees or fight in them? It didn't take me too long to realize I didn't like the role society had planned for me.

When it came time for me to start dating, it intrigued me that this was the way to become accepted. In high school I became bored with boys and related trivialities; wanting a strong mind as well as body, I got into a mind trip.

The mind trip came about the same time I decided I was queer. The superiority complex I developed as a defense against middle-class and heterosexual people seemed to me justifiable.

It was justified because they [my schoolmates], with all their middle-class behavior, showed themselves to be totally ignorant. Not only were they ignorant of the kinds of problems I had (an alcoholic father who beat me and a mother made spiritless by him), but they were ignorant of the privileges their social position gave them. They simply took it for granted that some time in their lives they would go to college and to Europe, that a new suede coat would be provided for them in the fall. They never questioned why all these things would be done. They never realized the world was theirs for the asking. They would simply get married, have children, and get a new car every year, and have good Christmases. They'd watch TV versions of poverty and say, "Those poor, underprivileged people."

The only way my relationship with my heterosexual schoolmates changed was that I grew to hate them more. I wanted to completely isolate myself from them, so I joined an all-girls gang. We went around beating up people and shoplifting. I also refused to shave my armpits or my legs, bathe, or comb my hair. Instead of wearing nylons and flats, I wore crew socks and sneakers. I did everything possible to make myself unattractive to my straight schoolmates.

As I approached the end of an ugly high school career and prepared to enter an ugly college career, my feelings of isolation from straight women came more to the front. I became frustrated with my state of forced celibacy. The only contact I had with other gay people was through idiot books I read—like psychology books—which filled my head with all sorts of shit about what gay people were like. It was really hard all my life to keep from thinking I was crazy, because those books and everyone around me told me I was, and often! But I never really thought that.

When I first came to Boston, it was my first real vacation from celibacy (and independence). I immediately proceeded into this really dependent relationship—which was fucked up.

Since the books I'd read told me there was a "butch" and a "femme," I identified with the "butch" role, and so I was "butch" in bed, but I really didn't control the relationship. I was tough, but so was she. Now I look on "butch" and "femme" as being the same as "sadist" and "masochist." They have a symbolic relationship in which one is strong and the other weak, and they both get off on it.

After this relationship I slept with lots of women. Finally I began a relationship with a woman who was the first person I've ever trusted. Since the beginning of that relationship she and I have both slept with several other women, so I can't say I'm unfulfilled sexually. I also feel fulfilled emotionally and intellectually, since our ongoing relationship has seen much equal dialogue.

I've explained quite a bit now about where my head is at. I love lots of women—my sisters. I may act "macho" at times, but I think being "macho" in some ways is right on.

The movement, by insulating itself with rhetoric, which is a middle-class thing, has insulated itself from me. It has no way of knowing who I am. What I want to say to the movement is: "Here I am. I'm a *Woman,* and you have to identify with me because of that. I'm going to trash you if I have to, because I love you."

My sisters have to deal with class and race, especially their own white, middle-class values. They must realize that they still have those values.

The lower (working) class will make the revolution. My sisters must become grassroots, learn to survive, before they can say they believe in themselves as revolutionaries. My sisters must believe in themselves. Only then will they be totally strong. And my sisters need to be totally strong, because they must make the revolution.

* * *

Dearest,
　　I am spending your
middle-class
　　　no money
　　　　on the street
20¢ will buy you what,
　　exactly.

　　Food for my body,
Lest my soul perish.
　I am oppressed, lady
Who flies her freak flag
from the antenna of
her Peugeot, Who can
afford the co-op & to
shout "Right On!"

I am,
　　Poor first
　　Gay second
　　　and
　　Woman third

　　　　Fuck your selfish rhetoric.
　　When you get the Power
　　I will be waiting
　　still for freedom,
　　　and
　　　Panhandling my ass off
　　　For you, my white-ass
　　Honey,
　　　Just for your church
　　　　Supper, Amen.

JESSE BUSHWACK SAVAGE

LESBIAN MOTHERS

In a society that is afraid of lesbians and wants to shelter its children from "queers," being a lesbian mother is very hard. Telling friends and relatives about being gay can be hard for anyone, but if you're a mother, they can try to put added guilt on you. They say, "What are you doing to the children? What will they think of you? What will their friends think?" Many gay mothers are torn between wanting to be openly gay and feeling protective of their kids in an uptight world. A father can make it hard too, whether the mother and children are still living with him or not. Nell's fourteen-year-old daughter says, "I don't feel any pressure from my mother to be gay, and my friends feel good about her, but I do feel pressure from my father not to be gay."

It isn't only people we know who give lesbian mothers and their children trouble. They often hear conversations and see graffiti that put down "dykes" and "faggots." Television and books are heavily antihomosexual. Even friends call each other "faggot" to be insulting. It's hard for them not to be affected by this.

If you have unchallenged custody, and your children can get to know your lesbian friends and lovers, they can come to their own conclusions about their mother's gayness. In the end, our being open and unapologetic is probably the best way to help our kids not to be ashamed of us.

JOAN. I feel good about being openly gay around my kids. They accept my affection for other women very naturally.

NELL. My kids watched my "coming out" over a year's time. First I went to gay meetings, and then I talked a lot to them about my feelings and fears, and finally I made love with a woman. On the morning afterward, when the kids came in and found us in bed together, one of them whispered to me, "Did you make love?" I laughed and said yes, and she said, "Well—finally!" They all know that I feel very open and proud about being a lesbian, and they accept it in the same way I do. I don't care whether or not they turn out to be gay, but at least they won't be afraid of gayness or think of it as sick or mysterious. They'll know that lesbians are strong and loving women.

For unmarried gay mothers another challenge is raising sons without men. Nell feels that her hardest problem is finding unoppressive men for her son to spend time with. He will be the only male in his house next year, and he doesn't see his father very much. Nell doesn't feel that he needs men as models. She wants his sense of values to be learned from her lesbian friends. But she does feel that he needs male company to keep from feeling isolated and lonely in her women's world. A boy's insecurity can start very young. Nan's year-and-a-half-old son spent the summer with her on a lesbian farm. He seldom saw men. One day he saw two men swimming nude, and he immediately took off his clothes and started playing with his penis. He was clearly identifying as male, and apparently was relieved to find somebody like him.

Most people think that homosexuals should be kept away from children. Lesbians who want to work with kids have to stay in the closet if they want jobs as teachers, nurses, pediatricians, counselors, baby-sitters, community workers, and so on. And often people deny the love and need between children and their mother's female lover. One gay woman helped to raise her lover's child for seven years, beginning with the pregnancy. Once, when the natural mother had to go to the hospital, her parents came at four o'clock in the morning and took the child a thousand miles away so that he wouldn't be left in the care of their lesbian daughter's lover. They kept him for several months. Years later the mother died,

and the grandparents again immediately took the child. The mother's lover, who was at least as close to him as his mother had been, was never allowed to see him after that. If she had been the father, the grandparents could not have treated her in that way or dismissed so coldly the close relationship she had with the boy.

Gay women who would like to have children of their own but don't want to have sex with men find it almost impossible. Artificial insemination and adoption are not permitted to open lesbians, so they are forced to be bisexual. Many lesbians are married to men.

LOLLIE. I'm married, with two kids. Frank and I are good friends. We were never passionate lovers; we were two frustrated lonely misfits who liked each other. I had always been drawn to women but had found only one who wasn't afraid to have a relationship with another woman. I felt terrific with her until she lost interest. Rejections were really getting to me. Frank and I started living together; I eventually got pregnant, and then married him. I'd really wanted to be a mother, and I didn't want to do this alone. Having kids was tremendously absorbing, but now they are older and much more independent, and I'm feeling that maybe I could stop denying my desire to be involved with a woman. But it's so complicated. When I feel attracted to a woman I panic. I'm very doubtful that anything can work out between us. I don't want to mess up the people in my family. I get along well with Frank. We share child care and other jobs. We believe in allowing each other lots of autonomy. The kids seem very happy with things the way they are. I feel really good about that, and I'm scared of changing anything. I have to convince myself that my needs are as important as anyone's in this house.

JOAN. It is hard. But staying in the marriage can be absurd and schizophrenic. I tried to and felt trapped. I wanted to be with women and love women, but my husband needed me. So I kept sleeping with him while fantasizing that I was making love to women. I tried to detach myself from him. Being with him was degrading and made me feel unreal, like acting a lie. Finally I met other lesbians, and with their support I felt strong enough to get out of the marriage.

Many gay women are afraid to reach out to others. They may make a phone call to Daughters of Bilitis once or twice, and nothing else. Or they relate to other lesbians secretly. They don't tell their husbands where they're going. Then they have to live with the constant fear of being caught. Either way it's a lonely trap.

Look! Women are the source of life! Blood-lined bellies, soft-thighed nourishers of a billion million infants—wild, moon-ridden, moon-driven creatures of such lushness that a thousand wars have not burned us out—that's who we are—that's where we're coming from—the mysterious, wondrous ones whom men know almost nothing about. When two of us are suddenly made able to see into each other, there is no course, no end for that journey. The earth trembles before our collision as we walk a path this side of loneliness, this side of what can be known through words alone—that side of revolution and madness—and everywhere love.

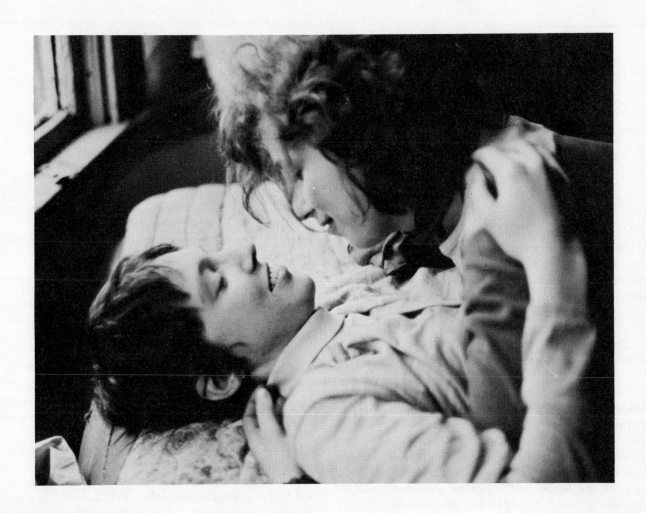

6
Nutrition and the Food We Eat

INTRODUCTION

It is especially important for us to know about good nutrition. It is one of the basic ways we care for our bodies; it is perhaps the most important preventive medicine; and eating well makes us feel better. Also, as women we often find ourselves responsible for the diets of others, especially children. To learn more about nutrition and pregnancy see the pregnancy chapters.

Good nutrition isn't just a simple matter of knowing what's good for us and then eating well. There are huge obstacles and problems.

* * *

Whenever Jimmy asks me for a marshmallow, I feel conflicted about what to do. I don't want to give it to him, since it's bad for his teeth and has so many preservatives in it. But if I say no, he cries and argues and puts up a stink for half an hour. Sometimes I just don't want all the hassle. So I'll explain why marshmallows are bad for him, but then let him eat them anyway if he still wants to.

* * *

I hear so much these days about chemicals and preservatives and food processing that sometimes I feel that there's nothing healthy left to eat. Everything is either artificially colored or has some huge DDT residue in it or has all the vitamins processed out—I just want to give up. And then I have the problem of liking all these horrible things. If they're all around me and much cheaper than those expensive organic health foods, and they taste good to me, why shouldn't I eat them?

* * *

Wintertime is long and full of colds and fevers in my house. I know we and the kids could eat better. But I'm scared to start thinking about good, nutritious foods because planning, shopping, and cooking for meals is all up to me in this household, and I don't have lots of time,

I've got other things to do, and things like frozen or canned foods are what I already know how to buy and cook. I somehow think it would take so long to relearn all this, it would be expensive, and then I'd have to start persuading my family to go along with the change.

* * *

The health-food nuts make me feel guilty all the time about the food my family eats, but I just don't think it would be any fun to live on soybeans and wheat germ. Is it possible to go halfway?

* * *

We feel it is important not to condemn ourselves for eating the way we do. Certain changes in our diets would clearly be more healthful, but it's not so easy to make the switch. It helps to find out about foods that are both satisfying and nutritious.

Should we take vitamins and supplements, or are they a waste, maybe even harmful?* How much protein is enough? Is meat protein necessary, is it even healthy for us? It is important to remember that nutrition is a controversial science and that we will find arguments both for and against many ideas or suggestions.

THE NECESSARY NUTRIENTS

Food gives our bodies the materials for growth and repair, and also provides the energy for all our activities. There are three main elements of food that we need: carbohydrates, fats, and protein. For body processes we

---

*Evidence shows that very large amounts of vitamin C (ascorbic acid) can form microscopic crystals in the urine and possibly cause kidney stones. On the other hand, large dosages of C cause the extra ascorbic acid in our body to spill over into the urine, where it appears to prevent the formation of cancer-causing breakdown substances. Some "experts" think this extra C prevents the return of cancerous tumors of the urinary bladder. Certain other vitamins, notably A and D, can definitely be harmful in very large dosages.

Nutrient	Chief Functions	Important Sources
Sodium, chlorine, fluorine, and other trace minerals. Most of our diets now contain too much sodium, largely because of sodium compounds used in processed foods and excessive use of table salt.	Varying functions, many of them not well understood. Fluorine is especially important from birth to six months. It helps to prevent tooth decay by hardening tooth enamel.	Meat, cheese, eggs, seafood, green leafy vegetables, fluoridated waters, sea salt.
Water Most people need 6–7 glasses of fluid (water, tea, juice, etc.) a day to keep good water balance in the body.	Not really a nutrient, but an essential part of all tissues. Often supplies important minerals, such as calcium and fluorine.	
Roughage (cellulose)	Also not a nutrient, but important for stimulating the intestinal muscles and encouraging the growth of certain intestinal bacteria. Keeps teeth clean and gums healthy.	Fruits, vegetables, whole-grain bread and cereals.

About Protein

There is great disagreement about how much protein is necessary. The 1968 revision of the *Recommended Dietary Allowances* of the National Research Council–National Academy of Sciences (NRC-NAS) suggests 55 grams of protein per day for a 128-pound woman or adolescent girl. For a 154-pound man the figure is 65 grams. Many doctors and nutritionists also recommend these amounts, but considerable research indicates that our protein needs may be less.

It is important to know the quality as well as the quantity of the protein we eat. Ideally, protein should be "complete," that is, it should contain all eight of the essential amino acids* and in the right proportions. Meat, eggs, and dairy products (milk, cheese, yogurt, etc.) contain "complete" proteins. Generally, other foods contain "incomplete" proteins, which are lacking in essential amino acids or have poorer amino-acid proportions. Soybeans, wheat germ, and nutritional yeast (brewer's yeast), though good protein sources, are "incomplete" in this sense.

There is, however, a simple way to make up first-rate, "complete" protein without using meat, eggs, or dairy products: "By combining different proteins in appropriate ways, vegetable proteins cannot be distinguished

nutritionally from those of animal origin."* All we have to do is combine foods so that the essential amino acids lacking in one food are present in another food eaten with it at the same time (amino acids don't wait around for each other and can only work together).

One good protein combination is beans and rice. When eaten separately, 1½ cups of beans and 4 cups of rice provide as much usable† protein as 13¼ ounces of steak. But when eaten at the same time, as in any common beans-and-rice dish, the same amounts provide as much usable protein as 19 ounces of steak. This represents a 43 percent increase in usable protein, simply because the beans and rice were eaten together! Other good protein combinations are bread with milk or cheese, or lentil soup with nonspongy whole-wheat bread.

When we are trying to lose weight, we want to get the most protein for the fewest calories.‡ Fish, cottage cheese, and skim milk are especially good for dieting, since they have relatively few calories compared with their usable protein. The following chart compares the "calorie cost" of different foods.

*These are the protein "building blocks" our bodies cannot make from other substances and must get directly from the food we eat.

*R. Bressani and M. Béhar, in *Proceedings of the 6th International Congress of Nutrition*, edited by E. and S. Livingstone (Edinburgh, 1964), p. 182.
†"Usable" protein represents the amount of protein we actually absorb and retain in our bodies. We can "use" anywhere from 50–95 percent of the protein we eat, depending upon the food. *Diet for a Small Planet* describes protein usability in more detail.
‡A calorie is a measure of energy often expressed in terms of heat.

CALORIE "COST" PER GRAM OF USABLE PROTEIN*

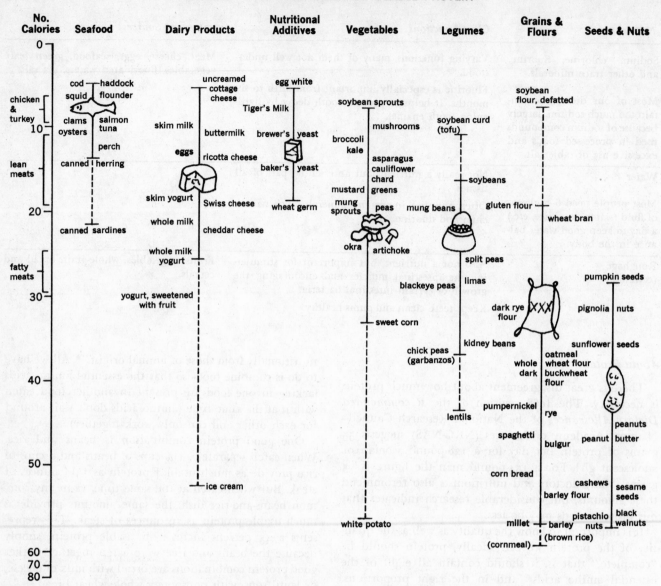

*From *Diet for a Small Planet*.

It is exciting for those of us who must feed both ourselves and others as well as possible on a limited budget to find out that meat isn't necessary for a good diet. We also know that meat protein is a very highly concentrated source of pesticide residue (especially animal livers), and that livestock is a very inefficient protein-maker compared with plant crops.†

Fats and Oils

Today we hear a lot about polyunsaturated fats, hydrogenated products, and low-cholesterol foods. Since cholesterol is closely linked to heart disease, a major killer in this country striking a growing number of

†This is important when we think about the world food shortage and realize that *half* the good, harvested agricultural land in America is used for crops fed to livestock.

women, it is important to understand more about the fat we eat.

First of all, fats and oils can come from either plants or animals. Fatty acids, which make up the main part of fats, are chains of carbon atoms with many hydrogen and fewer oxygen atoms added on. Whenever any of the carbon atoms in these chains are connected by double bonds (C=C), the fat is called unsaturated. Fatty acids that have two or more double bonds are said to be highly unsaturated, or polyunsaturated. These fats are almost always liquid oils of vegetable origin (such as corn, soybean, and safflower oils).

Saturated fats do not have double bonds and harden at room temperature. Most animal fat is saturated (beef, lamb, ham, and many dairy products). Saturated vegetable fats are found in many solid shortenings (Crisco and Spry, for example), coconut oil, cocoa butter, and palm oil (used in store-bought cookies, pie fillings, and nondairy milk and cream substitutes).

Hydrogenation refers to a process of changing liquid, unsaturated fats to solid fats ($C=C$ double bonds are broken by adding on hydrogen atoms to the chain). Some products are completely hydrogenated (hardened), some partially hydrogenated (some table margarines, for instance).

One important reason for knowing all this has to do with cholesterol, a waxy substance found in animal fats (in meats, egg yolks, and butter) and used in many of our body's chemical processes. Our bodies both make cholesterol and get it from the fats we eat. Everyone needs a certain amount for good health, but too much cholesterol in the circulation can cause heart and blood-vessel diseases. Cholesterol deposits can form in the lining of artery walls, eventually blocking off the artery channels completely. When this happens in a major artery of the heart muscle, the result is a heart attack. Although women tend to be protected from heart disease by their estrogen, more and more women now get heart disease, probably because of their diets.

How, then, do we cut down on the cholesterol in our blood? One way is to eat fewer animal fats. Another way is to avoid hardened (hydrogenated) vegetable fats. Probably most important, we should have enough vegetable oils high in polyunsaturated fatty acids. These "essential" acids lower our level of blood cholesterol considerably, though the exact mechanism is unclear. Linoleic acid, the most common fatty acid, is especially abundant in safflower, soybean, and sunflower-seed oils.

Apparently, the type of fat we eat may be more important than the total amount. If we want to keep a low cholesterol level, our diets should have a high ratio of polyunsaturates to saturated fats. That is, more of the fat we eat should be polyunsaturated, less of it should be saturated. One way of doing this is to substitute polyunsaturated margarines* for butter. Another way is to cook and bake with liquid vegetable oils (except olive oil, which is only mono-unsaturated) instead of margarine and butter.

Carbohydrates (Sugar and Starches)

Along with the little boy at the beginning of the chapter, many of us also want that marshmallow. We Americans eat huge quantities of sugar and spend a lot of money on candy bars and sodas. While some sugar is essential, most of us eat too much of it and from the wrong sources. We may never give up these sources en-

*Read the labels! Margarines that are partially hydrogenated are higher in polyunsaturates. Many cheap margarines are completely hydrogenated, and thus contain saturated fats. Some even contain butter.

tirely, but it helps to know healthier ways to satisfy our cravings for sugar.

Sugar is necessary for energy, but we get plenty of it naturally from fruits, vegetables, and milk. We also get sugar from breaking down starch foods such as breads, cereals, grains, and legumes. Eating concentrated amounts of sugar (found in various sweets and beverages)* is harmful to us in the following ways:

It can create a low-blood-sugar level by overstimulating our body's production of insulin, which then causes the liver and muscles to withdraw too much sugar from the blood. This sugar is stored as glycogen (a form of starch easily changed back into sugar) or as fat. Thus we may at first feel peppy as sugar rushes into the bloodstream, but after a short while we feel tired out, irritable, even exhausted or nauseated from the resulting low-blood-sugar level.

The fat formed from excess sugar creates an extra burden on our bodies and makes us feel sluggish.

Sucrose (ordinary table sugar, also found naturally in some foods, such as honey) causes tooth decay.

Sugar destroys an appetite for other, healthier foods.

Eating lots of sugar foods may cause diabetes in people who would otherwise not contract the disease.

Dental Health

Many of us forget that good teeth are an important part of good health. Poor nutrition can cause dental disease just as it causes other diseases of the body. For example, foods containing a kind of sugar called sucrose cause tooth decay in the following way.

Certain types of bacteria found in almost everyone's saliva can use sucrose to make themselves a protective coating. This coating helps them cling to our teeth as a sticky substance called dental plaque, which keeps our saliva from washing them away. These bacteria, tiny organisms known as streptococci, then multiply very quickly and produce large amounts of acids, enzymes, and poisons. These substances drip on or between the teeth, damaging the enamel and irritating the gums.

The most important way to prevent this decay is to brush our teeth daily to remove the plaque ("a clean tooth does not decay"). What we eat is next most important. Try to avoid foods with sucrose, especially between meals and at bedtime. Also, try to brush your teeth after eating sucrose-containing foods. Whenever possible, eat foods that act like a toothbrush (raw carrot sticks, apples, oranges, celery sticks, etc.). In this way your diet can play an important part in dental care.

---

*This includes raw sugar, honey, molasses, and other sweeteners.

In addition to sugar, coffee and cigarettes have the same effect on blood-sugar level. Some people try to get rid of their sluggish, low-blood-sugar condition by drinking more coffee or smoking more cigarettes. But every temporary lift is inevitably followed by fatigue, irritability, or headaches.

Try to eat some protein along with the sugar foods you do eat—for example, drink some milk along with a sweet snack. Protein is digested slowly and helps to keep sugar from being absorbed too rapidly into the bloodstream. To feel well throughout the day it is particularly important to have some protein for breakfast. (See the nutrient chart for good sources of protein.)

PROBLEMS WITH THE FOOD AND AGRICULTURE INDUSTRIES

"It's almost impossible to get my kids to eat well with all that advertising on TV for junk foods. If I don't get their favorite sugar-coated cereal, they keep pestering me until I do. Why can't there be more advertising for healthier foods?" The answer is fairly simple. Since the food industry is mainly interested in making more and more profit, it advertises those products that make the most money. Unfortunately, we, as well as our chil-

dren, have succumbed to this advertising and have in many cases adapted our tastes to the foods best suited for mass production, rapid turnover, and longer shelf-life. In other words, we have been conditioned to like the foods that give the food industry the most profit. Since most of us won't suddenly change all our eating habits, the food industry will probably continue advertising as it has been. However, we can learn about which highly advertised foods are best (or least harmful) for us and start to buy more of these products. (See "Some Valuable Suggestions" below.

"It's crazy the way food prices are skyrocketing. Pretty soon I won't be able to get enough to eat for me and the kids, let alone get enough nutritious food." The high cost of food is frightening. According to a representative of Merck Chemical Company, it "has been established that 35% of the retail cost of food is being paid by the consumer for convenience features . . . ready-to-eat breakfast cereals, instant foods, soup mixes, cake mixes . . . etc."* Many of us are angry about paying thirty-five cents out of every dollar for "conveniences" that often save us only ten minutes and damage our health in addition.

Also upsetting is the fact that we often have to pay twice—first to have important natural nutrients removed from our food, then to have a few of those nutrients

Food Pollution, p. 66.

General Foods Plant, Woburn, Massachusetts

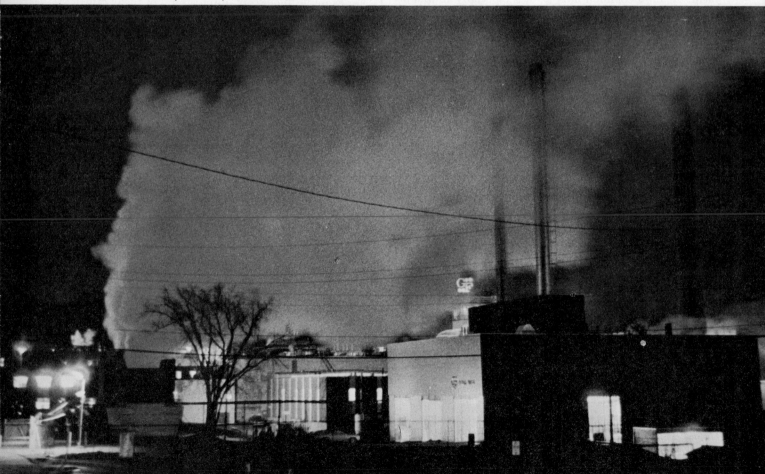

restored. (Food companies call this "adding nutrients," but it's really just partially replacing what was originally there and has been removed.) For example, during the processing of white flour, polished rice, and refined cereals the B complex of vitamins is totally removed. Only six of the B vitamins are now being put back in, but we are told by well-known experts like Dr. Frederick Stare that these are the key vitamins. Dr. Stare, by the way, who is a member of the faculty of the Harvard School of Public Health, wrote a syndicated column on nutrition while serving as a paid consultant to one of the nation's largest food corporations.) In fact, all the B vitamins are key vitamins, and it does little good to restore only six of them.*

"I don't understand how they get away with it. Can't the government do anything about all these additives and food colorings and pesticides and chemical fertilizers?" Government agencies such as the Food and Drug Administration (FDA) and the U.S. Department of Agriculture (USDA) have been largely ineffective, mainly because the food industry has so much control over them. Seventy percent of all food standards and regulations are proposed by the food industry itself.† And during meetings when the FDA makes important decisions about food standards, food industry representatives are often the only others present. Because of such industrial control, cola beverages don't have to label their caffeine content (which many people don't know about), some products don't have to label their fat content, and many potentially dangerous chemicals continue to be used. Also, our food is further contaminated by the agricultural industry's use of chemical fertilizers and pesticides.

Even a former commissioner of the FDA (Herbert Ley) has recognized that agency's ineffectiveness: "The thing that bugs me is that the people think the FDA is protecting them—it isn't. What the FDA is doing and what the public thinks it's doing are as different as night and day."‡ This is especially upsetting, since we are discovering more and more that the effects of chemicals are cumulative, that we store up these chemicals over the years until enough is present to seriously affect our bodies.

SOME VALUABLE SUGGESTIONS

Whenever you can, make your own soups and whole-grain breads. They contain far more nutrients than

Ibid., pp. 60–61.
†*The Chemical Feast*, p. 64.
‡Quoted in *New York Times*, December 31, 1969.

canned soups and spongy, store-bought breads.

Use cast-iron skillets and pans when cooking. They are an important source of readily absorbed iron, which is needed by women especially.

When cooking vegetables, use only a little water and keep the pot tightly covered. Also, try to save water in which vegetables have been cooked for stews, soups, sauces, broths, and so on. Many vitamins are lost to the air (oxidize) or dissolve in water—save them when possible.

Make sure fresh food is really fresh. Old vegetables may have fewer vitamins than frozen or canned ones.

Read labels to know what you are buying. Even though all the ingredients may not be listed, the ones that are must be listed in order of quantity, the first ingredient used in greatest quantity.

If you take any supplementing fat-soluble vitamins (A, D, and E), it is important to eat or drink some fat-containing food (milk, for example) along with the vitamin. This ensures absorption of the vitamin.

B_{12} is not found in vegetable products (except for certain seaweeds), so vegetarians should eat some eggs or dairy products (or take a supplement). B_{12} deficiency can result in anemia and nerve damage.

If your children pester you for junk foods, try out more nutritious substitutes that might satisfy them equally well. Many children like Granola as much as the popular, vitamin-robbed cereals. And popcorn is far better than many sweet snacks, which cause tooth decay as well as provide little nutritional value. Also, one way to avoid buying processed meats (bologna, salami, hot dogs, etc.) is to buy a large ham, bake it, slice it thin, and store it in the refrigerator for sandwich meat.

CONCLUSION

One very important concern for women is how we relate to food. Often we find ourselves using food as a reward for both ourselves and our children, or we turn to food when we are unhappy, frustrated, tense, or anxious (much as we might turn to cigarettes). Such situations usually involve very complex emotions, and would require a much longer discussion than possible here. Also, we feel tremendous pressures from our society to stay "thin and beautiful" and to diet, if need be, to maintain these thin standards. Such standards usually have little to do with our physical and emotional well-being, so we often find ourselves trying to look attractive at the expense of our over-all health. Some of us have found it helpful to discuss issues of women and weight with other women, who almost invariably share the same problems. By supporting one another it is sometimes possible for us to resist the tremendous pressures we resent so much. At least we can begin to feel stronger about what we believe in and what we want for ourselves.

For some of us who want to change our eating patterns it is often difficult to find inexpensive alternatives to what is offered in the local supermarket. Most supermarkets carry only hydrogenated peanut butter (with 7 percent sugar added) and foods that are almost always treated with chemicals. To find preservative-free foods we may have to go to a natural-food store, where prices are often high.

We need to make a united demand that our larger stores offer us healthier choices and carry more chemical-free foods. Such foods do not have to be more expensive than other foods. We should also demand that fruits and vegetables not be prepackaged, so that we can examine their quality.

We can also get control over our food selection by joining or starting food co-ops. Co-ops can get good food very cheaply. They can deal directly with natural-food wholesalers to get whole-grain breads, unhydrogenated peanut butter, and other preservative-free products. Co-ops are more likely to get what you want, unlike the local Safeway or A&P. Even a few families in the same neighborhood can work cooperatively by taking turns in baking bread for all the families in the group or in going to a nearby farmer's market, where foods are sold in bulk. If someone has a backyard, a group of people could plant an organic garden and thus be sure of pesticide-free vegetables.

Putting pressure on our congressmen to support strict food-regulation legislation will probably do little to improve the quality of our food. Every now and then a dangerous additive or pesticide might be banned, especially when dedicated groups such as Ralph Nader's or the Environmental Defense Fund win a hard-fought legal battle. But after DDT is banned, the agriculture business will find something else to replace it, and after Citrus Red #2 is gone, the food industry will find another harmful red food coloring. Even if the FDA really began to protect us, the food and drug industries would probably not take long to gain control of the agency once again.

Unfortunately, our system hasn't worked and isn't working now. Money seems to rule everything in our economy, including politics. The success we have in making more healthful foods available to us most likely will not come from winning legal battles (as least for a long time) but from joining with others around us to put pressure on local supermarkets, boycott harmful foods (and let the manufacturers know about it), join food co-ops, grow our own gardens, and help spread accurate information about food and nutrition. For all of us, being in control of our bodies also means choosing what we put into them.

FURTHER READINGS

Davis, Adele, *Let's Eat Right to Keep Fit* and *Let's Get Well*. New York: Harcourt, Brace and World, 1954.
   Both are interesting and contain fairly accurate information, though frequent recommendations to take vitamin pills are somewhat questionable.

Hunter, Beatrice T. *Gardening Without Poisons*. Berkeley: Berkeley Medallion Books, 1971.
   A good general guide to organic gardening.

Lappé, Frances M. *Diet for a Small Planet*. New York: Ballantine Books, 1971.
   Gives excellent evidence that meat is an inefficient, sometimes dangerous, source of protein. Tells how to produce high-quality vegetable protein, and includes many good recipes.

Marine, Gene, and Judith Van Allen. *Food Pollution*. New York: Holt, Rinehart & Winston, 1972.
   Excellent description of the food and agriculture industries' irresponsibility and the government's failure to protect us from the profit-seeking food corporations.

Present Knowledge in Nutrition. New York: The Nutrition Foundation, 1967.
   Prepared from articles written for *Nutrition Reviews;* covers recent findings about various nutrients.

Price, Weston A. *Nutrition and Physical Degeneracy*. Los Angeles: American Academy of Nutrition, 1950.

Rorty, James, and Norman N. Philip. *Tomorrow's Food: The Coming Revolution in Nutrition*. Englewood Cliffs, N.J.: Prentice-Hall, 1947; rev. 1956.

Sherman, Henry C. *The Nutritional Improvement of Life*. New York: Columbia University Press, 1950.

Tatkon, Daniel. *The Great Vitamin Hoax*. New York: Macmillan Co., 1968.

Turner, James S. *The Chemical Feast*. New York: Grossman Pubs., 1970.

Winter, Ruth. *Poisons in Your Food*. New York: Crown, 1969.

Your Money's Worth in Foods. USDA publication (Home and Garden Bulletin #183).
   Includes many bits of "consumer wisdom," ways to save money when we shop, etc. Order from the Superintendent of Documents, U.S. Government Printing Office, Washington, D.C. 20402 (25 cents).

7
Women in Motion

How can I explain it? It gets to you, it is you! We have this notion that mind and body are separate—but how can you feel good in the head, really, if your body's like a limp rag? Before, my body would embarrass me—do clumsy things, because there wasn't a lot of muscular control, or it wouldn't do much at all. Now that I exercise, I'm happier about my body, it acts and reacts in ways that please me—it's stronger, more real, more energetic. It's like being three-dimensional instead of two-dimensional; it makes me feel more complete, more whole.

We all know the need for good nutrition, adequate rest, and regular exercise. They keep our body systems functioning in good order, improve muscle tone (including the heart), and protect our bodies better against injury and susceptibility to disease, especially as we age. A healthy body also helps keep our minds balanced and alert, and vice versa. The well-known symptoms of nervous tension—headaches, insomnia, indigestion—have affected most of us at one time or another. Yet instead of using natural preventatives like exercise and healthy food, we rely heavily on artificial means, which may be harmful—aspirin, tranquilizers, antacid.

The Eisenhower and Kennedy years saw a new emphasis on physical fitness. Concern developed because so many American men failed their army physicals and because a major research study revealed that American children did very poorly, compared with their European peers, on strength and flexibility tests.* So everyone's need for exercise became pressing.

WHY WE DON'T GET THE EXERCISE WE NEED

In agricultural societies or rural areas the concept of exercise is fairly meaningless.† The substance of peoples' lives is strenuous physical labor, with women doing as many (or more) of the heavy tasks as men. Today in America most people live in urban or suburban areas. Here working-class people—especially blacks, but whites too—do the hard physical labor. Still, a growing majority of jobs—not just middle-class ones—require little physical effort although they may be extremely tiring.

Women, even more so than men, tend to use energy in a way that leaves us exhausted. Our lives are busy, even frenetic, yet the moving around we do is often repetitive motion that doesn't use our bodies completely.

*Kraus-Weber test, referred to in an article by John F. Kennedy, *Sports Illustrated*, December 26, 1960, pp. 15–16.
†Physically active games and dance, however, have been a part of almost every society from the beginning of human life. Most of them were "religious or utilitarian in origin," but as time went on, some were performed "primarily for relaxation and recreation" (Deobold B. Van Dalen and Bruce L. Bennett, *A World History of Physical Education: Cultural, Philosophical, Comparative*, Englewood Cliffs, N.Y.: Prentice-Hall, 1971, p. 5).

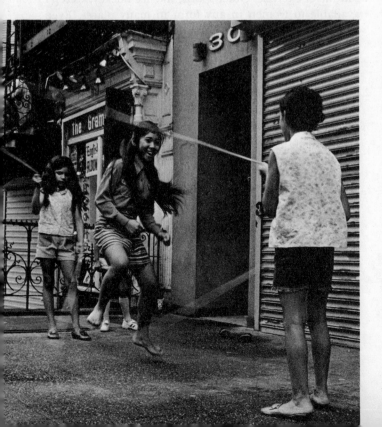

Think of how we spend our time:

as housewives doing repetitive household chores;

as mothers chasing around after kids;

at jobs—in offices or factories in stationary positions requiring painful ways of bending and/or endless hours of sitting that often result in poor posture and back trouble, or in hospitals, or as waitresses on our feet all day.

Getting the exercise we need is in many ways harder for us than for men. When men decide to get exercise (if they have the time and money) they can usually find facilities—a gym or YMCA, private clubs, steam baths, or athletic leagues. In contrast, the facilities available to women are much more limited. Many cities don't have YWCAs, and even schools sometimes lack gyms for women—the girls have to use the boys' gym. Jill's story is typical: "A group of us were looking for a place to play basketball occasionally. We couldn't find any public place. School gyms close at night—or are reserved for league competition—and college gyms are restricted to students or faculty."

Even when facilities are available, they are often not free. You have to pay to join a health club, a suburban country club, or a city Y. (If you're a mother, you often have the additional cost of child care.) Most cities do have free parks, but as one of the girls in our neighborhood complained, "The boys take over, and if we're lucky, they'll let us play once in a while."

Finally, there's a problem of time. Thirty-eight percent of American women (or 31.5 million females) are a part of the labor force. Many also have families and therefore another job waiting for them when they get home. For a mother it is especially difficult to make time for some form of regular exercise unless, of course, it's done with her kids. "Exercise tends to get tacked on," says Mimi, a mother of three. "When my life gets very busy, it's often the first thing to go even though I feel better when I'm exercising." In this respect single women have it easier.

Still, when time, money, and the opportunity exist, a strikingly small number of women incorporate exercise into their daily lives. There are reasons other than the ones we've listed. Social reasons. Many of us have to fight against the prejudiced ideas that women can't do certain things and that we shouldn't do certain things.*

*These prejudices affect most deeply middle- and upper-class women. Precapitalist and capitalist exploitation has never seen anything wrong with driving black and working-class women as hard as men. Sojourner Truth's famous outburst makes that abundantly clear: "The man over there says that women need to be helped into carriages and lifted over ditches, and to have the best place everywhere. Nobody ever helps me into carriages or over puddles or gives me the best place . . . and ain't I a woman? Look at my arm! I have ploughed and planted and gathered into barns, and no man could head me . . . and ain't I a woman? I could work as much and eat as much as a man when I could get it—and bear the lash as well . . . and ain't I a woman?" (From a speech to the Women's Rights Convention, Akron, Ohio, 1851.)

How many of us have had more than one of the following comments hurled at us?

"Strong women aren't feminine—muscles will scare away the boys."

"Well, aren't *you* a little tomboy!"

"Sweating is unladylike."

"The boys won't like you if you beat them at baseball."

"Hey, that one with the knee guards looks like a dyke."

"Ah, you throw like a girl."

From early childhood on, many women are discouraged, subtly and sometimes not so subtly, from participating in strenuous physical activity. We get the idea from our parents, our schools, our neighborhoods, and society. From infancy on, baby girls are pampered and treated more delicately than boy babies. A woman we know sometimes introduced her baby girl as Danny. The adults who met "Danny" encouraged her to play actively without worrying about a few bumps or even tears. But when she was introduced as Sara, people were more protective of her. No wonder many girls grow up scared to try out things with their bodies. In a recent questionnaire directed to women studying karate, many women wrote that as little girls they had been encouraged to go outside and run around, or to dance or swim during the summer, but rarely to pursue athletics seriously.

In schools, especially in the past, physical education programs often weren't required for women. When they were, less was expected of them. Our team sports often had softer rules—a women's regulation basketball court was formerly one-third the size of a men's standard court, which made for a much slower game. Some gym programs for women bog down into a needlessly boring routine of exercise. Other sports, like ice hockey, weren't available to women in any form in many places. Even neighborhood streets are usually the boy's turf. Growing up to believe that physical coordination is a male characteristic, boys will teach each other athletic skills but won't do the same with girls. Joanne told us: "Sometimes the boys would let me join their stickball games, but if several of us girls wanted to play, they would chase us away." And organized sports is mostly a male world —from the professional level down to neighborhood little leagues.

As we pass into and through adolescence, the pressures on us to be "popular with the boys" reach epidemic proportions and often quench still further our desire to exercise strenuously. We're warned not to compete with boys or they won't like us, so we become cheerleaders to the boys' teams. We give up learning athletic skills in favor of learning to swing our hips. We're taught that popularity depends on "femininity": muscles on a woman are considered unattractive—to men, of course. Alice told us: "When I started studying karate my boyfriend got real upset: he was afraid I'd get muscular and not be his slim little lady anymore. But that's his problem. I feel good now, and I'm not so afraid of a bruise or two anymore."

For some women the threat of being unpopular with the boys or looking "unfeminine" is an empty one. Those women tend to grow up active and tough. But for most women who have been brought up to consider male approval primary, such threats are intimidating, and they prevent many of us from developing our physical potential. Cheryl's example is not unusual: "I was real good at ball games. The boys fought to have me on their team. When I got married—at sixteen—Jim was jealous of the other men and wouldn't let me play ball anymore. So I just sat around."

There's also the threat that we'll injure ourselves if we try to do something too strenuous. A female dance student was frightened that a leg-lifting exercise might damage her uterus. Many women have been taught that physical activity during menstruation is dangerous. Uncomfortable perhaps, but not at all dangerous. Women in fact do all kinds of heavy work without injury to their reproductive organs or any other part of themselves. Nell described arguments she had with her husband: "Peter gets angry at me for moving furniture. 'You'll hurt yourself,' he says. He doesn't know how many heavy things I lift—like our thirty-pound son! I think he's scared that my being stronger will make me less dependent on him." It is lack of muscular development that makes some activities or jobs risky for women now, *not* some inherent weakness in the female body. With routine, sensible exercise, we can depend on our bodies to be more powerful and flexible, quicker and less prone to injury.

A final deterrent to doing vigorous exercise is the clothing that we're expected to wear, which constricts and abuses our bodies in some pretty striking ways:

High heels damage our feet permanently. Our entire foot is meant to hit the ground—our arches are shock absorbers, and that function can't be carried out if half our foot is in the air. High heels also force our weight forward, making balance difficult, which is awkward as well as dangerous. Tight low-heeled shoes cramp our bones and prevent our feet from breathing. The paper-thin soles on many women's shoes not only give our feet no protection against the cold in winter, but the lack of cushioning between the hard ground and our feet causes tired legs.

Tight belts and collars, corsets and girdles, overly tight panty hose, and other restrictive garments impede our breathing, circulation and digestion.

The bra debate goes on. The breasts consist of glandular connective tissue with muscles behind. Some people argue that wearing no bra helps strengthen those muscles and keeps the breasts high and firm. (It's certainly comfortable for small-breasted women.) Others argue that

going braless causes the connective tissue to break down and will eventually lead to sagging breasts. That's all we know!

Other clothing is functionally limiting, though not necessarily damaging:

Real short skirts make it difficult to lean over or bend down, not to mention the fact that they invite attack or lecherous comments on the street.

Real long skirts bind one's legs and make it difficult to move or run on the streets.

Bikini bathing suits are impractical except for lying passively in the sun: the straps are often cutting or the tops fall off easily.

Women's pants discourage us from exercising in places where there are no public toilets. It turns into a whole humiliating production to take down your pants in public if you have to piss.

THINGS ARE BEGINNING TO CHANGE

Some of this is beginning to change. The changes are most apparent in the area of clothing. In recent years many women have become as concerned with comfort and practicality as with style and appearance. Increasingly women wear pants; they're easier to move in, warmer in cold weather, and greater protection against the eyes of men on the street. Even at secretarial or receptionist jobs, for example, where women are expected to look "ladylike," the right to wear pants has been won. More women have begun to design and make their own clothes. A woman we know designed a pair of pants with a zipper going from the front to the back of the crotch. You just unzip the pants and pee standing up—no need to take down your pants!

There are similar trends in footwear—away from the binding, pointy, high-off-the-ground shoes toward healthier styles: sandals, moccasins, sneakers, various kinds of boots, all of which keep the feet closer to the ground and allow them to live. (Go barefoot when and where possible.)

There has been a general increase in public athletic facilities—more public swimming pools, skating rinks, and even tennis courts. YWCA programs have been expanded, and college and public school programs have improved. Rules for organized sports have been changed as the various collegiate authorities have recognized that women can play a harder, faster game than they believed possible. For example, women now use the same regulation-size court for basketball as men do. New areas are opening up: for example, some communities have ice hockey leagues for women.

Crucial to all this is the growing interest among women in more physical activity. It's no longer unusual to see women jogging along tracks where only men used to run. There's a growing demand for self-defense classes among women.We're also beginning to develop a pride in female athletes whom we'd never heard about, because, as in many other areas, that part of our history has been ignored or suppressed. Babe Didrikson Zaharias, for example, did just about everything—the javelin throw, the 888-meter hurdle, high jump, basketball —superbly, winning countless medals and championships. Or Florence Chadwick, an American, swam the English Channel three times, both ways—in 1950, 1951, and 1955.

As we start to enter a field that has been predominantly male, we realize how little we know about female anatomy. What little we do know often focuses on sexuality and reproduction. Our general anatomy is similar to men's: we're both spinal creatures with legs, arms, muscles, and brains. There are undeniable differences, though, besides the obvious sexual ones.*

The basic difference in terms of muscle mass is hormonal. The major male hormone is testosterone; in women it's estrogen and progesterone. At puberty estrogen slows down a girl's growth, while testosterone does not immediately do the same for boys. This difference causes men to be larger, squarer, and more muscular

*We don't know how much these differences hold true for different races or societies, past or present. Westerners tend to be larger than eastern peoples, but we don't know about the differences between women and men in other parts of the world.

than we are, particularly across the shoulders. Most women won't be able to lift as much weight as most men, though many of us are stronger than men. Our bones usually weigh less than men's since they're carrying less muscle, and we generally have 10 percent more body fat.

Men have larger rib cages than women, which allows them to take deeper breaths, providing greater endurance in running.

The pelvic bone is shaped differently in men and women: it rises at a different angle. As a result, we have more lateral flexibility (which allows childbearing), but possibly less speed in running.

Women usually have smaller hands than men, which may affect our ability to grab and hold onto things like basketballs or footballs.

These physical differences can be compensated for:

Skill often matters more than strength; when this is the case, women can excel. For example, one acknowledged star of the British Olympic Equestrian team is a woman. In the self-defense or martial arts a 120-pound woman can throw a 250-pound man.

Reflex also counts a lot. Many activities depend on an ability to respond swiftly and accurately. Examples include gymnastics, the self-defense arts, tennis.

Endurance: it has been proved statistically that women are healthier from birth and their average life span is five years longer than men's.Women can surely build up endurance to become really outstanding in swimming, hiking, jogging. A study of long-distance drivers showed that the women's capacity for alertness increased 10 percent with time, whereas the men's fell off 11 percent. This ability to endure and remain sharp has obvious implications for physical performance.

And, of course, the belief that we can do it, whatever the form of motion, if training is serious and regular, is critical. There is no doubt that the present gap between women's and men's ability to use their bodies fully will be greatly reduced. It is NOT a matter of innate male ability, despite what many of us are taught. Natural skill, of course, varies from person to person, but we all have the capacity to learn. General health and age will influence that capacity. A woman with a good balanced diet will have more energy than someone who lives on Coke and potato chips. Speed is usually a function of age. But, older women: don't for a minute believe that you can't be strong and healthy and learn to develop your body. (See "Some Final Advice," p. 90).

In recent years many of us have begun to recognize our own physical potential. We are interested in, even inspired by, the women who excel at sports. But given the American world of athletics, based as it is on the most aggressive, dog-eat-dog patterns of male competitiveness and greedily engaged in marketing the successful athlete like any other product in our society, we do

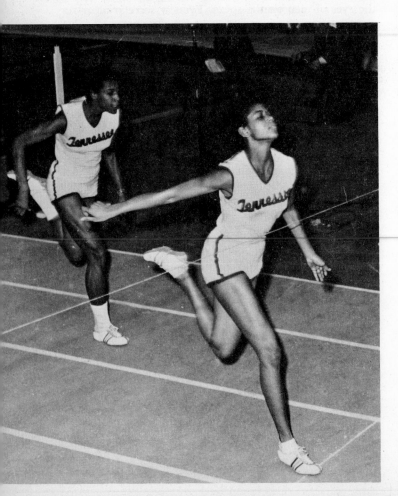

Wilma Rudolph Equaling Her World Record
in the Indoor 60-Yard Dash

not want to see women triumphing over women in ugly, masculine ways. Instead of turning talented people into superstars, we favor providing opportunity and encouragement for all. We feel it essential that we develop ourselves, to be the best we can, each and every woman. We want to be concerned with how we feel, not just how we look. That means a healthy glowing body that uses its resources well.

CHOOSING AN EXERCISE: SOME GUIDELINES AND SOME BENEFITS

We can learn to throw a ball or swim or climb a tree. It's up to us to decide, not our doctors, husbands, boyfriends, or girl friends. What's important is finding a kind and amount of exercise that's right for each of us, for our bodies, our minds. This will vary from woman to woman, but here are some general criteria:

Select an exercise that stretches and strengthens the entire body—arms, legs, torso, neck.

Pick an activity that feels good, that gives pleasure.

Select something that allows you to pace yourself, with which you can work at enlarging your own capacity, both in the frequency and intensity with which you do it.

For some of us it'll be important to find an activity that can be done at home.

The total exercises, like running or swimming, are the best, because they use and therefore develop many different muscles and at the same time keep the bodily systems healthy, as well as expand their working ability. Forty to fifty percent of body weight is muscle. Bulging muscles alone won't create good health, but the more solid the muscle—not loose and flabby—the better we'll feel: everyday tasks will be much easier, less tiring. In other parts of the world women do vigorous physical labor, while here we often rely on men to lift heavy items or even open jars. Strong muscles do promote a generally more healthy body: strong back muscles reduce the likelihood of back problems; strong abdominal muscles are necessary for holding internal organs in place and often make childbirth less painful. Not to mention the greater independence we'll feel.

A total physical activity will make you pant. One woman we knew was afraid that panting meant her body was breaking down. In fact the opposite is true. That kind of exertion will help breathing: working harder, you'll begin to breathe more slowly, deeply, and more regularly. Your lungs will develop a larger capacity for air. With strenuous exercise, blood that is ordinarily pooled in the organs of the body is drawn into circulation; the heart has to pump this increased amount of liquid around faster; over time this means that the heart, a muscle, will strengthen and be able to pump

out a greater volume of blood with fewer strokes. The contractions and relaxations of the muscles, especially in the legs, which have been called a second heart, will squeeze the veins, particularly helping the blood return upward to the heart. Increased circulation ensures that all the muscles and organs get a continually fresh supply of blood, which is essential to their survival and well-being.

Total exercise also helps our attitude toward food and improves our digestive process. It regularizes eating habits: we eat more if we need to, but it helps curb the compulsive eating that is a problem for so many women. The movement of the body and its muscles speeds up the peristaltic (wavelike) action of the digestive organs and therefore the elimination processes as well. People who exercise regularly are less prone to constipation and kidney stones.

Obviously, physical activity will alleviate certain kinds of tension. Mental tension and physical tension are intimately related. Vigorous exercise will help both body and mind relax. We are not suggesting exercise as a cure-all, as a substitute for changing this oppressive society into a human one we can live in, but we are saying that we need exercise to relieve the harmful effects of all the frustration, anxiety, and anger we experience daily. Exercising regularly will help us sleep better (as long as we don't jog a mile just before bedtime). If your body has good tone and doesn't slouch, your mind will surely function better. Learning and practicing many sports is not only a physical exercise but is also mentally stimulating since it requires concentration, memorization, and creative thinking about how to move the way we want to.

Jogging, as we have said, is one of the best forms of exercise. A mile run in the morning will make you feel better all day long. Do it any place—in the country, along a river, in parks, or even around the block. Wear comfortable, loose-fitting clothes and sturdy, flexible shoes.

Especially in the city, try to run in the early morning or late evening, when the air is least polluted by traffic and industry. We realize this may be a problem, especially at night because of dangerous streets. Find company to run with if you can—it is safer and also less lonely.

Build up slowly: start at a slow pace and gradually increase speed and distance. At first walk, then jog, then walk again. As you get stronger, vary periods of slow running with periods of sprinting. This alternation is very good for circulation.

Move your feet naturally (toes pointing straight ahead, though) and let your arms swing, the left arm moving with the right leg and the right arm with the left leg. Try to relax, especially your neck and shoulders.

Stay off pavements, if possible, because the shock of your feet constantly hitting such hard surfaces may result in inflammation of the muscle tissue or cause the calf muscles to be torn away from the bone. An additional benefit of running is that it helps varicose veins by pumping the blood up from the legs.

If you can't run outside, do it inside—even while doing other things, like talking on the phone. Some people enjoy running to music. One woman we met jogs while watching TV: "You can run right through a movie once you get into it," she told us.

If you don't feel strong enough to try running, then begin to build up strength by walking daily. Move briskly, with strong strides, using your entire leg.

Bicycling is a great exercise, especially for the legs. Replace as many car trips with a bicycle as time and distance will allow.

Skiing is another vigorous activity that uses the entire body while improving control and balance. And it's tremendously exhilarating as well. There are disadvantages, however: it's both seasonal and expensive.

Swimming is another excellent general conditioner. Try to swim at least several times weekly. Start each session with one, four, or ten laps, whatever feels comfortable, and build up by pushing yourself to do at least one more lap than you think you can.

Group Sports are also great exercise if done regularly. Basketball, hockey, tennis, baseball, handball, and other ball games will build coordination, endurance, and improve agility. Certain techniques can be practiced alone, while the whole game requires others. This takes a bit of getting people together, but it's worth it—a fast, hard game is good for the spirit as well as the body.

Self-Defense Arts are increasingly popular with women and can be excellent forms of exercise. Judo, Aikido, karate, and Tae Kwon Do have the added advantage of teaching us how to defend ourselves. Warm-ups for these skills can include running, stretching, weight lifting for arm development, while the various techniques (punching, kicking, throwing) rely on timing, speed, and accuracy rather than brute strength, which makes them ideal for women. Like group sports, the self-defense arts improve balance, coordination, control, and of course endurance; in addition, they sharpen your mental capacities—you learn to be decisive, to develop a plan of attack quickly, both offensively and defensively.

Yoga is not just for Eastern mystics and American hippies. Many women of all ages have found yoga rewarding. It develops muscle tone and control, produces limberness and flexibility, and helps you learn how to relax. After doing yoga for a while many women feel reunited with their bodies.

Dance can also be a strenuous form of exercise, especially when done regularly and in a disciplined way. Any form of dance will strengthen and stretch your muscles, teach you muscular control, and improve coordination and balance. As a creative art it also encourages physical expression—without words—of emotions and moods.

Working at Home, there are many exercises you can do to develop strength and build up flexibility. Some suggestions:

Strengthening exercises include push-ups, leg lifts, sit-ups. If you have lower back trouble, keep your back rounded while doing leg lifts or sit ups in order to avoid hyperextension of the back. The Royal Canadian Air Force manual suggests a variety of stretching exercises. Get the combined women's and men's manual and begin with the women's exercises, building up gradually to the men's, which are more demanding.

Use dumbbells to build up arm muscles. There is a series of ten exercises, to be done with three-pound weights, available in most sporting-goods stores. Start with 10 each, build up to 15, then 20. They may be boring as repetitious activity tends to be, but don't cheat; they won't help unless you do them vigorously.

Jumping rope is excellent exercise and doesn't take up much room. Try to jump steadily for a minute, pause to catch your breath, and jump another minute. Repeat three or four times. Or try doing the jumping-jack exercise shown in the illustrations.

Reassess the physical work you do during the day and make each motion using muscles so as to develop but not strain them. Try to build up both sides of your body equally; don't favor the strong side. We women tend to leave heavy household work for men—painting, lifting, trash removal. We could choose to do these tasks and get more exercise than we otherwise would.

What about the home exercisers being sold now? Chin-up bars, hand grippers, stationary bicycles can be fun and useful. But why spend a lot of money on gimmicks when there are ways of using just your body to get the same benefits? It's better to save your money for healthy foods or real athletic facilities or camping trips or decent hiking shoes.

None of these physical activities is an either-or proposition. Running is a total exercise because it is so good for all your body systems and your leg muscles, but you may want to supplement it with the dumbbell routine to develop your arms. Yoga is fine for stretching and building muscle, but you still need the benefits that come from vigorous sweating and panting. Whatever you do, you should do it regularly. Short periods of frequent practice are better than fewer longer ones. Try to spend fifteen minutes each morning exercising. It's bound to improve your entire day.

As you're thinking about what to do, you'll have to decide whether to work alone or in a group. If in a group, then with all women or a mixed group? Many forms of exercise or sports can be practiced alone: running, swimming, karate, working out at a gym, yoga, dance. Many of us lack the discipline to work by our-

SOME SUGGESTED ARM EXERCISES

Stand with your feet shoulder width apart and feet pointing straight ahead. In each exercise (except #1) make sure you complete the motion of one arm—that is, return it to starting position—before moving the other arm. Don't let your arms just flop back to starting position: use your muscles to pull the arms back down.

1. Starting with arms hanging at sides, twist wrists simultaneously with an abrupt back-and-forth motion.

2. Arms at sides, fists facing forward (palms down), lift just your forearms up and down: left arm up, down, then right arm up, down. One arm should return to starting position before other arm is lifted. Alternate arms.

3. Same as #2, but with palms facing upward, fists facing backward.

4. Elbows bent, fists at shoulder height. Straighten one arm directly above shoulder, bring hand back down, raise other arm, lower. Continue, alternating arms.

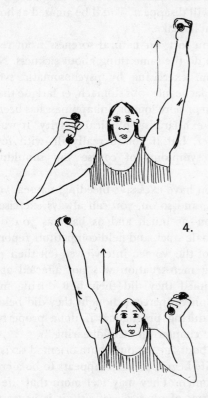

4.

5. Arms straight out to the side at shoulder height, palms facing upward. Bring one hand in to shoulder, moving only forearm and keeping elbow at same place. Straighten arm to starting position, and bend other arm. Straighten. Continue, alternating arms.

6. Arms at sides, palms facing downward. Lift one arm straight in front to shoulder height. Lower arm. Raise other arm, then lower. Continue, alternating.

7. Arms at sides, lift left hand to underarm, return to starting position. Lift right hand, and return. Continue, alternating arms.

8. Arms at sides. Lift left arm (straight) to the side, shoulder height, return. Lift right arm, return. Continue, alternating.

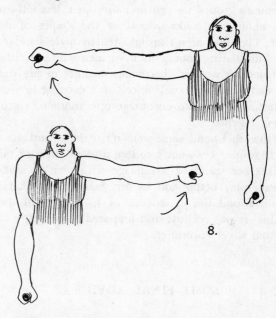

8.

9. Arms straight out to the side at shoulder height, fists facing forward. Bring left fist to shoulder, moving just the forearm, and return to starting position. Repeat with right arm. Continue, alternating.

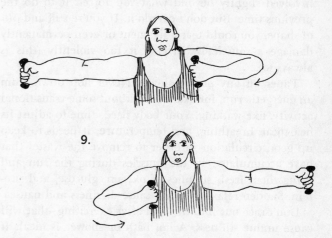

9.

10. Arms at sides. Simultaneously, bend both arms at the elbow and swing right arm in front of the stomach, with hand reaching toward the shoulder, and left arm in back reaching high. Swing arms back to the sides and alternate arms: this time left arm in front and right arm in back.

selves, at least at first. Others of us get lonely or bored. Exercising to music may help some.

Especially in the initial learning stages of many skills, some organized instruction is necessary. In addition to providing technical information, a group can also provide support and encouragement. Women we know studying yoga agreed that they needed the discipline of a class situation when they began; as their skills and confidence grew, they found it easier to practice alone. In women's groups we can be more open, less self-conscious about our awkwardness or the shapes of our bodies. There we aren't intimidated by male standards or by humiliating comments from men who are either threatened by women's becoming stronger or are only interested in us as sexual objects. It's exciting to work together as women, to encourage one another to grow stronger together.

On the other hand, some women cite the advantages of mixed groups. A women's college athletic director said she likes her teams to scrimmage with men—it makes the team play better and harder. Some female karate students found the experience of sparring with men valuable—it was realistic and prepared them better for an actual street encounter.

SOME FINAL ADVICE

Now that you're about to begin your exercise program, here is some final advice and a few cautions:

Start slowly and build up, in general and during each session. Muscle growth comes from pushing each muscle involved slightly beyond what you forced it to do the previous time. But don't overdo it. If you're stiff and out of shape, you could tear a ligament or even permanently damage a muscle by driving it too violently (this is always so).

Taper off any period slowly. Never flop down from an energetic run, for example, without some transitional activity, like walking. Your body needs time to adjust its heartbeat, breathing, and temperature; it needs to keep up good circulation in order to remove the wastes that have accumulated in the muscles during the run and bring them fresh supplies of oxygen, glucose, and protein. Sudden relaxation may cause dizziness and nausea.

Don't race out into the cold after exercising—that will cause undue stiffness. A hot bath or shower is ideal: it will relax your body, keep circulation up, and clean your body after all the sweating. If you have access to steam baths or a sauna, that's a wonderful treat.

Don't eat heavily before exercising. The stomach requires a large blood supply to digest food, and exercise diverts the blood from the stomach to other muscles. The stomach's attempts to function actively on less blood than it needs may cause pain. Make sure to eat a variety of healthy foods to meet the demands of greater physical activity and particularly to replace the calcium, sodium chloride, and iodine lost through sweating. Except under extreme conditions, you don't need to take salt pills. At the same time try to cut down on cigarettes, alcohol, and harmful drugs.

Get plenty of rest. You'll probably need more once you start working your body harder, and you'll probably sleep better too. See if you can sleep or rest on your back or side on a moderately hard, flat surface, using only a thin pillow.

Expect some stiffness. If you're really pushing your muscles, they're bound to hurt the following day. But don't pamper yourself and stop. The best remedy is moderate exercise: that will increase circulation, which will help carry away accumulated lactic acid causing the stiffness. A hot bath, heat, or massage applied to a particular muscle are also helpful. Heat and massage are relaxants; they also dilate the blood vessels, speeding waste removal. As you keep exercising, your body will gradually become accustomed to working harder and the discomfort will disappear. You'll be amazed at how much progress you'll make.

Just as you sort out natural soreness from real pain, you need to do the same thing about sickness. Never be put off from exercising by psychosomatic symptoms. Many a headache, nervous stomach, or fatigue that comes from tension or boredom or unhappiness has been driven off by some exhilarating physical activity. It won't hurt a cold either, but if you're really ill—with fever and other such symptoms—of course you shouldn't push yourself.

Unless you have excessive bleeding, nausea, vomiting, bad cramps, and so on, you can always exercise during menstruation—as much and as hard as you desire. A study of female track and field competitors reported that 63 percent of the women interviewed felt their performance during menstruation was not affected at all; 29 percent claimed they did their best during menstruation; while only 8 percent thought they did below par.*

Exercise during pregnancy, if done properly, is excellent. (See chapter on "Childbearing.")

A word about age. In our youth-oriented sexist society the line "Life begins at forty" appears to be a cruel joke to many women. They may feel more that life ends at forty. In terms of physical activity, it is never too late. If you are over thirty and haven't exercised for a long time, begin gradually. At any age you can build up strength, endurance, and coordination—it just will take a little longer, but it will come, provided the determination is there. Remember that marathon champions have

*From a report by J. Kral and E. Markalous, cited in *Injury in Sport*, by J. R. Armstrong and W. E. Tucker (London: Staples Press, 1964), p. 118.

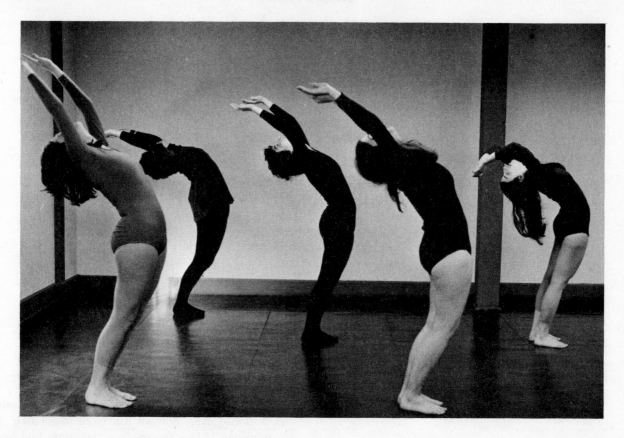

their best years between thirty-five and forty-five (as opposed to sprinters, who peak at a much younger age). A fifty-year-old woman we know jogs three miles a day. A sixty-two-year-old woman we met recently began doing yoga and loves it: "I haven't felt so young and energetic in years!" she told us. "My over-all health is much better, and it's such a welcome relief from housework."

Be patient! It will be hard work and perhaps discouraging at first. You may come home exhausted and dripping wet from jogging one block. You may be frustrated by not being able to make your muscles work the way you want them to at the beginning.

But exercise can help change our lives. It has already given many of us new energy, new confidence, and greater independence. "I have more respect for my body. It belongs to me now." "Dance has developed my muscles and stretch. It's beautiful to become aware of my capabilities, to grow." "Karate has made me feel stronger, more alive, more independent. I can run and dance and even climb a tree. Some days I feel like I could fly."

We have in the past accepted limitations on what our bodies can do. But we women are beginning to take our lives into our own hands a little in countless other ways—demanding job equality, free childcare and abortion, nonsexist advertising and education, and coming out as lesbians. And that means also demanding better neighborhood athletic facilities free to all and well-rounded programs for girls in our schools.

We need to love our bodies and treat them well. Where would we be without them?

8
Rape and Self-Defense

RAPE

RAPE is sexual intercourse without consent, or violent sexual aggression by a man (or men) against a woman (or child). Rape causes mental and physical damage.

WHOSE FAULT IS RAPE?

Because of the persistent myth that most women secretly want to be raped, and thus get what they want, a woman is usually blamed for her rape. Men are often excused for their sexual aggressiveness because of their "uncontrollable" sex drive. (This, too, is a myth. In Menachim Amir's study* of 646 rape cases it was found that 71 percent of the rapes were planned. This premeditation reflects something quite different from a spontaneous, "uncontrollable" urge.)

Basically, rape is the fault of our cultural emphasis on "sex and violence," now an American idiom like "love and marriage." Many newspapers, magazines, and movies encourage people to groove on sadism by graphically illustrating incidents of sexual violence.

*Patterns in Forcible Rape (University of Chicago Press, 1971).

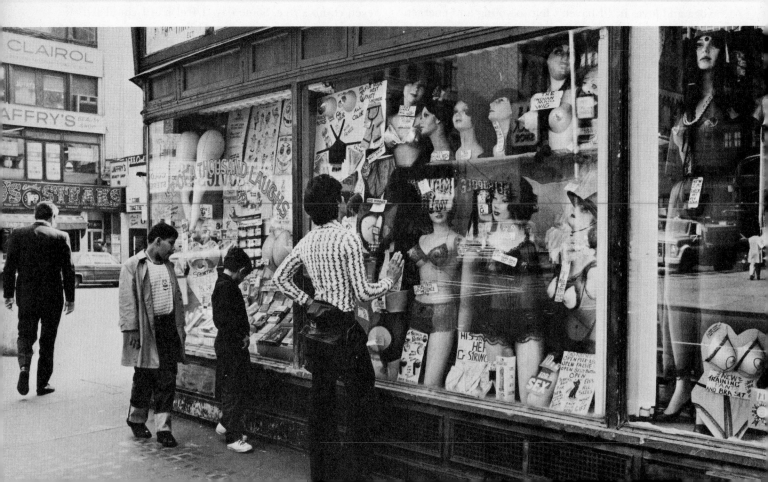

RAPE AND RACE

It is a common but false assumption that most rapes are by black men against white women. In Amir's Philadelphia study, 93 percent of all rapes were carried out by black men against black women or white men against white women. Only 4 percent were white men against black women and *only 3 percent were black men against white women.*

RAPE AND THE LAW

Officials estimate that there are four to ten times more rapes committed than reported. Why? The legal system represents the white, male-dominated status quo, and rape cases are no exception. A woman who wants to prosecute for rape can usually expect little help from either the police or the courts. Often in rape trials the defense tries to show or suggest that a woman has a "bad reputation," to put on trial her character rather than the offense of the defendant. (This is not the case in robbery trials, for example.) She will often be assumed to be lying, she will have to face the rapist again, and she will have to relive the rape.

Some detectives view rape charges as a woman's revenge: "If she thinks she's pregnant, she'll go for a rape charge" or "The prostitute's check bounced, so she claimed she's been raped . . . ho, ho, ho."

When a woman doesn't resist, but instead succumbs to being raped in order to avoid being both raped and severely beaten, she is often assumed to have consented. In one case we know about a detective took the woman aside to proposition her himself (he probably expected her to "consent" again).

WHAT WE CAN DO AS WOMEN

"But if you don't prosecute, what do you do with your anger?" asked a woman at a conference on rape in New York. Someday we will have women rape squads and will be so strong that we won't be attacked as much. Someday we will have free medical care and more sympathetic doctors. Someday we will be able to retaliate, to either send rapists to rehabilitation centers (not prisons) or humiliate them by beating them up.

But what can we do now? Being mentally and physically prepared may help us not to panic. Talking with other women about their experiences may be useful. Having thought about what we would do if raped (Would I try to talk to the guy? About what? Should I call the police? Would I fight?) may really help a lot.

Each rapist is different, but some women have tried talking to their attacker, have tried somehow to make contact. One woman screamed at a guy to say something, anything, so she'd know he was human. He started talking about where he grew up and what his life had been like, after which he raped her anally so she wouldn't get pregnant. Another woman managed to talk a rapist out of murdering her. You shouldn't expect to talk yourself out of rape, but establishing human contact may keep worse things from happening.

Sometimes knowing ways to fight (such as some judo or karate techniques) can give us confidence and help us to defend ourselves. Too often we don't feel able or aren't willing to hurt another person. We experience paralysis instead. One woman who was being choked to death saw a knife within reach but couldn't bring herself even then to stab the guy who was trying to kill her. On the other hand, another woman fought off an attacker who had succeeded in killing other women and she survived eighteen stab wounds.

Some hints from *Stop Rape,* a pamphlet put out by a women's group in Detroit: If you're being attacked in an apartment, building, or hotel, don't yell "Help," yell "Fire!" If you're in an elevator, press the emergency button. If you're being followed on the street, go up to a nearby house (break a window if necessary).

Learn to recognize car and license plates. If you hitchhike, make sure the doors have handles on the inside and know how to get out of the car quickly.

Knives are dangerous to use against someone stronger than you since they can be turned against you. But if you want to use one, hold it down around your hips and use it underhand, not overhand. Practice kicking—you can reach farther with a kick. If you have one punch to land, make it count. Try distracting the attacker's attention first—throw something, a tissue or a glove. *Don't Be Afraid to Hurt Someone Who's Hurting You.*

WHAT TO DO IF YOU HAVE BEEN RAPED

If you have been raped, you should immediately go to a hospital or doctor. Your concerns are three:

1. Venereal disease. Most hospitals will give rape victims preventive penicillin.

2. Pregnancy. You can wait until six weeks after your last period, get a pregnancy test, and arrange for an abortion if necessary. Less anxiety is involved if you take

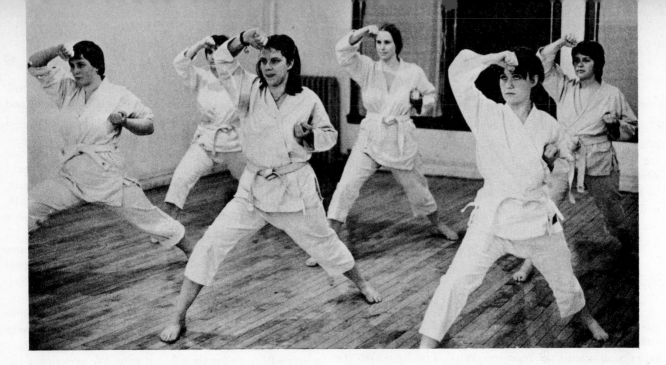

estrogen, which, if taken within twenty-four hours of intercourse, will prevent implantation of the fertilized egg. The estrogen drug (diethylstilbestrol is most commonly prescribed) makes you nauseated and uncomfortable for the five days you take it and may have unknown side effects. These factors have to be weighed against the dangers and anxiety of pregnancy.

3. Lacerations. If you are bruised, cut, or even just generally shaken up, you may want to get a checkup.

If you want to prosecute, you need to call the police immediately; don't change clothes or take a shower and wash away the "evidence." You should be prepared to feel as though the police are raping you again. They will interrogate you, make you go through every detail of the action (which side did your pants zip on, where did he touch you, etc.), and in general make the experience very humiliating.

In some cities only the city hospital will see you, and you may have to wait two to three hours before a gynecologist shows up. Since the gynecologist will probably be a male, he may have little regard for the revulsion that you might feel at being handled by a man just after being raped.

If you've been raped, call a friend for help. If a local women's center has formed a rape squad,* call them. Women who have been raped and have talked about it afterward are apt to feel less guilty and ashamed, because they could express their anger and discuss the crime as something that happens to many women, than those who keep it a secret they have to carry alone. We must help one another to feel and express this anger, since failure to do so can have serious consequences. One woman who was raped was severely depressed for six months until she could finally express her rage at what had been done to her.

It is not the police, the courts, or men who will stop rape. Women will stop rape.

*A group of women who assist rape victims, go with them to the hospital, possibly offers some protection against rape threats.

SELF-DEFENSE

Developing a healthy body makes us happier, more complete people—as long as we're alive, that is. In this violent society, learning to protect ourselves from male attack is an integral part of our physical and psychological health. A reported rape occurs every seven minutes in America—at about the same frequency as births of baby girls. Then there are the sex murders of women, many more than the sensational ones by men like the Boston Strangler or Richard Speck. Every woman—whether or not she is the victim of one of these vicious crimes—knows the fear of dark deserted streets, strange noises in the middle of the night, obscene phone calls, and the everyday humiliation of dirty remarks and gestures on the streets.

LEARNING TO PROTECT OURSELVES

For too long most of us have had to rely on men, money, or luck for a limited kind of "protection." Some of us, particularly working class women, learn how to take care of ourselves while growing up—we have no choice. We're often exposed to more physical violence than middle and upper class women and sometimes forced into situations where we learn to use our arms and legs and to take pain—at home, in schools, on the streets. Many others of us are reared in highly protective environments where fighting is discouraged. As a result we feel incredibly helpless and vulnerable and even go so far as to question our right to defend ourselves.

We believe it's essential that all women begin to take the right to self-defense seriously. An earlier chapter dealt with the need to build up strength and endurance and the ways to accomplish this. That strength alone, however, will not teach us how to fight. Most women are terribly afraid of pain and violence: they are afraid both of hitting and being hit. We don't know how much pain we can take; many of us panic at the mere suggestion of being hit. On the other hand, we have little sense of the potential power in our own bodies—we don't know our own strength.

SELF-DEFENSE TRAINING

We encourage all women to learn some basic techniques of self-defense that include actual fighting. There are several possibilities. If you have time and money you can get formal instruction in a school. Check the yellow pages under "judo" or "karate" for schools in your area. Some YWCAs have self-defense classes, which are usually cheaper. In some areas women's groups are setting up free self-defense classes that are open to all women. Or you could set up your own class with some friends and try to find a woman with some experience to help you occasionally. Failing that, get a couple of books on self-defense and try to learn some techniques from the pictures and description.

There are many martial arts to choose from. Judo utilizes throwing, grappling, and choking techniques. It also teaches you to wrestle.

Aikido is similar to judo in that it relies on the motion of the attacker. You wait for the attack and use the attacker's body motion against him by pulling, twisting, throwing. It is a purely defensive art.

We have found Tae Kwon Do, or Korean karate, a most satisfactory form of self-defense for women. It teaches us to mobilize our entire body as effectively as possible, utilizing a variety of striking techniques, with special emphasis on kicks. That is important, since most women's legs are more developed than our arms, and we can kick farther than we can punch. Tae Kwon Do always combines a defensive motion (like a block) with an unarmed fighting technique (a kick, punch, or strike) that allows you to control a sphere around you. As you learn the techniques you can begin to utilize them in sparring—actual fighting situations. The general body conditioning will build up your leg muscles tremendously, so you will move solidly with new self-assurance, which is in itself a deterrent to men on the prowl.

A warning for those of you who are looking for a formal school: make sure to find one that takes women seriously, or try to set up an all-female class. Many male instructors provide a watered-down version of karate that allows no bodily contact and stresses get-away gimmicks. Others cruelly say, "If you think you can do this as well as a man, try this . . . ," and are physically brutal. Watch out also for ugly competitiveness where only the best get better or the women are played off against each other.

SOME THINGS YOU CAN DO

Whether you enroll in a formal class or set up informal training, begin right now to think about self-defense. It is a skill that can be learned, although it is a long process that will require discipline and regular practice. But it is also a matter of common sense and learning to think strategically. Practice with friends. Think through possible situations. What would you do if someone came up and grabbed you from behind? How would you respond if someone approached you while you were in a telephone booth? Suppose a man's hand started creeping up your knee on a subway. Take turns playing the attacked and the attacker in each situation. Work at breaking out of holds or wrestling on the floor. It's also important to spar with each other—punching and kicking (not too hard) to help break down some of the fears and inhibitions women have against striking out and getting hit. If you practice with a friend you're much less likely to panic in a real attack situation, since you will have prepared yourself and built up some confidence in your ability to fight back. Fear is a deadly emotion that may keep you from remembering what you can do.

Any woman can use the following techniques (while observing a few precautions):

On the street, especially at night and in unfamiliar surroundings, be alert at all times. If a bad or potentially bad situation starts developing, the safest response is to run unless you're really confident about being able to defend yourself. Head for a store, building, or lighted area where people are likely to be.

If you're caught by surprise and don't think you can run away, look around for something to hit with or

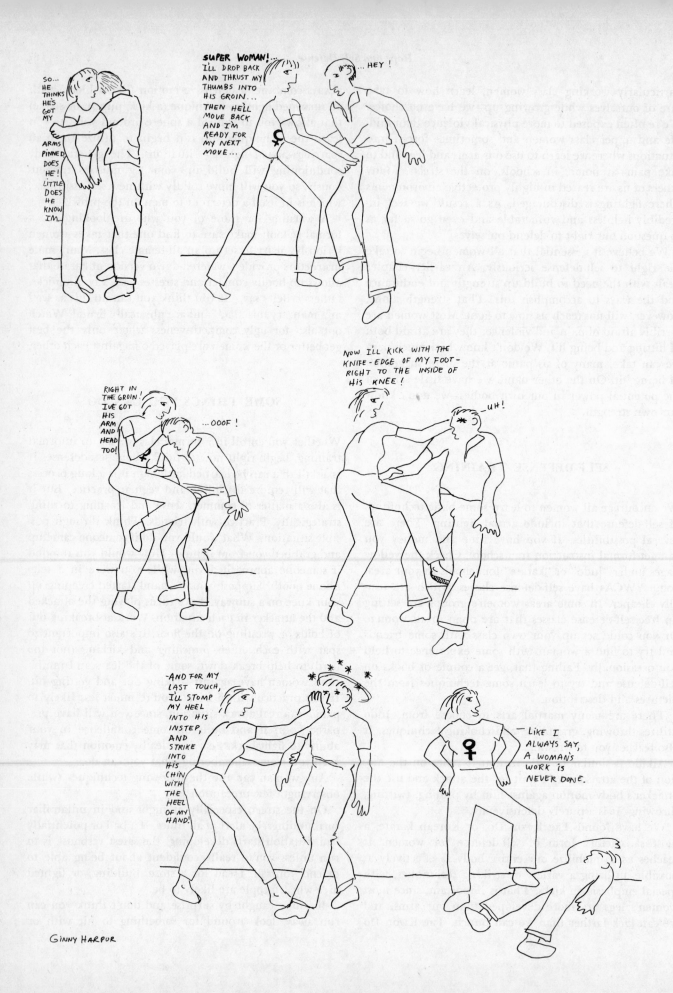

throw—a bottle, chair, a brick or rock. Think creatively about what you're wearing or carrying. A belt buckle, hard shoes, a heavy pocketbook, or an umbrella can all become makeshift weapons. Some women feel good about carrying for ready use (not tucked away in the depths of a handbag or knapsack) a pepper shaker; an artificial plastic lemon filled with lemon juice, vinegar, or other burning substance; or a deodorant spray. The problem with any of these is that you have to be really quick to use them. If you hesitate, the attacker has time to grab the object from you and perhaps use it against you. On the other hand, we know women who have successfully warded off attack by a toss of the pepper shaker, and were able to escape. Other weapons, such as knives and guns, require training or practice to be used safely and effectively. Check with your local police department about the legality of carrying knives, guns, or even mace sprays on your person, or keeping them in your apartment or house.

At home know what's around that you could use in an emergency—rolling pin, hammer, baseball bat, fireplace poker, knife, brick, broom or anything else that is effective. And don't be embarrassed to sleep with one nearby if it makes you feel better.

If you're grabbed from the front, the most effective response is a fast and hard knee to the attacker's groin. This never fails, and you don't need a Charles Atlas physique to make it work. If your arms are free, use them: chop or punch at his head—temples, eyes, right under the ears, mouth, nose. Or bite.

If you're grabbed from behind, move your hips so you can drive your elbow back into the attacker's solar plexus (the sensitive region of the stomach under the breast bone and between the last ribs), then finish him off with a blow to the groin with the back or side of your fist.

Whatever you do, do it quickly and with all the strength you can muster. Remember, in dangerous situations we often respond with a power we didn't know we had, because the level of adrenalin rises in our bodies, speeding up our reflexes and giving us an unbelievable spurt of strength and energy. As you counterattack, let out a yell—not a scream for help, but a loud, blood-curdling battle cry. This will give you a psychological boost and will scare your attacker, throwing him off guard and helping your chances for escape. Once you're free of his grasp, don't hang around to see how he is. *Run. Fast.*

Your use of these techniques depends upon your being able to move quickly and effectively. Clothes often inhibit movement. It's easier to defend yourself if you're wearing pants (not too tight) and shoes that stay on your feet when you kick and run. Clothes like these attract less of the kind of attention that may provoke attack and will also give you more confidence in your ability to take care of yourself.

If you're hitchhiking—and that's often the only form of transportation available—much of the same general advice is applicable. Avoid late-night hitching, or do it in pairs; and try to steer clear of less populated areas. Be careful. Don't get into the back seat unless there's a back door. Be cautious about cars that have more than one man and no women. Remember, you can refuse rides, and you absolutely should if your instincts tell you that an offer may lead to trouble. If trouble develops, you can hit with fists, elbows, knees; scream and cause lots of commotion and then try to get out of the car. Assess the situation—the car speed, the amount of traffic—and do what you decide is best—quickly.

To begin to deal with the danger that confronts us on the streets and in our homes all women should start demanding (as some already have): better-lighted streets; good, frequent public transportation all night long; the right to keep dogs in our apartments; the safest locks for doors and windows installed at the landlord's expense (which should be a part of the housing code in every town and city); specially trained women to go with police on rape calls; some way of forcing police to prosecute rapists (they almost never will unless a forty-year-old man rapes an eight-year-old child); a change in the penalties for rape so juries will convict (they are so high now that most juries—usually male—don't convict); at least some women on all rape juries; self-defense courses at our places of work (especially where women are on graveyard shifts, like in restaurants, hospitals, the phone company) and in our communities. These classes should be free and should teach women how to develop and use their bodies for their protection.

Through learning self-defense we will be on our way to becoming less vulnerable and more self-reliant women. A woman black belt and teacher of Tae Kwon Do expressed it well: "Learning self-defense has given me a greater choice in deciding and doing what I want. I don't feel so much a prisoner of my body. I feel like a being of a bigger world." And as we spread that skill around, and begin to defend each other, we will be on the way toward ending that oppression that will stop only when it becomes as dangerous to attack a woman as it is to attack another man.

9
Venereal Disease

THE PROBLEM

IN SPITE of the fact that prevention is possible and adequate treatment is available, venereal disease is a major problem in the United States today. VD, especially gonorrhea, is spreading alarmingly fast among people of all ages and occupations. It threatens women, in the many cases in which it goes undetected, with pelvic inflammatory disease (often requiring major abdominal surgery), sterility, subfertility, stillbirth, miscarriages, the birth of diseased children. This public health scandal exists primarily because people at all levels of responsibility have been too moralistic or too ashamed about sex to research methods of prevention and to spread information about available methods of prevention and cure.

The two most common venereal diseases are syphilis and gonorrhea. In 1971 the U.S. Public Health Service (PHS) figures showed over 23,000 newly reported cases of syphilis and over 624,000 cases of gonorrhea, an increase of about 6 percent over the previous year. These figures are estimated by PHS to represent only part of the actual incidence of the two diseases. Recently Dr. John D. Millar of the Public Health Service estimated that a total of 2.25 million people in this country—among them 640,000 women—have gonorrhea.* This discrepancy between reported and estimated figures is due mostly to two causes. First, many people who have these diseases do not know they need to seek or feel uncomfortable getting medical help. Second, private physicians report only a small percentage (20 percent or less) of their cases even though required to do so by law.

Syphilis and Gonorrhea—How They Spread

Syphilis and gonorrhea are different diseases, but since they are both acquired through sexual contact with a person who has one or both of them, they are classified as venereal diseases. ("Venereal" means relating to sexual intercourse.) Each is caused by a different microorganism

*Lawrence Altman, "Gonorrhea Tests Urged for Women," *New York Times,* December 20, 1971, p. 19.

(bacterium). These bacteria live best in a warm, moist environment, and when taken from this environment to a drier, cooler one, they die in a very short time. They may also be killed by extreme heat. Stories of syphilis or gonorrhea being picked up from toilet seats, door knobs, towels, dishes, and other objects are not true. People acquire VD only through intimate contact with other people who have the disease. Live syphilis and gonorrhea bacteria must be deposited directly on warm, moist surfaces, such as the linings of the genitals or the lining of the mouth or throat, or on a break in the skin. Sexual intercourse with a person who has a venereal disease provides ideal conditions for the transfer of these bacteria.

Syphilis is often spread through sores on any part of the body. (See syphilis symptoms below.) Gonorrhea can be spread through anal intercourse or through fellatio, from a man's penis to a woman's tonsils. The discharge from the penis carries enough bacteria to spread the disease via the hands, especially to the eyes. Gonorrhea is not spread from mouth to mouth or from mouth to penis or from vagina to mouth, as through cunnilingus, or, on the fingers, from the vagina to other body parts.

Prevention—General

Despite the fact that most of the literature on VD (including a lot of this chapter) stresses treatment and cure of VD, it is becoming clearer and clearer that prevention is not only possible but also the only hope for wiping out VD in this country. This fact can be shown by some simple calculations.*

*Even though two million people could be treated (and cured) for gonorrhea in the next year, gonorrhea would still be an epidemic at the end of the year. However, if only 25 percent of those people exposed to gonorrhea were to use some preventive measure during all of next year, the incidence of gonorrhea at the end of the year would be reduced by 96 percent! Consider this: In January, given two million gonorrhea carriers, instead of two million more people catching gonorrhea, there would be only one and a half million people catching it. In February, instead of one and a half million more people catching gonorrhea, there would be only 1,120,000. And so on. By the end of December, under 100,000 people would be catching gonorrhea from another infected person. This is a reduction of about 96 percent.

VD is not a disease that you have only once, like chicken pox, and to which you are forever after immune. You can have VD as many times as you are exposed to it, and there is no vaccine currently available to prevent someone from getting VD. However, a gonorrhea vaccine has recently been tested* and may be available in the near future. If one partner has VD, there is no *sure* way to prevent the transfer of bacteria to the other partner during sexual intercourse, but there are a number of effective preventive measures we should all know about.

Some of these preventive measures have been known for many decades, and even used with success during wartime experiments.† Until very recently information about these measures has been suppressed for several reasons:

Some VD preventive measures (e.g., certain contraceptive foams, jellies and creams, and condoms) are also forms of birth control. Earlier in this century many people, especially leaders of society, were morally opposed to contraception.

Our culture has needed the fear of VD to limit sexual activity outside of marriage, especially the "promiscuity" of young people and women. With the advent of widespread birth control, which eliminated the fear of pregnancy, fear of VD became the last effective deterrent to complete "sexual license."

Following are some useful ways you can help to prevent VD:

Using contraceptive foam, certain creams (Cooper Cream, Ortho Creme), and certain jellies (Certane Vaginal Jelly, Ortho-Gynol Jelly, Milex Crescent Jelly, Koromex A Vaginal Jelly, Preceptin Gel). Also, Lorophyn vaginal suppositories (*not* a contraceptive) are effective. Many of us have been surprised to find out that these contraceptive measures are also effective preventors of VD and hope that this information will no longer be suppressed. Though common knowledge among scientists for many years, only recently has this information been published.‡ (Check "Birth Control" chapter for relative effectiveness of these products.)

Using condoms. This method was commonly used by soldiers during wartime and is a very effective VD preventor.§ The condom must be put on before the penis touches the partner's vagina or anus. Of course, a condom doesn't protect against infection from syphilitic sores that are not on the genitals.

Using the morning-after pill for VD (different from the morning-after pill for birth control). This pill provides an adequate dose of penicillin or one of the tetracyclines to prevent the contraction of VD immediately after exposure to an infected person. You need a prescription for this and may have trouble finding a doctor who is willing to provide such prevention for VD. A free clinic might be a good place to find such a doctor. The idea of using a small amount of penicillin for VD prophylaxis (prevention) is not yet widely accepted among public health officials. We must push for research into this important area.

Using the "short arm" inspection. This technique, known by prostitutes and in the military, involves examining the penis *before it becomes erect* (before the man is sexually aroused). You pull back the foreskin if he is uncircumcised, then squeeze the penis as in masturbation. (For the exact technique, check with any urologist or internist.) A drop or two of liquid indicates the presence of an infection. Since these drops can be confused with the drops of semen that may come out when the man first gets aroused, one must use use this technique carefully. As a general rule, especially since some people show no symptoms, for your complete protection it makes sense to use a condom and/or a vaginal spermicide.

Treatment—General

VD is not difficult to cure in the early stages of the illness if a doctor or clinic is consulted for treatment. But the treatment plan that is prescribed must be followed strictly or there is a chance that some of the active bacteria will remain and cause further bodily damage. Therefore it is extremely important to know the early symptoms of both syphilis and gonorrhea, and to realize that if there is even the slightest possibility that you have VD, you should seek medical advice promptly.

Most states have VD clinics where you can get blood tests and penicillin free of charge. At these clinics they usually ask you for the names of any people you have had sexual relations with since you got the disease, so they can contact those people and give them treatment. (This is called case-finding.) They keep all names secret, and it's usually a good idea to cooperate with them. But if you don't want to give the clinic people names, then it's your responsibility to get in touch with anyone you had sexual contact with. It might mean life or death for those involved.

Where to get testing and treatment for cheap or for free: call your state's Division of Public Health, a local

---

*Louis Greenberg, MD, paper delivered at Second International Venereal Disease Symposium, April 13, 1972, St. Louis, Missouri.

†Thomas H. Sternberg, Ernest B. Howard, Leonard A. Dewey, and Paul Padget, "Venereal Diseases," in *Preventive Medicine in World War II*, Volume 5 (Communicable Diseases), Washington, D.C., Office of the Surgeon General, Department of the Army.

‡Singh et al., "Studies on the development of a vaginal preparation providing both prophylaxis against venereal disease and other genital infections and contraception," *British Journal of Venereal Disease* (1972) 48, p. 57. The above list of contraceptives, changed from that of the original study, represents the most recent unpublished research of the Singh group.

§Randolph Cautley, Gilbert W. Beebe, and Robert Latou Dickinson, "Rubber Sheaths as Venereal Disease Prophylactics," in *American Journal of the Medical Sciences* 195: 155–63 (1938). A. C. Gelatte in *U.S. Naval Medical Bulletin* 30: 460 (1932).

hot line, Planned Parenthood, or a local hospital. If you don't trust your local hospital to keep your treatment confidential, try a larger hospital in a nearby city, where VD cases are often handled in a special VD clinic or in another clinic like the skin clinic. Almost all minors can be treated without parental permission. See below, "Protect Yourself—Protect Others," for more information.

SYPHILIS

Syphilis is caused by a small spiral-shaped bacterium called a spirochete. Once these bacteria have entered the body through intimate sexual or physical contact, the disease goes through four stages.

Symptoms of Syphilis

Primary. The first sign is usually a sore called a chancre (pronounced "shanker"). It may look like a pimple, a blister, or an open sore. It is usually painless. It probably will show up any time from nine to ninety days after the bacteria enter the body. This sore usually appears on or near the place where the bacteria enter, usually the genitals. However, it may appear on the fingers, lips, breast, anus, or mouth. At this primary stage it is very infectious, since the chancre is full of bacteria, which can be easily spread to others. Sometimes the chancre never develops or is hidden inside the body, giving no evidence of the disease. This is particularly true for women, in whom the sore frequently develops inside the vagina or hidden inside the folds of the labia. In any case, the sore will go away by itself whether or not the person gets treatment. But the bacteria are still in the body, increasing and spreading.

Secondary. The next stage occurs anywhere from a few weeks to six months later. It usually lasts three to six months, but sometimes the symptoms of this stage can come and go for several years. By this time the bacteria have spread all through the body, and there are many possible symptoms. A rash may appear over the entire body or just on the hands and feet. Sores may appear in the mouth. Joints may become swollen or painful, and bones may hurt. There may be a sore throat, mild fever, or headache (all flu symptoms). Patches of hair may fall out. An infectious raised area may appear around the genitals and anus.

This is the most infectious stage of the disease. It can be spread by simple physical contact, including kissing, because bacteria are present in the open syphilitic sores on any part of the body. And this is also the stage in which syphilis imitates other diseases. Sometimes the symptoms are so mild that they go unnoticed. Again, the symptoms disappear, but the bacteria remain active in the body.

Latent. During this stage, which may last ten or twenty years, there are no outward signs. However, the bacteria may be invading inner organs, including the heart and brain. In the first few years of the latent stage the disease may still be infectious, but after that it usually isn't.

Late. In this stage the serious effects of the latent stage appear. Depending on which organs the bacteria have attacked, a person may develop serious heart disease, crippling, blindness, or mental incapacity. Out of every hundred untreated syphilitics twenty-three people will be killed or incapacitated in this late stage of the disease.

Diagnosis of Syphilis

Syphilis can be diagnosed and treated at any time. Early in the primary stages a doctor can look for subtle secondary symptoms (like swollen lymph glands around the groin), or analyze some of the pus from the chancre if one has developed. Very soon after (usually within a week or two after the chancre has formed, though it may take longer), the spirochetes will be in the bloodstream, and they will show up in a blood test. From then on, through all the stages, a blood test will reveal the infection. It is usually best to have at least two blood tests several weeks apart, even if the first one is negative, because sometimes mistakes happen. The syphilis blood test is often given when a person is tested for gonorrhea, and just as a check in many situations, as for marriage. However, it could be used a lot more than it is now.

Treatment and Test for Cure of Syphilis

The treatment for syphilis is penicillin or another antibiotic like tetracycline for those allergic to penicillin. It may be one high dose or a series of smaller doses for a short period of time. It's just that simple. Again, it's important to have at least two follow-up blood tests as checks to be sure the treatment has been complete, since sometimes people have relapses. But the main thing to remember is that the first three stages of syphilis can be completely cured, and that even in late syphilis the destructive effects can be stopped from going any further.

Syphilis and Pregnancy

If a pregnant woman has syphilis, she can pass the bacteria on to her unborn baby. The bacteria attack the fetus just as they do an adult, and the child may be born dead or with important tissues deformed or diseased. But if the mother's syphilis is treated before the eighteenth week of pregnancy, the fetus will probably not be infected at all. (Even after the fetus has gotten syphilis, penicillin shots will stop the disease, but cannot repair damage that has already been done.) Therefore it is very important that every pregnant woman get a blood test for syphilis as soon as she knows she is pregnant. Thus, if she has the disease, she can be treated for it before she gives it to her child. She should have the test repeated during pregnancy whenever she thinks she may have been re-exposed to syphilis.

GONORRHEA

Gonorrhea is caused by a bacterium shaped like a coffee bean, called a gonococcus, which works its way gradually along the passageways of the genital organs. This disease can be transmitted to another person at all stages. Unlike syphilis, which can go all through the body, gonorrhea is essentially a disease of the genitourinary organs. It can also travel through the bloodstream and cause infection in the valves of the heart, acute arthritis, meningitis, blindness, or even death. In women the disease is more likely to persist and spread than in men, because the cervix becomes inflamed and the endocervical glands drain poorly, not allowing the bacteria and pus to be passed out of the body.

Your method of birth control may affect how easily you can catch gonorrhea and how easily you can get rid of it. Since the pill usually makes the vagina more alkaline than normal, a more favorable environment for the bacteria is created, increasing to almost 100 percent the possibility of a successful infection. The environment created by the pill also seems to help the spread of gonorrhea into the fallopian tubes, even as soon as two or three weeks after infection. An intrauterine device (IUD) seems to serve as a focus of the infection, making the disease more difficult to treat. If the infection does not respond to treatment, the IUD is often removed during treatment, and then reinserted when treatment has been successful. (Also, see "Prevention," above.)

Symptoms of Gonorrhea

Gonorrhea is often asymptomatic (without symptoms) in women. A recent study of women receiving regular pelvic examinations showed that 80 percent of the women found to have gonorrhea were asymptomatic carriers.* Since the cervix and vagina are basically sensitive only to pressure, the infection is not felt. The minority of women who do develop symptoms do so anywhere from two days to three weeks after exposure. They develop a vaginal discharge or have painful urination or both. Often women attribute these symptoms to other routine gynecological problems or to the use of birth-control methods, such as the pill. As the disease spreads

*Lawrence K. Altman, "Gonorrhea Tests Urged for Women," *New York Times*, December 20, 1971, p. 19.

up the uterus and fallopian tubes, a woman may start to have severe pain on one or both sides of her lower abdomen. She may also have vomiting and fever. If a woman has a mild case of gonorrhea, she may feel the same symptoms in much milder form over several months. Her menstrual periods may become irregular. These symptoms should not be ignored since they may indicate one of the most severe complications resulting from untreated gonorrhea—salpingitis. This is scarring and infection of the fallopian tubes. Repeated episodes can result in pelvic inflammatory disease and sterility. Remember that gonorrhea can also be spread from a man's penis to a woman's throat, infecting her tonsils and giving her a chronic sore throat. The rectum and anus may also be irritated.

While the symptoms in a man (see chart at end of chapter) are usually disturbing enough for him to seek medical attention,* a woman usually remains ignorant of her infection until she is alerted by an infected male with whom she has had sexual relations, or is traced by a public health service case-finder as a named sex contact, or until her own infection has spread, causing sufficient pain to prompt her to see a doctor.

Testing and Diagnosis of Gonorrhea

In detecting gonorrhea the slide tests for men are accurate, while for women they are not. There are two types of tests for gonorrhea that are currently used: the gram stain and the culture. In the gram-stain test a smear of the discharge is placed on a slide, stained with a special dye, and examined for gonorrhea bacteria under a microscope. This method, though 99 percent reliable for men, is highly unreliable for women. Other organisms can easily mask the gonococcal bacteria. Although it is still the only method used in many places, it should not be used without the second test—the culture test. The culture test also involves taking a smear of the discharge. But before it is examined it is inoculated on a special culture plate and incubated under special laboratory conditions for several days in an attempt to let the gonorrhea bacteria (if there are any) multiply. This allows the bacteria to be detected more easily. A modified culture test (Clinicult) is now also available for doctors or other testers who don't have ready access to a laboratory.

It is important to emphasize that even the culture test can be inaccurate for both men and women. Accuracy depends greatly on which sites are chosen to take the culture from. Ideally, the four sites most commonly infected in a woman—the cervix, urethra, vagina, and rectum—should be cultured, but rarely is this feasible. If a

*There has been an alarming recent increase in the number of asymptomatic males, that is, men who have gonorrhea without feeling any symptoms. The rate is probably about 5 percent of those infected.

single site is chosen for culture, the cervix should be selected, since a single cervical culture will detect approximately 82 percent of infected women. Studies have indicated that about 50 percent of infected women show an infection in the anal canal. Therefore, to maximize the chances of detecting gonorrhea in women, a culture specimen should be obtained from both the cervix and rectum or urethra. Even if sites are cultured, however, 6–9 percent of infected women may not be diagnosed at any one visit.[*] One explanation for the insensitivity of the culture method is that the gonococcus organism often dies en route from the clinic or doctor's office to the laboratory, thereby resulting in a false negative result for a woman who is in fact infected. This contributes to the unreliability of the test. There is some evidence that there is a greater chance of detecting gonorrhea during menstruation.

Treatment for Gonorrhea

The normal treatment for gonorrhea is high-dosage injections of penicillin. Syphilis treatment is a lower dose over a longer period of time. Other antibiotics such as tetracycline are available if a person cannot take penicillin. However, treatment is not as easy as it sounds. Because gonorrhea bacteria have the ability to build up resistance to penicillin, strains of gonorrhea have developed which require higher dosages of penicillin treatment. There are currently at least two thousand such resistant strains known.[†] One way they seem to develop is when a low dosage of antibiotics is taken for protection against the disease. This happened in South Vietnam when women, forced to earn a living through prostitution, tried to protect themselves. A low dosage may not be strong enough to kill the gonococcal bacteria, but it provides an environment in which the bacteria can adapt to varying levels of the antibiotic. Taking the treatment for gonorrhea in full at the prescribed time intervals maintains a high enough level of antibiotic in the bloodstream to prevent resistant strains from developing. The dosages required, however, are still far lower than those commonly used for several other kinds of infection.

As a result of the development of resistant strains, the Public Health Service has increased its recommended dose of penicillin four times in the past ten years, with the dose for women now at the maximum injectable amount at one time (4.8 million units) and the dose for men at half that. Some recommend a dose of 6 million units for women.[‡] Recently a gonorrhea-specific antibiotic, spectinomycin (generic name), or Trobisin (brand name), has been developed. It is normally used only against strains that are difficult to treat, since it is much more expensive than penicillin and thus less readily available. Another method uses oral probenecid, which retards urinary excretion of penicillin and thus maintains the high level of penicillin in the bloodstream for a long enough period of time to accomplish a cure. This does not minimize the problem of diagnosing gonorrhea in women and developing a test that tells a woman when she has been cured, nor does it minimize the danger of taking such high-potency drugs.

Test for Cure of Gonorrhea

It is important that every woman treated for gonorrhea have at least two negative culture tests before being considered cured. (The culture test, as mentioned before, is not always totally accurate or reliable.) Retreatment with double the initial dosage of penicillin or another drug is indicated if follow-up cultures remain positive. Because the average doctor lacks the complicated laboratory facilities for diagnosing VD, he often treats patients who suspect an infection without making a laboratory diagnosis. Such a procedure is particularly unsafe for women who must rely on laboratory tests for assurance of cure and also because of the danger of taking high dosages of penicillin or other antibiotics. The need for a mass screening blood test for the diagnosis of gonorrhea, particularly in women, is more than obvious.

The diagnosis and cure of gonorrhea in women thus becomes largely hit or miss, depending on the type of laboratory facilities at the disposal of her doctor, the thoroughness of the examination, the condition of the culture—all factors considerably beyond her control. The unreliability of present diagnostic devices is but another impediment to any successful control of gonorrhea in this country. What is more important for the individual woman, however, is the fact that unreliable tests for gonorrhea mean the disease can go undiagnosed and therefore untreated until serious damage is done.

Pregnancy and Gonorrhea

A pregnant woman with untreated gonorrhea can infect her baby with the disease as it passes through the birth canal. In past years many babies were born blind because of gonococcal conjunctivitis. All states now require the eyes of newborns to be treated with silver nitrate or penicillin drops in order to cure this disease if it is present. Unless there has been severe damage to the cornea, treatment of the infected newborn's eyes can usually prevent permanent visual damage. What is particularly disturbing, however, is the reported rise in cases of gonococcal conjunctivitis over the past ten years.[*] The increase is attributed to the increasing prevalence

---

[*]Health Organizing Collective, "Venereal Disease," p. 3.

[†]A. J. Dazall-Ward, "Venereal Diseases: New Problems for the Physician and the Community," *Disease-a-Month* (January 1971), p. 22 (Chicago, Year Book Medical Publishers, Inc.).

[‡]"Gonorrhea—Treatment in the Female," ACOG Technical Bulletin, No. 6 (February 1972) (American College of Obstetricians and Gynecologists, 79 West Monroe Street, Chicago, Ill. 60603).

[*]Health Organizing Collective, "Venereal Disease," p. 4.

OTHER VENEREAL DISEASES

Other diseases besides syphilis and gonorrhea are transmitted by sexual contact. These, however, comprise only about 1 percent of the total amount of VD. One of the more common of these is herpes simplex, type II. This virus, which causes blisters on the genitals, is similar to the virus that causes cold sores. There is no known cure for this disease, but it is worth checking to make sure it is not anything else. Another disease, condyloma acuminatum, is caused by a wart virus. It produces lesions of the sexual organs, often looking like cancer. The response of this disease to treatment is capricious, and recurrence is common. Other venereal diseases less frequently seen in this country include chancroid, granuloma inguinale, and lymphogranuloma venereum. These can all be treated.

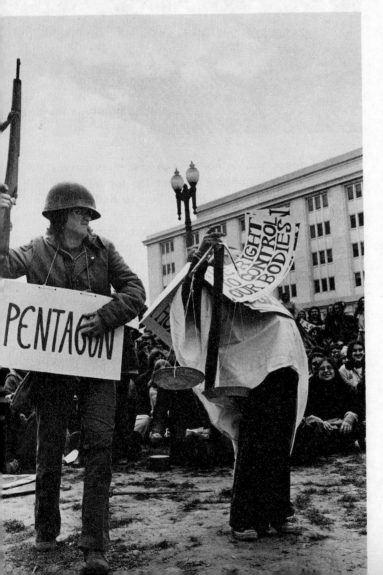

THE POLITICS OF VENEREAL DISEASE

If we look carefully at the history of venereal disease, we find that it seems to be tied to times and places in which rape and prostitution are very common. During times of wars and invasions many men are sent to foreign countries, where they don't have to worry about the laws or social pressure they would feel back home. Outright rape becomes a common occurrence and prostitution begins to grow. Syphilis was initially taken to China by white explorers from Europe. The first big epidemic in Europe was spread from Italy, where the French and Italian soldiers were fighting a long-drawn-out war and raping the local women. In South Vietnam in recent years the U.S. troops have nearly destroyed all normal life and work. Prostitution flourishes where troops are stationed because there are so many women and children with no other means of support. In fact, one nearly penicillin-resistant strain of gonorrhea that originated in Vietnam has been called "Vietnam Rose" by doctors in this country. Perhaps a better name would be "American Invader."

The PHS is charged with the control program for VD in the United States. This involves testing for VD and follow-up investigations to locate sex partners and others whom a person might have infected. In half the states the law requires that positive results of lab tests for VD be sent to the health commissioner, who must then get in touch with the tested person's doctor or clinic to determine if the disease actually exists. Many private doctors, however, do not report VD cases to the PHS for follow-up even though this means they may be endangering the lives of the contacts under the guise of saving their patients from embarrassment. Considering the techniques and general attitude of the PHS, this is understandable. Their methods of probing are not always purely medical, but often have moral overtones. A lot of the people who are supposedly helping to stamp out VD are really much more interested in stamping out "illegal" sex. However, laws are changing. In almost every state now minors can be treated without parental knowledge. Still, private doctors sometimes send the bill to the patient's parents if not told otherwise.

In 1969, of a total of almost $12 million of federal funds appropriated by Congress for the entire PHS VD-control program, little more than $500,000 was reserved for the new gonorrhea-control program. These token federal funds were channeled into special studies in gonorrhea control that concentrated, not on research, but on improving the traditional case-finding and treatment method, which had already proved to be a very limited and ineffective approach to the control of gonorrhea. The gross inadequacy of federal funds allocated in this area over the past years is partly responsible for the unmanageability of gonorrhea in this country.

Up to now gonorrhea has not been treated as a dangerous epidemic because its severest consequences were found mostly in poor (black, brown, and white) communities where there is still no adequate health care available. Sterility from gonorrhea is a type of population control that whites tolerate for Third World people. No one in authority was ready to put money into researching and eliminating a disease that most severely affected the poor, whatever their color. But the extent of the epidemic is beginning to make legislators grudgingly acknowledge that larger research and treatment programs are essential. Nevertheless, only a little over $30 million was appropriated for 1972.

Whereas vaccines have been developed for polio, measles, and other infectious diseases, there is no preventive vaccine yet for any venereal disease. A simple screening test for gonorrhea is being worked on by the Federal Venereal Disease Program (Center for Disease Control) in Atlanta, Georgia, but effective tests are not expected for at least a year. There is no other major research facility for venereal disease in the country.

A number of clinics have made the blood test for syphilis a routine part of an ob-gyn examination for some time, and many are just starting to give gonorrhea tests routinely, with some government encouragement. Even so, there is a shortage of VD clinics.

VD tests and thorough, readable, educational information should be part of every family-planning clinic and health facility and educational facility. Educational programs with follow-up treatment can work. In China a nationwide campaign, reaching even remote villages, has educated the people to the symptoms of both diseases and the importance of curing them. The campaign to educate and to treat people was so successful that the teaching hospitals in Peking have difficulty in finding cases to show students.*

PROTECT YOURSELF—PROTECT OTHERS

If you notice any symptoms of VD in yourself, no matter how mild, you should go to a doctor or a clinic at once. (Turn to the last section of this chapter for a concise checklist of VD symptoms.) Don't panic or feel guilty or embarrassed. Clinics and state departments of communicable diseases (VD division) can be helpful for answering questions over the phone. In many places there are clinics to which you can go for free treatment and tests, or you can go to a private doctor if you have the money (probably $20–$30). In forty-eight states, if

*China! Inside the People's Republic, Committee of Concerned Asian Scholars, Bantam (New York, 1972), pp. 55–59.

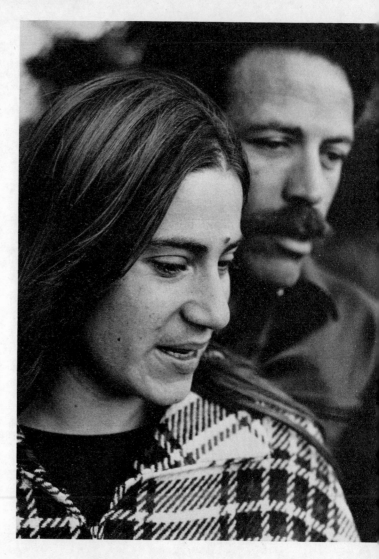

you are a minor, you do not have to have your parents' permission to be examined and treated for VD. (See above, "Treatment—General," for how to find a good place for testing and treatment.)

If you have sexual relations with someone, try to find out if there is any chance that your partner has VD or has been exposed to VD recently. Don't be embarrassed to ask. If two people care about each other they should certainly be looking out for each other's health.

If you find out you have VD, don't have sexual relations with anyone until you are well. If you had intercourse with someone when you had VD but didn't know it, you should tell that person right away so that he or she can get treatment. It is especially important in such cases for men to tell women that they might be infected with gonorrhea, because the woman probably wouldn't notice any symptoms in herself until the disease has already done a lot of damage.

Don't depend on one test only. If the first test for gonorrhea or syphilis doesn't show anything, make sure the doctor takes another one to be safe. Women should make sure the doctor takes smears from at least the cervix and the anus or urethra. Don't just accept whatever he says. Some doctors aren't careful enough—and it's your life, not his.

Since it is so difficult for a woman to tell if she has VD (especially gonorrhea), she should be routinely tested for it during general physical exams and gynecological examinations. Even if you are sure that you have had no contact with someone infected with VD, you may be saving other women's lives by demanding that your doctor routinely give you and every other woman tests for VD without attached moral judgment.

	GONORRHEA	SYPHILIS
Causative Agent:	*Neisseria gonorrhoeae*	*Treponema pallidum*
Mode of Spread:	Sexual intercourse Oral or anal contact In the birth canal Accidental infection of eyes from discharge	Sexual intercourse Oral or anal contact Through the placenta
Incubation Period:	1–14 days	9–90 days
Symptoms:	*Male:* Painful urination Urethral discharge Frequent urination Anal infection—often no symptoms *Female:* Often no symptoms Increased discharge Frequent urination, with late symptoms of fever, chills, pain, and abdominal cramps Sore throat after fellatio	*Primary:* Chancre (painless sore) *Secondary:* Rash Flu-like syndrome Mouth sores Patchy balding Eye inflammation *Latent:* No symptoms *Late:* Heart disease Deafness Muscle incoordination Blindness Insanity Paralysis Death
Diagnosis:	*Male:* History of exposure Microscopic examination of discharge with isolation of organism *Female:* History of exposure Culture with isolation of organism	History of exposure Examination of fluid from chancre, or Blood tests (after early primary stage) Lumbar puncture
Treatment:	Penicillin substitute Penicillin substitute Spectinomycin (Trobisin)	Penicillin Penicillin substitute
Slang:	Clap, morning drop, the whites, a dose, pox, lucs, siff, Old Joe, strain, gleet	

IMPORTANT INFORMATION ABOUT PENICILLIN TREATMENT

Whenever you get penicillin treatment for any disease, don't drink alcoholic beverages for forty-eight hours. They reduce the effectiveness of penicillin.

If you are allergic to penicillin, ask the doctor to use another antibiotic, such as tetracycline. Tetracycline, however, can cause tooth discoloration in a child if it is used during the second half of pregnancy. You may develop an allergy to penicillin when you are treated, since you are receiving such a large dose at one time. If you have any unusual symptoms after the treatment, especially if your throat or face begins to swell, return immediately to the doctor or clinic. The reaction can be fatal unless treated quickly. You also have a one in 3,000–4,000 chance of having a "bad trip" for twenty to thirty minutes from procaine penicillin (not other kinds). If this happens you become agitated and excited and resist efforts to restrain you.*

*ACOG Bulletin No. 6.

FURTHER READINGS

Brecher, Edward. As yet unpublished work by author of *An Analysis of Human Sexual Response.* Emphasizes prevention.

Grover, John W., with Dick Grace. *The ABC's of VD.* Englewood Cliffs, N.J.: Prentice-Hall, 1971.
  Chatty, comprehensive, positive. Only a few minor slips into moralism. Skip the Foreword.

Massachusetts State Public Health Department, Venereal Disease Division.
  Much information was learned from or checked with people in Massachusetts for accuracy. Very open and helpful. Your own state VD department is probably also a good place to contact for information. VD clinics (sometimes part of other clinics) are good information sources.

U.S. Department of Health, Education and Welfare, Public Health Service, Communicable Disease Center, Venereal Disease Branch, Atlanta, Ga.
  This group has some publications, including a medically comprehensive book, *Syphilis: A Synopsis.* Contact HEW in Atlanta for the book.

VD Handbook, by the Birth Control Handbook/VD Handbook Collective. Excellent. For single copies, send 25¢ for mailing and handling costs to The Collective, P.O. Box 1000, Station G, Montreal 130, Quebec, Canada.

Venereal Disease. Health Organizing Collective of New York Women's Health and Abortion Project, 36 W. 22 Street, New York, N.Y. 10010.
  Important VD facts for women and the political context of difficulties in treating it. This group puts out a small series of women's health pamphlets for 10 cents each.

10
Birth Control

INTRODUCTION

LET'S SAY YOU want to have sexual relations with a man and you don't want a baby right now—or maybe ever. You want to be able to enjoy sex without worrying about pregnancy. You don't want to have to spend anxious days every month waiting for your period. For most women it is easy to get pregnant: each month for over thirty years your body gets ready carefully and in detail for you to get pregnant. A man has 300 million or more sperm on call at any moment. But you are the one who gets pregnant, not he. You need birth control—good birth control: an effective, safe, cheap, and easily available method of avoiding pregnancy. In 1973 there are some good birth-control methods to use. But they are not perfectly effective, they are not always available, and they tend to put the burden of choice, acquisition, use, maintenance, and risk on the woman instead of on the man and the woman together.

As we each try to find and to obtain a birth-control method that is good for us, we may run up against one or more of the obstacles that exist in our society: repressive laws in some states; antisex attitudes in churches, schools, and families; poor publicity about sources of birth-control care; misleading or inadequate information from profit-oriented drug companies—and even from doctors; difficulty in getting back-up abortions when a birth-control method fails; or, simply but critically, the high cost of medical examinations and contraceptive ("against conception") materials, such as pills or jellies. We must work hard politically to get rid of every one of these obstacles, for they assault and endanger the right of women to decide whether and when we will have children.

But even now most people who are willing to persist can get some kind of birth control. (See the list of organizations on p. 137 for help if you have trouble getting birth control in your community.) However, as we try to

separate sex from pregnancy, we can run into another set of obstacles that is more personal and at times just as difficult—the attitudes of our boyfriends or husbands, and attitudes we ourselves hold about birth control and sex. This introduction will try to prepare you to use the sections on birth-control methods with an understanding of both the external ways in which our society may make it hard for you to get birth control and the internal attitudes that may influence you and make it hard for you to make a reasonable and realistic choice.

Birth-Control Information and Sex Information

Particularly for young and single people, such information is restricted in this country by the influence of a strongly antisex morality that has roots not only in the Catholic Church but also in many other conservative American churches and in the puritanical shame about sex that has a hold on so many of us. In some places these attitudes still have a hold on public policy. Until the March 1972 Supreme Court decision on the Bill Baird case it was illegal in Massachusetts to prescribe or sell birth control to single women. In some places birth control cannot be publicized; in some states teen-agers cannot yet get medical birth-control care without parental permission. There is rarely a clear and positive public policy of spreading information and free contraceptives to all who want them, including young people. The only places where we consistently see assertive birth-control programs are ghetto areas. This is a touchy thing, for while poor women do want to be able to control their pregnancies, it is hard to accept elaborate birth-control programs for the poor when women, men, and children have so many unmet needs for basic health care—for childbirth, for control of disease, for preventive care.*

*For more on this important issue see Toni Cade's anthology, *Black Woman* (New York: Signet, 1970).

Medical Institutions and Birth Control

Drug companies, doctors, and clinics have a lot of control over our choice and acquisition of birth-control methods. See the "Women and Health Care" chapter of this book for a more general critique of the American health-care system.

Much of the available information about effectiveness, safety, possibility of side effects, and reversibility of the different contraceptives is researched and published by the drug companies, who are interested primarily in sales. The prescription task force of the Department of Health, Education and Welfare estimated that in 1968 the drug companies spent $4,500 per physician per year on advertising and promotion of all drugs.* Each company quotes the highest possible effectiveness rate for its product. IUD (intrauterine device) salesman say, "Just put it in and you'll never have to worry about pregnancy again"—a slight exaggeration considering the 2–4 percent failure rate. The companies have tended to be irresponsible about side effects. The 1970 Senate hearings on the pill revealed that the drug companies had sought little feedback from doctors or pill takers about side effects and complications. Until the FDA (Food and Drug Administration) cracked down and demanded that the patient be told more specifics, the flower-covered patient pamphlets tended to leave out known side effects and to gloss over known risks. There is great need for independent research on birth-control methods: It has been shown that many of the "independent" studies so favorable to the pill have been done by scientists and doctors actually financed by drug company grants.† So we have to be careful where we get our information.

What about the doctors? Most of us, unable to get enough trustworthy information about birth control, have depended on our doctors to choose what's best for us. But our doctors themselves often do not or cannot learn all they should. Much of the information they get is from the drug companies or from magazines partly financed by drug company advertisements. And what the doctors do know, they often do not take the time or the trouble to pass on. Doctors are trained to treat us as patients, not people; they give us reassurance rather than the information we need. They assume we don't want to know (and many women in the past have not wanted to know), or they scoff at our ability to handle the information. An eminent Boston gynecologist, witness for G. D. Searle (the major birth-control pill manu-

facturer), said at the 1970 congressional pill hearings that he didn't tell his patients of all the potential risks and side effects of the pill because, "Well, if you tell them they might get headaches, they will get headaches."*

Some doctors let themselves get overly busy, others are just plain irresponsible. These doctors will put a woman on pills without carefully examining her, will put in an IUD without explaining that it has a failure rate, or will send a woman home with a diaphragm without letting her practice putting it in so that she'll know what it feels like when it is in right. Many don't arrange to have nurses or paramedical counselors fill in what they themselves neglect to say. This kind of sloppy care can be given both in private offices and in clinics, where the crowd and bustle can make it extra hard for a woman to ask all the questions she needs to ask. (Planned Parenthood and some other clinics are more careful.)

What to do? It seems that women all over the country are walking out of doctors' offices and clinics with methods of birth control that they have not really thought about or clearly chosen and that they are not absolutely sure how to use. No wonder so many of us get pregnant when we don't want to, even though we are supposedly practicing birth control.

We must learn for ourselves and teach each other about every available method of birth control. We have to know enough to recognize when a doctor is not examining enough or explaining enough or demonstrating enough. When we are at doctors' offices or at clinics we have to be responsible enough to ourselves to ask questions and make sure that they are answered. We can't take the place of doctors, but we have to demand to know what is pertinent to our health and safety.

Where to look for the information we need to have? This chapter and some of the books recommended in the bibliography (especially the McGill booklet) try to give an impartial and honest view of the available methods of birth control. Medical journals sometimes print reports on failure rates, side effects, and other relevant factors. The British government's Committee on Safety of Drugs has run a careful study on estrogen levels in birth-control pills (see p. 117), and we can learn from them things that our Food and Drug Administration does not have time or money to go into. We can get some limited guidelines from the FDA. (See the IUD section for a recent FDA decision on the Copper-T device.) A most valuable source of information is our friends. In the past, women have been embarrassed about birth control and have spoken of it only in whispers, spreading scary stories about Cousin Sally's gory side

*Health-Pac *Bulletin* (March 1970) p. 12. (Published by the Health Policy Advisory Center, Inc., 17 Murray Street, New York, N. Y., 10007.)
†*Loc. cit.*

Loc. cit.

effects. But by speaking openly and by carefully comparing experiences and knowledge, we women can learn a great deal to guide us in our own choice of birth-control methods, and we can also support each other in forcing laws, doctors, clinics, and drug companies to make vital changes in practice and attitudes.

Abortion and Birth Control

The need for abortions will stop when birth-control methods are improved and made universally available. Until then, however, *we must have abortion as a back-up measure for women whose birth-control methods fail.* Few doctors recognize their responsibility to terminate a pregnancy that results from an IUD failure or from the accidental slipping of a properly used diaphragm. This situation makes many of us keep taking pills longer than we really want to.

Men and Birth Control

One of the most important influences on the way we practice birth control is the attitude of the men we sleep with. Ideally, if two people want to have sex, they are close enough to each other to be able to avoid misunderstandings or bad feelings about birth control. This isn't always true, primarily because—despite the fact that it takes a man and a woman to make a baby—today the prevention is mostly up to the woman. One reason is that we women have a more personal interest in preventing pregnancy than men do, for we bear the children, and in this society we are in large measure responsible for raising them. Second, today's most effective birth-control methods are for women to use; condoms, withdrawal, and rhythm, methods that depend on the man or on the man and woman together, do not work nearly as well as the pill, the IUD, or the diaphragm.* And research on male contraceptives goes slowly, in part, we suspect, because men like leaving it to us. (See "Future Methods," p. 136.)

Total responsibility for birth control, which today falls on the woman, is a burden in many ways. We must make the arrangements, see a doctor, get examined, go to the drugstore, and usually pay for the supplies. With the pill or the IUD, it is our bodies that feel the side effects, and, more seriously, our bodies that take what-

---

*Ironically, the burden of total responsibility for birth control is a recent one. For the centuries before the invention of the diaphragm in 1882, women had to depend on men (condoms, withdrawal) to keep them from getting pregnant (and on crude abortion and infanticide as frequently needed back-up methods). The diaphragm was a breakthrough because it was an effective method that women could use. With the diaphragm a woman was more in control of her body than she had ever been before.

ever risks are involved. The way most couples use the diaphragm the woman must not only be sure to have the diaphragm and enough cream or jelly right at hand but she must also disappear into the bathroom and put it in by herself. When we ask a man to use a rubber as even only a temporary alternative, he often resists: condoms are a drag, he tells us—he can't feel intercourse fully with a condom on. Total responsibility for birth control reinforces limiting stereotypes of male and female sexual response: not worrying as much about pregnancy, a man can relax and enjoy sex at times when the woman is too anxious to let go. Total responsibility means that if we don't have some kind of birth control and we are pressed to have intercourse, it is up to us to say no; it means that if we have sex without birth control it is our fault if we get pregnant.

Many couples do not even talk much about birth control. The man assumes the woman has taken care of everything, the woman protects herself as best she can (perhaps resenting this situation and repressing her anger), they have intercourse, and she hopes she won't get pregnant. No matter how good the sex is between them, his unwillingness to share in the prevention of pregnancy lurks in the back of her mind, particularly if there are other inequalities in their relationship. She can't help but wonder: If he thinks birth control is my business, what will he think if my birth-control method fails and I get pregnant? If he decides that pregnancy is my business too, then he is free to leave or to withdraw from me emotionally. The birth-control issue, then, highlights a central aspect of our vulnerability—our dependence on men not to let us down.

A reasonable and supportive man who feels that he naturally shares in the responsibility for avoiding pregnancy can make the burdens of birth control a lot lighter. When there is no good birth control available, he can control his desire for intercourse in the same way that you control yours; he can explore other kinds of sex play with you. He can use condoms some of the time. He can get a vasectomy (see p. 136) if you are a long-term couple wanting no or no more children. He can overcome his feeling that creams are gooey and repulsive and help put in the diaphragm, making it an enjoyable task. He can help pay for supplies. Even when you are using pills or an IUD, he can appreciate that you are running risks for your and his mutual pleasure; he can talk with you about your side effects instead of assuming they are your problem. It's his attitude that counts: it all comes down to whether he thinks preventing pregnancy is your job or his to share. If he shares it, then you're not alone. If he doesn't, you are more likely to get pregnant —without support, you are less likely to carry through with some kind of birth control and use it well.

Women and Birth Control

Many of us have found that some of the most stubborn obstacles to our use of birth control come from inside ourselves. For some of us Catholicism, and for many others the lurking puritanism in our culture, have made us grow up ashamed of our sexuality. To obtain birth control is to admit that we are going to have sexual relations with a man. If we feel ambivalent about whether having sex is right or wrong, particularly if we are young and unmarried and going against the premarital sex taboo, it is hard to admit even to ourselves that we are doing it. So our tendency is to let sex happen in passion or in "love," but not to premeditate it, not to learn in advance what we need to do to prevent pregnancy.

Some of us are also too romantic about sex to use birth control very well. Romance about sex is probably a way we have of dealing with our ambivalence as to whether sex is good or bad: sex is beautiful, sex is spontaneous and uncontrollable, sex is spiritual, sex is anything but two bodies fertile with egg and sperm wanting to get together and make babies. So when we get into making love with someone, it seems somehow too clinical and unromantic to talk about pills, creams, condoms, applicators, fertile days, and so on. Drugstores require no doctor's prescription to sell us a virtually 100 percent effective method of birth control—foam for the woman and condoms for the man, which, if used together, protect us almost perfectly. But for some reason, even when we know about foam and condoms, we have a hard time interrupting a romantic and instinctive sexual flow to get up and go to buy them or, once they've been bought, to get them out and use them. It is hard to know how to deal with this. We need a great deal of common sense, self-control, mutual support—and we don't always have them.

Another attitude that keeps us from using birth control every time, or using the method that is best for us, is one of reluctance to inconvenience the man. If you are just starting to sleep with him, you hesitate to suggest that you postpone making love until you are using some kind of protection, for fear that he might decide not to sleep with you at all. You don't want to turn him off by suggesting that he use a rubber. If it is a long-term relationship, in which you are using anything but pills or an IUD, you are apologetic about the interruption to insert foam or diaphragm, or you shy away from insisting that he use a condom some of the time. One woman told us that shortly after marriage she learned that her husband was putting the condom on too late in intercourse to be perfectly safe, but for several months she used extra birth-control foam rather than insist to him that he was doing it wrong. Maybe anticipation of these

problems makes you keep taking pills beyond the time you wanted to stop. Many women trying to practice the rhythm method have a hard time saying no during their fertile times because they are afraid their men will get angry or will seek satisfaction somewhere else. This fear of displeasing the man is a measure of the inequality in our relationship with him. It runs deep in many of us; it keeps us from asking for the kind of touching or timing we need in sex; and it keeps us from imposing our need to use birth control every time, and the need to use a method that pleases us as well as it pleases him.

There's another reason why we don't always use birth control when we should—that familiar and human self-delusion, the feeling that "it won't happen to me." If we have never been pregnant, or if all our pregnancies have been planned ones, it is somehow hard to connect with the fact that we might get caught. For many of us our sex education has been so poor that we don't have a really clear idea of how pregnancy happens anyway. The egg and the sperm are not a reality to us. There is also the sense of playing a game with our bodies, seeing how far we can go before that persistent natural reproductive process catches up with us. There is also, for someone who has never been pregnant, an unconscious curiosity as to whether she can get pregnant at all, a need to prove to herself that she is not sterile.

There are many other psychological and even pathological reasons why some of us get pregnant even in situations in which birth control is fairly easily available. The point of mentioning some of these reasons here is that if you are having sexual relations with a man and you are not using a good means of birth control, you should try to understand why and do what you can about it—or else you may get pregnant when you don't want to. Sometimes the reasons are external, in society; but sometimes they are internal, caused by society's attitudes, but internalized and accepted by ourselves. We must reject our society's puritan attitudes and believe that what we are doing is right, that our sexuality is a valuable part of us which we have every right to express, that we have a right to pleasurable and worry-free sex, that we are an equal partner in sex with needs that we are entitled to assert. Until we accept ourselves as healthily sexual, we will have trouble using birth control. And the external obstacles to obtaining birth control will continue to exist until sufficient numbers of us feel good enough about our sexuality to fight publicly for effective, safe, easily available methods for both men and women to use.

Birth Control and Sexual Availability

The near-perfect effectiveness of the pill and the IUD can bring increased pressure on a woman to have intercourse with any man who wants it, or to do it with her husband or long-term lover any time he wants to whether she wants to or not. We used to be able to say, "No, I can't, I might get pregnant." Now we have to be more honest and say, "No, I don't want to." This takes strength, and we don't all have it all the time. If both men and women can get used to saying "I don't want to this time" without being apologetic or scared, and if both men and women can get used to hearing this said without being threatened or feeling rejected, then sexual relations will probably be a lot better and more satisfying for both sexes.

CONCEPTION—THE PROCESS TO BE INTERRUPTED

Conception takes place when a sperm from the man's penis, ejaculated into the woman's vagina during sexual intercourse (or onto the lips of her vagina during sex play), swims with its millions of fellow sperm up her vagina, through the cervical opening, through her uterus, and up to the outer third of a fallopian tube, where it finds an egg and enters (fertilizes) it. The fertilized egg in 4–5 days travels down the fallopian tube to the uterus, where it looks for a good place to implant in the uterine lining. If it arrives at such a place, it becomes attached to the lining and starts to grow. Unless the woman has a miscarriage or an abortion, about nine months later she will give birth to a baby.

The egg: The chapter on "The Anatomy and Physiology of Reproduction and Sexuality" (pp. 12–22) describes the monthly cycle in which the egg ripens in and bursts out of the ovary, and in which the woman's uterus

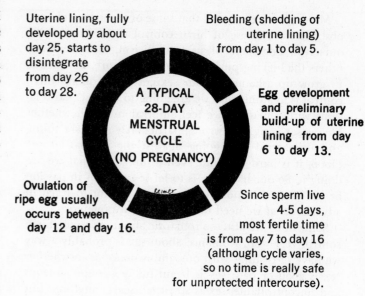

MONTHLY FERTILITY CYCLE

Uterine lining, fully developed by about day 25, starts to disintegrate from day 26 to day 28.

Bleeding (shedding of uterine lining) from day 1 to day 5.

A TYPICAL 28-DAY MENSTRUAL CYCLE (NO PREGNANCY)

Egg development and preliminary build-up of uterine lining from day 6 to day 13.

Ovulation of ripe egg usually occurs between day 12 and day 16.

Since sperm live 4-5 days, most fertile time is from day 7 to day 16 (although cycle varies, so no time is really safe for unprotected intercourse).

prepares a lining of nutritious tissue to feed a fertilized egg. The egg bursts out of the ovary at mid-cycle (halfway between menstrual periods—see "Rhythm," pp. 132–34) and can be fertilized for only about 12 to 24 hours.

The sperm: Here are a few important facts about sperm. For more information see *Conception, Birth and Contraception,* by Demarest and Sciarra, and *Boys and Sex,* by Wardell Pomeroy (New York: Dell, 1968).

Sperm are made in the man's testicles ("balls") and are stored in the epididymis.

Sexual stimulation makes blood pour into openings (cavernous tissue) inside the penis, causing the penis to get stiff, hard, erect. A few sperm can come out in the

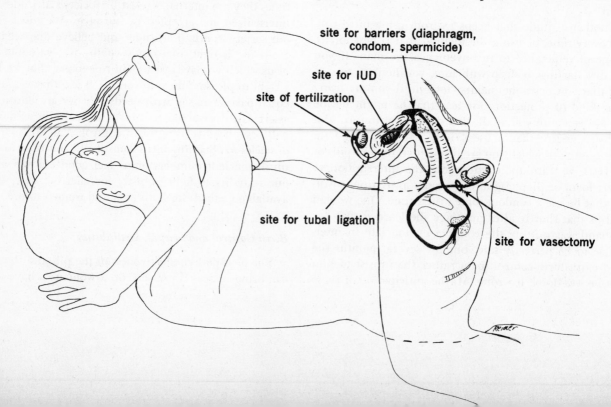

site for barriers (diaphragm, condom, spermicide)

site for IUD

site of fertilization

site for tubal ligation

site for vasectomy

drops of liquid that come from the penis soon after the erection occurs. Continued sexual stimulation usually makes the man have an orgasm. Just before orgasm the sperm travel up the vas deferens and wait in the seminal vesicles. At orgasm they pass into the prostate gland, where they are picked up by about a teaspoonful of seminal fluid and are propelled out of the urethra by rhythmic contractions which are very pleasurable to the man.

About 300–500 million sperm come out in one ejaculation. So many will die on the long hard trip up to the egg that this great number are needed for nature to be sure that reproduction will indeed go on.

Sperm come out fast, usually headed straight for the entrance to the cervical canal. They swim fast too—an inch in 8 minutes—so a sperm may reach an egg in an hour and a half.

The vagina is a hostile environment for sperm, so sperm in the vagina die in about 8 hours. But once sperm get to the uterus they can live for 4–5 days.

BIRTH-CONTROL PILLS

How They Work

To get a foundation for a clear understanding of how birth-control pills work, you should read the section on menstruation in the chapter on "The Anatomy and Physiology of Reproduction and Sexuality" (pp. 18–22) if you have not already done so. It describes what hormones are and how the menstrual hormones, estrogen and progesterone, guide a woman's monthly menstrual cycle. For a more detailed and complete description of the menstrual hormones, see the Appendix to that chapter, p. 21–22. Read the Appendix now if you want to, or wait until you have some time to concentrate on it. You can understand how the pills work without knowing the various parts of the menstrual cycle in as much detail as is given there.

The way the pills work to prevent pregnancy is outlined in simple form on the chart on p. 112. The chart puts the menstrual cycle and the pill cycle side by side. It shows how the pills interrupt your menstrual cycle by introducing synthetic versions of the menstrual hormones, estrogen and progesterone, at times different from those when they usually appear in your cycle.

Currently used birth-control pills prevent pregnancy primarily by inhibiting the development of the egg in the ovary. On the fifth day of your cycle (see chart), the low estrogen level usually triggers your pituitary gland to send out FSH, a hormonal message that starts an egg developing in one of your ovaries. The pill gives you just enough synthetic estrogen to raise your estrogen level high enough to keep that message from being sent. So, during a month when you are on the pill your ovaries remain inactive, and there is no egg to be fertilized by sperm. This is the same procedure by which a woman's body avoids unnecessary menstrual cycles when she is pregnant: the fetus puts estrogen into her blood, thereby inhibiting FSH. So in a way, using much lower levels

BIRTH-CONTROL PILLS. Middle sample is a 28-day pill.

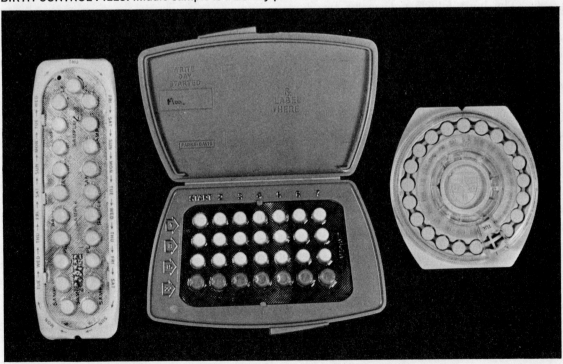

WOMAN'S MENSTRUAL CYCLE AND THE WAY THE 21-DAY BIRTH CONTROL PILL AFFECTS THAT CYCLE TO PREVENT PREGNANCY

Normal Menstrual Cycle	*With the Pill*
DAY 1. Menstrual period begins.	DAY 1. Menstrual period begins.
DAY 5. An egg in a follicle (pocket, sac) in one of your ovaries starts to ripen. The egg starts developing in response to a hormonal message (FSH) from your pituitary gland, which in turn has been triggered by the low level of *estrogen* (an ovarian hormone) at the time of your period.	DAY 5. Take your first pill. In the pill, you take two hormones every day: *estrogen* and *progesterone*. *Estrogen*: In the pill, you take more *estrogen* than there usually is in your body on Day 5—just enough to stop the usual message from your pituitary gland (FSH) for an egg to develop. By taking this amount of *estrogen* every day for 21 days, you avoid having an egg develop at all that month. Your ovaries remain inactive. There is no egg to be fertilized by sperm.
DAYS 5–14. The follicle in which the egg is developing makes first a little, then more and more *estrogen*: 1. *Estrogen* stimulates the lining of your uterus to get thicker in preparation for pregnancy. 2. As estrogen increases, it slows down and then cuts off FSH, the pituitary gland's message for an egg to develop (to avoid having more than one menstrual cycle at a time).	*Progesterone*: A little *progesterone* every day, instead of a lot from Days 14–26, provides two vital back-up effects: 1. Keeps plug of mucus in your cervix thick and dry, so sperm have a hard time getting through; 2. Keeps the lining of your uterus from developing properly so that if an egg does ripen (if *estrogen* level of pill is too low for you, or if you forget a pill) and a sperm does make it through the cervical mucus and fertilizes the egg, the fertilized egg will not be able to find a good place on the lining to implant.
DAY 14. Ovulation: *estrogen* reaches a high enough level to cut off the pituitary's egg development hormone (FSH) and to stimulate a hormone which triggers egg release (LH). Ripe egg bursts from ovary, starts 6½-day trip down fallopian tube to uterus. Fertilization by sperm from the man must occur in first 24 hours.	
DAYS 14–26. The burst follicle now makes two hormones for about 12 days: *Estrogen* continues. *Progesterone*, which reaches a peak about day 20: 1. makes plug of mucus in your cervix get thick and dry, a barrier to sperm; 2. stimulates the lining of your uterus to get very thick and to secrete a sugary substance which will feed a fertilized egg if pregnancy occurred this month.	
DAYS 26–27–28. If pregnancy did not occur, ovary's manufacture of estrogen and progesterone slows down to very low level. The lining of your uterus, which needs the stimulation and support of these hormones, starts to disintegrate.	DAY 26. Take your last pill. DAYS 27–28. Sudden drop in *estrogen* and *progesterone* makes the lining of your uterus start to disintegrate.
DAY 29–Day 1. Menstrual period begins. Low level of *estrogen* (see Day 26) will in a few days stimulate pituitary's egg development hormone (FSH) to start a new cycle.	DAY 29–Day 1. Menstrual period begins. Your period is lighter than normal, because of effect #2 of *progesterone* in the pill.

of estrogen, the pill simulates pregnancy, and some of the pill's side effects are like those of early pregnancy. If ovulation occurs, it is because you have been given too low a dose of estrogen in your pill to inhibit your own FSH level.

Synthetic progesterone is used differently in the two major kinds of pill. With the sequential pill you take pure estrogen for 15–16 days, then a combination of estrogen and progesterone for 5 days. This schedule is more like that of your regular menstrual hormones, but is less effective in preventing pregnancy because all it does is inhibit ovulation. The combination pill, described in the chart, combines estrogen and progesterone for the entire 20 or 21 days. The addition of progesterone every day provides two back-up effects: increased thickness of cervical mucus makes a barrier to sperm, and improper development of the uterine lining makes implantation impossible should ovulation and fertilization occur.

For purposes of birth control, then, *combination pills are best.* Combination pills are better also in regard to safety and side effects: they generally need to use less estrogen, and the estrogen they do contain is consistently counterbalanced by progesterone. (Estrogen has been linked to most of the major and many of the minor side effects of the pill.)

COMBINATION PILLS

Description

Small pills that are taken for 20 or 21 days each month. Synthetic estrogen and progesterone are combined in each pill. You take one pill each day. During the days that you are not taking pills your period usually comes. The 28-day pill is a combination pill for women who have trouble remembering an on-and-off pill regimen, and would do better taking a pill each day. Twenty-one pills contain hormones, seven are placebos.

Effectiveness

The combined-agent pills have a 0.5 percent pregnancy rate. Pregnancy can occur if you forget to take your pill for two or more days, if you try to juggle your pill schedule, if you don't use a back-up method of birth control for your first packet of pills, and occasionally when you change from one brand of pill to another (if you change to avoid side effects, use another method for one month to be safe).

EFFECTIVENESS OF BIRTH-CONTROL METHODS

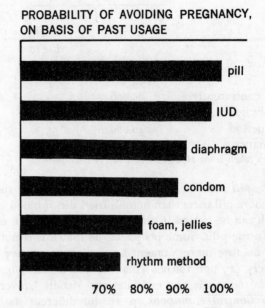

PROBABILITY OF AVOIDING PREGNANCY, ON BASIS OF PAST USAGE

- pill
- IUD
- diaphragm
- condom
- foam, jellies
- rhythm method

70% 80% 90% 100%

Reversibility

If you want to become pregnant, stop taking pills at the end of a packet. Your ovaries have been inactive while you were on the pill, and it may be a few months before they start functioning regularly again. Your first nonpill periods, for instance, will probably be a week or two late. But if you ovulated regularly before taking the pill, you will probably start ovulating again, and 90 percent of women become pregnant within a year after stopping pills. If ovulation and menstruation do not start within six months, they can be made to start, if there are no additional problems, by the use of clomiphene citrate (brand name, Clomid: of course like many drugs Clomid has its own possible side effects). Since 15 percent of couples are temporarily or permanently infertile anyway, it is difficult to tell whether the pill actually causes permanent infertility. Most doctors think not.

Safety

Many of us are uneasy about taking a hormone-affecting medication every day for months and years since its effects have not been conclusively tested and since it has been in wide use for only fifteen years. Yet many of us choose to take whatever risks are involved because we absolutely don't want to get pregnant. What price do we pay for such perfect protection against pregnancy?

RISK OF DEATH WITH VARIOUS CONTRACEPTIVE METHODS

| | | Women age 20–34 years (1,000,000 users/year) | | | Women age 35–44 years (1,000,000 users/year) | | |
		Deaths due to pregnancy	Deaths due to method	TOTAL	Deaths due to pregnancy	Deaths due to method	TOTAL
Method	Pregnancies						
IUD	30,000	7	unknown		17	unknown	
Oral contraceptives	5,000	1	13	14	3	34	37
Diaphragm	120,000	27	0	27	69	0	69
Safe period	240,000	55	0	55	135	0	135
Pregnancy	1,000,000	228	—	228	576	—	576

Figures taken from McGill *Birth Control Handbook*

The pill and blood clots. English surveys* have shown that more pill users than nonpill users die of blood clots, which can be caused in susceptible women by the estrogen in the pills. Some people argue that this is not too bad, because more women die during pregnancy and delivery (25 per 100,000) than of blood clots on pills (3 per 100,000 is one estimate; see McGill University, *Birth Control Handbook*, p. 19, for different statistics and a breakdown according to age). But this argument is not entirely reassuring. As one woman wrote us from New York, "I have trouble with the comparison of death rates. I don't think that most women choose a birth-control method with death rates in mind. And the fact that the risk of death is indeed a consideration is indicative of just how lousy the situation is." We must find a birth-control method that is both perfect and safe at the same time. For now, if you want to use pills, consider that only a very small percentage of pill users actually die of blood clots; be sure you see a careful doctor before you begin and while you are taking pills; and make sure that the doctor checks your susceptibility to blood clots as thoroughly as possible. (See section below, "Who Should Not Use the Pill.")

The pill and cancer. There has been no proof that the pills cause cancer. The pill does cause polyps (nonmalignant tumors) to grow in the lining of the cervix in some women, and causes changes in the cervical cells of others. Neither of these conditions is apparently precancerous, but some doctors feel that not enough long-term studies have been made to prove absolutely that such effects are not an indication of precancerous conditions. It is known that estrogen can aggravate existing cancer, so for your safety be sure you are carefully checked—pelvic and breast examination and Pap smear—before you start taking pills and every six months to a year while you are taking them. If a close member of your family has had

*The British Dunlop Committee Report, *British Medical Journal*, April, 1968.

breast cancer, many doctors will not prescribe pills for you. If you do use pills with this family history, be extra careful—get a checkup every three months, and learn to examine your own breasts for lumps.

The pill and your children. There seems to be no relationship between infant sexual abnormalities and the pill, although this is another area in which not enough long-term studies have been made. Children who find pills and eat them might become nauseated but won't be seriously hurt.

That is some of the information available to us when we try to make a decision about using pills, but a lot of what we hear is contradictory. We are confused and alarmed by "pill scares," such as the one caused by exaggerated press reports of the 1970 Senate hearings on the pill. Thousands of women went off the pill in a panic that spring, and who knows how many got pregnant. Whom should we listen to in this controversy? Opponents of the pill include some very intelligent and concerned people, professionals and non-professionals alike. One of the pill's most vocal opponents is Barbara Seaman, author of *The Doctors' Case Against the Pill*. In her book she cites case history after case history in which the pill can be suspected of having caused injury and death. In most of the cases the woman who died or suffered had not been examined carefully enough by the doctor who prescribed pills for her, had not had checkups while taking the pill, or had not been told that there was some risk involved in taking it. Others had too long ignored pains that were in fact warning signals, and had sought help too late. But some of the deaths seem to have been unpredictable and unpreventable.

Perhaps a majority of gynecologists in this country take a positive stand and advocate use of the pill. The authors of the McGill *Birth Control Handbook*, an excellent and careful description of birth-control methods and their advantages and hazards, come out fairly pro-pill, with a strong feminist perspective. They assert that although there are many medications in use that are potentially dangerous, the pill receives extra attention because, "it is the first 100 percent contraceptive, the first drug to weaken male society's control over women. . . . Male chauvinism searches to introduce a new fear into women" (p. 20). They also point out that the dangers of the pill should be considered relative to the dangers of other drugs we take all the time (aspirin, for example), of air pollution and poisonous food additives, of just crossing a busy street.

We feel that both pro-pill and anti-pill people are saying important things. Having learned from both Mrs. Seaman and the McGill authors, we have set up the following reasoning for ourselves: Birth-control pills are dangerous for some women, and in other women can cause side effects that range from nuisances to major pains and changes. But many women have taken the pill with no apparent side effects at all. Also, 100 percent protection against pregnancy is a very important tool for many of us as we start to take control over our lives. Many women, therefore, will continue to use the pill.

We feel that every woman deserves to be able to make, and must make, an "informed decision" (Barbara Seaman's phrase) about using birth-control pills. She must know the risks, and she must know about other birth-control methods that she could use. If she chooses the pill, she must be able to see a responsible gynecologist or an internist who is well acquainted with birth-control pills. (See the section below, "How to Get Pills," for an idea of what the doctor should ask and check before giving a woman pills.)

How Long to Take the Pill

There is disagreement among doctors as to how long it is healthy to stay on the birth-control pill. Dr. Robert Kistner writes, in his pro-pill book *The Pill*, that, "the problem of infertility following use of the Pill occurs sufficiently often that many physicians recommend that younger women discontinue the Pill for short intervals periodically. This is particularly important in women who have not demonstrated their ability to become pregnant."* He plans to take women in this age group off pills for three or four months every two years. Dr. Elizabeth Connell, a knowledgeable doctor who has done a lot of research on the pill, told a seminar on methods of conception control at the New York University School of Medicine in the spring of 1971 that a woman could take the pills for ten years or more as long as she had periodic checkups. On an average, women today probably take the pill for three or four years and then stop for at least three months. If you stop, however, be sure you find out about other birth-control methods and choose one that you'll use every time—which can be hard once you've known the freedom that the pill gives.

*R. Kistner, *The Pill*, p. 87.

Who Should Not Use the Pill

The pills would be dangerous for certain women. To help the doctor in screening women who want to use the pill, the FDA requires the drug companies to publish a list of contraindications, or conditions that prohibit the use of the pill. The doctor should check a woman for each one of these contraindications:

Any disease or condition associated with poor blood circulation: thromboembolism (blood clotting), thrombophlebitis (clot in the veins of the legs), bad varicose veins, pulmonary embolism (blood clot in the lung), a stroke, retinal thrombosis (blood clot in the eye), heart disease or heart defect. The estrogen in the pill, like the estrogen in your body during pregnancy, is suspected of increasing your blood's tendency to clot. Clots that form in your blood vessels can occasionally break loose and travel to your heart, lung, or brain and cause death. This is more likely to happen in women over thirty-five years of age. There is also a nine times' greater risk of nonfatal thromboembolism for pill users.*

Hepatitis or other liver diseases. As the liver metabolizes the sex steroids (progesterone and estrogen), no one with liver disease should take pills until the disease is cleared up. A woman who tends to get jaundice during pregnancy should not use pills.

Undiagnosed abnormal genital bleeding.

Cancer of the breast or of the reproductive organs, and, in many cases, a family history of breast cancer. (See p. 114 for discussion of the pill and cancer.)

Lactation. Nursing mothers should not take the birth-control pill for two reasons. First, the pill tends to dry up the mother's supply of milk, especially if administered soon after she gives birth. Second and more important, it is suspected that some estrogen will come through into the milk. As estrogen has the effect of closing up the bony epiphyses and thereby inhibiting bone growth, it would be dangerous for the infant to take in any estrogen. Recent research has led some doctors to question whether a low-dosage pill would really dry up the milk supply, and whether estrogen would be present in amounts that could possibly affect bone growth. So, this is a controversial subject; for now, most nursing mothers do not take the pill.

Cystic fibrosis. Definitely no pills.

Who Can Use the Pill Conditionally

People with the following disorders or ailments can use the pill, but should do so only *under close medical supervision*.

Diabetes. The progesterone in the pills tends to bind the body's insulin and keep it out of circulation, just what a diabetic or an incipient diabetic doesn't need.

*McGill, *Birth Control Handbook*, p. 19.

Increasing numbers of doctors, however, have put diabetic women on the pill, figuring that since pregnancy can be fatal to a diabetic, the risk of the pill is worth it. They have found that the pill increases the diabetic woman's insulin requirements, so that she must have periodic blood tests to measure her blood-sugar count. If you are a diabetic, or if close relatives are diabetic, be sure you have these blood tests regularly if you go on the pill.

Migraine headaches. For reasons that are not yet completely understood, some women taking the pill develop or suffer increasingly serious migraines, throbbing headaches which result from spasms of the blood vessels in part of the brain. The danger is that if a woman tends to get migraines, which are one form of vascular spasm, she might be more likely while on the pill to suffer a more extreme and damaging form of vascular spasm like a stroke. So women with a tendency to migraines should use the pill with caution.

Epilepsy and asthma. Fluid retention caused by estrogenic pills (see section "Differences Among the Several Brands of Pill") can aggravate epilepsy and asthma. Low-estrogen pills should be used, diuretics can be taken, and the woman should stay under close medical supervision.

Circulatory conditions. A woman with high blood pressure or mild varicose veins must take pills with caution. (See above, "Who Should Not Use the Pill.")

Tendency to severe depression, or any serious psychiatric problem. Although premenstrual tension and depression are often relieved by the pill, certain pills will cause certain women to become very depressed.

Sickle-cell trait. There is increasing suspicion that women with sickle-cell trait may have a higher incidence of thromboembolic disorders resulting from the pill. Women with sickle-cell anemia should not take the pill. Black women planning to go on the pill, therefore, should have a sickle-cell test.

Age. Women over thirty-five run a statistically higher risk of thromboembolism and other complications when taking the pill. Since risks during pregnancy increase also, women over thirty-five should consider a combination method like IUD and foam, or the diaphragm and condoms, or sterilization—tubal ligation for them or vasectomy for the sex partner.

How to Get Pills

We have seen, above, that certain physical conditions would make birth-control pills very dangerous, so it is in our vital interest to have a doctor prescribe our pills. Don't borrow them from a friend. Be sure the doctor examines you carefully, including an internal pelvic exam, breast exam, Pap smear, blood-pressure, blood and urine tests. The interview should include questions about you and your family's medical history to find out whether you have a tendency toward breast cancer, blood clots, diabetes, migraines, and so on. Too many doctors prescribe birth-control pills hurriedly; it's up to you to make sure you are carefully checked for each one of the contraindications. When you are on pills you should see a doctor every six months to a year for the same tests and examinations.

How to Use Pills

With most pill regimens you start your first pill on the fifth day of your period, counting the day you start your period as day one. Some pills start on the first Sunday after your period comes. You take one pill each day at approximately the same time of day. If you feel nausea, take the pill with a meal or after a snack at bedtime. Here is an almost foolproof schedule: Take a pill at bedtime; check the packet each morning to make sure you've taken a pill the night before; and carry a spare packet of pills with you in case you get caught away from home. *Read the directions carefully*. With 20- and 21-day pills you take one pill a day for 20 or 21 days and then stop for a week or 8 days, during which time your period will come. With 28-day pills you never stop, and your period comes during the time that you are taking the seven different-colored pills.

If you forget a pill. Take the forgotten pill as soon as you remember it, and take the next pill at its appointed time, even if this means taking two pills in one day. If you forget two pills, take the forgotten pills as soon as you remember, then keep taking your pill every day but use an additional method of contraception (foam, condoms) for the rest of that cycle. If you forget three pills or more, withdrawal bleeding will probably begin, so act as though you are at the end of a cycle. Start a new packet of pills according to the directions for your particular type of pill (7 or 8 days from last pill taken), but use another method of birth control from the day you realized you forgot the pills through 10 days of the next cycle.

Protection. Your first packet of pills may not protect you perfectly, as an egg may have started to develop before day five, so to be safe use another method of birth control for at least the first two weeks. After your first month on pills you will be protected against pregnancy all month long, even during the days between packets.

Differences Among the Several Brands of Pills

If you choose to take the birth-control pill, how do you and the doctor determine which pill you should take? We should be aware that different pills have different kinds, strengths, and quantities of synthetic estrogen and progesterone in them. The first and firmest guideline for choice has been suggested by the British Committee on Safety of Drugs, which warns us that high-estrogen pills are more likely to give us blood clots. The committee advises that only products containing 0.05 mg or less of estrogen be used, that products containing 0.075 mg or more of estrogen are associated with a higher incidence of thromboembolic disorder. Pills with 0.05 mg of estrogen are: Ortho-Novum 1/50, Norinyl-1 (same as Ortho-Novum 1/50), Demulen 1, Demulen .5, Norlestrin 1, Norlestrin 2.5, Ovral. Pills with more than this recommended dose of estrogen are: Ortho-Novum 1/80, Ortho-Novum 2, Ovulen, Enovid-E, Enovid 5, Norinyl 2, and all sequential pills. Many doctors are still prescribing high-dosage estrogen pills either because they don't know about the report or because they disagree with it. Others prescribe higher-dosage estrogen pills if a woman has had bad side effects from a higher-dosage progesterone pill or if there is an indication that she will have them (see below). In these cases the doctor must be sure to inform the woman of the higher risk of blood clots.

The kind of side effects that a particular pill is likely to have is directly related to the amount and potency of the progesterone with relation to the estrogen in that pill. There are several kinds of synthetic progesterone, called progestins. Certain progestins, such as norethindrone (used in Ortho-Novum, Norlestrin, Norinyl, Norquen), tend to produce androgenic ("male") effects—for example, hairiness, scanty periods, acne, permanent weight gain. In a low-dosage estrogen pill in which the progestational potency is not counterbalanced by strong estrogenic effects the over-all effect of that pill will be androgenic. On the other hand, with pills in which the estrogen dominates, either because of a lower progestin-to-estrogen ratio or because of the use of a less potent progestin, the effects tend to be what are called estrogenic, or "female," such as heavier periods, fluid retention, breast swelling and tenderness.

The exact effects that a given pill will have on your body, if you experience side effects at all, depend on your normal estrogen and progesterone levels. These levels are hard to test accurately, but you and the doctor can judge them in a general way. For instance, if you have a lot of body hair and scanty menstrual periods, you can guess that in your normal nonpill body chemistry there is a predominance of progesterone over estrogen. A low-dosage estrogen pill like Ovral or Demulen, or a low-estrogen, high-potency-progestin pill like Ortho-Novum 1/50, or a high-dosage progestin pill like Norlestrin 2.5 is likely to accentuate your progesterone-related characteristics, and you might experience one or more of the progestin-excess symptoms—changed sex drive, poor vaginal lubrication, susceptibility to monilia vaginitis, breast enlargement, appetite increase and permanent weight gain, acne, depression, or fatigue. A more estrogenic pill (for example, Ovulen or Enovid-E) would be likely to balance your natural excess of progesterone, although it might increase your risk of blood clots (if it did more than make up for your normal lack of estrogen).

On the other hand, if you have heavy periods or large breasts that get tender before your period, or if you tend to retain fluid and often feel bloated, you are probably estrogen-sensitive or have a natural overbalance of estrogen in your system. A low-dosage estrogen or high-potency progestin pill would be good for you, whereas a high-estrogen pill would be likely to give you nausea, bloating, breast tenderness, leg cramps, chloasma (see p. 118), and heavy periods.

Today it is impossible to predict with complete accuracy what kind of effect, if any, a certain pill will have on you. So use these guidelines when you can, show them to the doctor, but if a doctor believes that a certain pill will be right for you, try it. You can switch if one of these effects shows up.

Possible Side Effects

The pill is a medication that enters your bloodstream and travels around your body affecting more than just your ovaries, and so you may experience some seemingly unrelated side effects. Remember the doctor who said, "If we tell women they might get headaches, they'll get headaches." Although this is a crude generalization, sometimes, particularly when we aren't sure we want to be taking the pill at all, we start to blame every mental and physical problem on the pill instead of looking for other causes as well. We have a right to know all the possible side effects of the pill, but we must keep in mind that a majority of women notice no side effects at all other than some nausea when beginning. Also, virtually all side effects are reversible—they will stop when the pills are stopped. And you may decide to put up with mild side effects rather than choose a less effective or less convenient method. If you get an unpleasant side effect from one brand of pill, you can switch to a different brand, and often the effect will disappear. If you do change brands, use an additional birth-control method (foam, condoms) for the first two weeks of the new brand.

Here are the side effects that you might notice. For a more detailed description, see p. 18 of the McGill *Birth Control Handbook*.

Nausea. The estrogen in the pill might make you feel sick to your stomach, just as a pregnant woman does while her body is getting used to the high level of estrogen that the developing fetus puts into her blood. Nausea usually goes away after two months; there is less if the pill is taken with a meal or just before bed; use antacid tablets for relief.

Fatigue. Another common symptom of pregnancy that can affect pill users is tiredness and lethargy, a side effect caused by progesterone. Fatigue usually lasts only two or three months while your body gets used to the different hormone level.

Change in menstrual flow. Your periods will be lighter with most pills (estrogenic pills cause more normal flow). Occasionally your flow will be very slight, or you will even miss a period. This doesn't mean that you are pregnant. If you miss a period two months in a row, consult a doctor.

Breakthrough bleeding, that is, vaginal staining between periods. If there isn't enough estrogen or progesterone in the pill to support the lining of your uterus at a given point in your cycle, a little of the lining will slough off. (This may also occur if you miss a pill.) It usually happens a week or so after you start the first month of pills. Often it clears up by the second or third cycle as your uterus gets used to the new level of hormones. Some women stop breakthrough bleeding by taking two pills a day for several days and then returning to the regular dosage for the rest of the month. If breakthrough bleeding doesn't stop after a few months, you may need to try different brands of pills until you find one that more closely corresponds to your own hormone levels. Breakthrough bleeding does not mean that the pill isn't working as a contraceptive.

Breast changes. Increased breast tenderness might occur, but usually lasts only a couple of cycles. This happens more often with estrogenic pills. Pills in which the progestin is dominant tend to cause breast enlargement, which may last as long as you are taking them.

Weight gain. Androgenic or progestin-dominant pills such as Ortho-Novum, Norlestrin, or Ovral can cause appetite increase and permanent weight gain because of the buildup of protein in muscular tissue. If you want to gain weight, this is helpful. Estrogenic pills (Enovid, sequentials, Ovulen) can cause fluid retention because of increased sodium. This effect is temporary and usually cyclic. Watch your salt intake, or change your brand of pill. Some people who retain fluid take a diuretic drug to stimulate their urine production, but diuretics have their own risks and side effects (rob body of potassium, for instance), so use them sparingly if at all.

Headaches and tension from fluid retention—an estrogenic effect. Some women develop bad migraines and have to change or even stop taking pills.

Rise in blood pressure in susceptible individuals.

Vaginitis. This can occur with any brand of pills. Vaginitis is a vaginal infection that may be caused by yeast, fungus, or bacteria. The pills increase the sugar and water content in the vagina, so that all atmospheric yeasts or bacteria (or fungi) find the vagina excellent to grow in. It does not always occur, but the point is that any of the pills could make the vagina more susceptible, particularly to monilia. Progestin-dominant combination pills are the most likely to cause this susceptibility. If you get recurrent vaginitis, you may have to discontinue taking the pill.

Increased susceptibility to venereal disease. For a long time we knew that the pill helped the spread of VD, because fewer men were using condoms to prevent pregnancy. But the link turns out to be more direct. In the same way that progesterone makes the vagina more susceptible to monilia, it seems to make it more susceptible to the gonococcus. One Boston doctor reported to us that women not on the pill tend to notice flare-ups of gonorrhea most often at the time of their period, which means that they were exposed to and caught the disease a few days before that, at the time in their cycle when progesterone was at its peak. A representative of the Massachusetts Department of Public Health, Venereal Diseases Office, told us in October 1971 that women on the combination pill are more likely to catch gonorrhea when exposed, and women on the pill who do get gonorrhea seem to develop dangerous pelvic inflammatory disease more quickly—in other words, the disease spreads up into the uterus and fallopian tubes more quickly. These are serious dangers. If you are taking pills, and either you or your sex partner are having intercourse with more than one person, remember that you are just about 100 percent susceptible to gonorrhea, and try to protect yourself. Wash carefully (both of you), use condoms and spermicide (see list under "Diaphragm") for protection against VD, and get yourself checked regularly by a doctor (you usually have to ask for VD tests). See the chapter on VD.

Change in intensity of sexual desire and response. Many women experience an increase in sexual desire as soon as their fear of pregnancy is removed. But increasing numbers of women on progestin-dominant, low-dosage estrogen pills are complaining of loss of sex drive, lack of vaginal lubrication, decreased sensitivity in their vulval tissues, and decreased ability to have orgasms. One Boston doctor told us that 25–50 percent of his patients who are on low-estrogen, progestin-dominant pills have these side effects to some degree. In fact, this doctor often uses a higher-dosage estrogen pill, such as Enovid-E or Ovulen, for women with these side effects, being sure to tell them that the higher dosage of estrogen means a higher risk of thromboembolism.

Chloasma, or changes in skin pigmentation, sometimes described as "giant freckles." Very rare. Occasionally permanent, but usually disappears or fades after pills are stopped.

Depression. Some women complain of increased irritability or a tendency to feel depressed on the pill. These are progesterone-related side effects, and they tend to get worse instead of improving with succeeding cycles.

Acne. A progestin-dominant pill can cause or increase skin oiliness in some women. An estrogenic pill can decrease acne.

Gum inflammation. New York Times, December 12, 1971: "The use of oral contraceptives has given dentists a new periodontal problem because, like pregnancy, the hormones in the pill foster the development of gum inflammation." Women on the pill should brush their teeth extra carefully, use dental floss regularly, and see a dentist every six months to a year.

Warning Signals

Any side effect that lasts more than two or three cycles should be reported to the doctor. More serious symptoms of adverse reactions are: severe pain and swelling in the legs, bad headache, blurred vision. These should be reported immediately, for they are signs of incipient thromboembolism, and if you are about to get blood clots you had better stop the pill. (Note on leg pain: some leg cramps might be caused by fluid retention induced by the estrogen in the pill. Don't confuse this with the severe leg pain of thromboembolism, but also don't hesitate to call a doctor if the leg cramps become painful.)

Responsibility

Birth-control pills are primarily the woman's responsibility. You see the doctor, get examined, remember to take the pill, feel the side effects, and run the risks. Hopefully, the man you sleep with understands this, is supportive, and agrees to use condoms for a while or put up with a less invisible means of birth control if you want to stop taking pills.

Advantages and Disadvantages of the Pill

ADVANTAGES

Almost complete protection against unwanted pregnancy.

Regularity of menstrual cycle—a period every 28 days.

Lighter flow during periods (with the combination pill). This effect pleases most women, bothers some.

Relief of premenstrual tension.

Fewer menstrual cramps or none at all.

An estrogenic pill will clear up acne for some women. The pill often brings a sense of well-being and a new enjoyment of sex because the fear of pregnancy is gone.

Taking the pill has no immediate physical relationship to lovemaking. This is especially relaxing if you are just starting to have intercourse and have a lot to learn about your body and his. Later on when you are more comfortable with sex and more able to communicate openly with your partner, a diaphragm or foam and condoms will not seem like such interruptions.

DISADVANTAGES

The disadvantages have been described under the section on side effects. The only other one is that you do have to remember to take a pill every day. Some women are too forgetful, or live lives that are too chaotic for them to remember to take a pill every day. Younger women living at home who have to hide their pills from their parents sometimes leave them behind or are unable to take them on time.

SEQUENTIAL PILLS

Most of the preceding information on combination birth-control pills applies to sequentials also. But there are some differences that make it foolish to use sequential pills for birth control except in the case of overreaction to the progesterone-related side effects of the combination pill. Here are some of the differences:

Description

Sequential pills, by using estrogen alone for 15–16 days and combined estrogen and progesterone for 5–6 days, inhibit the development of the egg in the ovary but do not provide the two progesterone-related back-up effects (see p. 111, "How They Work").

Effectiveness

Sequential pills are therefore less effective in preventing pregnancy than combination pills. Someone taking sequentials must be very careful not to miss a pill or even to vary the time of day when she takes it. Even when no pills are missed, there is a 1.5 percent pregnancy rate, because sometimes the estrogen level is just not high enough for a particular woman, and an egg develops despite the pills.

Safety

More cases of thromboembolism have been reported by women on sequentials.

Possible Side Effects

Sequentials, in which estrogen is unopposed by progesterone for the first part of the month, emphasize estrogenic effects such as nausea, bloating, breast tenderness, headaches, heavy periods.

Some sequentials—C-Quens, for example—have been taken off the market. Others are still sold. Some doctors use them to regulate a woman's menstrual cycle. Oracon is a sequential pill that is currently being prescribed for women who overreact to the daily progesterone in combination pills—for instance, for a woman with acne. If your doctor prescribes a sequential, 1) make sure it is necessary and 2) be sure not to forget a pill!

IUD, OR INTRAUTERINE DEVICE: COIL, LOOP, AND SHIELD

Description

Most IUDs are small white plastic (occasionally metal) devices of different shapes and sizes. They are placed semipermanently inside the uterus by a trained person—in this country usually a doctor. One or two strings extend into the upper vagina so you can check weekly that the device is still in place. Once the IUD is inserted, nothing needs to be done other than weekly checking, unless there are problems or you want to get pregnant. Removal must be done by a doctor.

How the IUD Works

No one is absolutely sure how the IUD works to prevent pregnancy. Centuries ago when camel drivers in the Middle East started out on a long journey across the desert, they would insert pebbles into the uterus of a female camel to keep her from becoming pregnant on the trip. Thus a foreign body in the uterus seems to prevent pregnancy most of the time. There are several current theories as to how:

The IUD, which touches the lining of the uterus at several points, irritates the lining and keeps it from developing properly, so a fertilized egg cannot find a good place to implant.

The IUD speeds up the peristaltic waves by which the fallopian tube moves the egg down toward the uterus. The egg's normal journey of 4–5 days gives the uterine lining time to become secretory under the influence of progesterone. (See the left side of the chart on page 112.) If the egg reaches the uterus too soon, the lining won't be ready.

Studies are being done to determine if the presence of

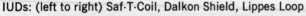

IUDs: (left to right) Saf-T-Coil, Dalkon Shield, Lippes Loop

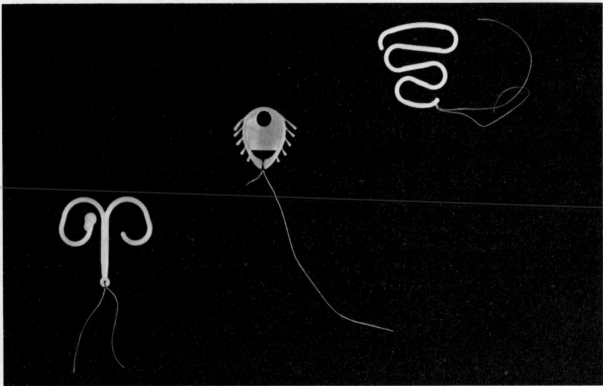

the IUD causes hormonal changes which cause the suppression of ovulation.

A fairly recent theory holds that the uterine wall responds to the foreign body by sending out macrophages —huge white blood cells—which try to get rid of the IUD, and failing that, devour egg or sperm or both. This is not an infection.

Some people find it a little unsettling that no one knows exactly how the IUD works. Others, uneasy with the pill's more generalized effects and the pregnancy rates of other methods, choose the IUD. At least the effects of the IUD are local—if something goes wrong, your uterus hurts and you seek medical help.

The Different Types of IUD

The original IUD was the Grafenberg ring; it and many similar closed devices, such as the Hall Stone Ring, are not in wide use today because of relatively high pregnancy and infection rates. The most commonly used devices today are the Lippes Loop and Saf-T-Coil. It has been found, however, that women who have never been pregnant can have a hard time tolerating the coil or the loop: a uterus that has not been stretched by pregnancy tends to react to one of these devices with cramping, backache, and expulsion. In the past three years doctors have been trying two new devices designed especially for use by the woman who has never been pregnant. The Majzlin Spring, a stainless steel device, has a low expulsion and low pregnancy rate, but it has caused considerable backache, calcium deposits, and inflammation of the uterine lining, and many doctors have found it very hard to remove, so it is not being used much any more. The Dalkon Shield is the most recent hope of never-pregnant women. In its first year and a half of wide usage the shield seems to have low expulsion and complication rates, but its pregnancy rate in women who have not been pregnant seems to be higher than expected. So there is no perfect IUD.

The most recently introduced IUD is the Copper-T, a T-shaped plastic device with a 200-sq-mm coil of copper wire around the stem. Copper is supposed to have antifertility effects. The FDA recently recalled the Copper-T from commercial use because it has not been proved not to introduce a harmful amount of copper into the bloodstream. One Boston doctor who is using the Copper-T experimentally said in March 1972 that in the sixty women who have received it from her since June 1971 there have been no expulsions, one failure, and no complaints of unusual side effects.

Effectiveness

Second only to the pill (and, some doctors feel, matched by the diaphragm when the diaphragm is used perfectly). The Saf-T-Coil and the Lippes Loop have about a 2 per-

cent pregnancy rate in women who have had a pregnancy. The Dalkon Shield is showing in 1972 a failure rate of about 3–4 percent in women who have not had a pregnancy.* (Drug company representatives tend to give a lower failure rate for their device.) For 100 percent protection some women use foam or condoms with the IUD, all the time if they feel particularly fertile, or for 7–10 days at mid-cycle (see "Rhythm" section, p. 133). Many Planned Parenthood clinics advise women to use a supplemental birth-control method for the first three months while using an IUD, as that is the time when conception seems to take place most often. Some doctors feel responsible for an IUD failure to the point that they will give you an abortion if your IUD fails. Question your doctor on this point. If you do become pregnant with the IUD in place, a miscarriage can be caused about 50 percent of the time simply by having the doctor remove the IUD.

Reversibility

Chances of becoming pregnant are the same as before using the IUD.

Safety

Major dangers are perforation and infection. Perforation of the uterus, occurring in one out of 2,500 women, has been found by the American Medical Association to be primarily the result of faulty insertion. Occasionally the IUD will slip out through a perforation into your abdominal cavity, so it is important to check the strings weekly (see section, "Possible Side Effects," p. 120) to make sure the device is in place. Infection flares up after insertion if the doctor does not maintain sterile conditions or if you have gonorrhea, severe vaginal infection, or pelvic inflammatory disease at the time of insertion. For your safety have yourself checked for VD before you get an IUD. While you have an IUD in place you run about a 5 percent higher risk of infection in vagina, uterus, tubes, ovaries (according to one Boston doctor). If you feel abdominal tenderness or pain with deep intercourse (when the penis goes in deep) report it to the doctor. If you catch gonorrhea while the IUD is in place, there is a chance that you won't be able to be cured until the IUD is removed. If you get pregnant with the IUD in place and go on with the pregnancy, there is no danger to the infant.

Who Should Not Use the IUD

Anyone with the following conditions: endometriosis, venereal disease, any vaginal or uterine infection, pelvic

*One Boston doctor believes that the shield fails only when it has not been placed deep enough in the uterus. He now uses a local anesthetic in the cervix to allow him to put the shield in deep enough without pain.

inflammatory disease, prohibitively small uterus, excessively heavy menstrual flow and/or cramping.

How to Get an IUD

Because of the risk of perforation, the IUD must be inserted by a well-trained person, which in this country usually means a doctor. Choose a doctor who has had some experience with IUDs and find out in advance which device she or he uses. Be sure you have a full pelvic and breast examination, Pap smear, and VD tests if necessary. The doctor does a sounding of the uterus to check its size and shape. The IUD can be put into a tipped uterus. If the uterus is small, as it is if you have had no pregnancies, you'll get a small IUD. (If it is too small, you won't be able to have one at all.) Just before insertion, the Saf-T-Coil and Lippes Loop are straightened out in a plastic tube like a straw; remember, the diameter of the cervical opening is the size of a thin straw. The doctor gently puts the tube into the vagina and up into the uterus through the cervix. Then the IUD is pushed through the tube and, being made of "memory plastic," springs into place within the uterus (except that it is put into your uterus instead of your vagina, it is similar to putting a tampon in place). The Dalkon Shield comes at the end of an applicator. No plunger is used; the applicator is twisted and pulled out, the shield remaining in place.

The process can hurt, sometimes a lot, because the uterus is stretched a bit by the device. You may have cramps during the insertion and for the rest of the day. Bring a friend with you if you can, and take aspirin beforehand, or a tranquilizer if they work for you, or try shallow panting to take your mind off it. The IUD can

stay in place for years but you should have it checked every six months to a year, at the time of your regular gynecological examination.

When to Get an IUD

Insertion while you have your period or just afterward is preferred because (1) it is a little easier at that time; (2) insertion can make you bleed; and (3) most important, doctors and clinics want to be sure you aren't pregnant, as an IUD insertion can cause a miscarriage. IUDs can also be inserted at the time of an abortion.

How to Check Your IUD

Squat, bringing your bottom down near your heels, and reach in your longest (clean) finger. The bathtub or shower is a good place. Bearing down while you are sitting on the toilet is another good way to bring your cervix within reach. You might be confused by the folds of your vagina, but when you reach your cervix you will know it, as it is harder and more substantial than anything else you'll touch. Find the dimple in your cervix; this is the entrance to your uterus, and the strings of the IUD should be sticking out a little way. Some days your uterus will be tipped in such a way that you can't reach the cervix or find the hole; try again the next day. If you cannot find the strings for a few days, or if you feel a bit of plastic protruding, call your doctor or clinic.

Possible Side Effects

Some women experience considerable bleeding, cramping and/or backache for the first few days after insertion.

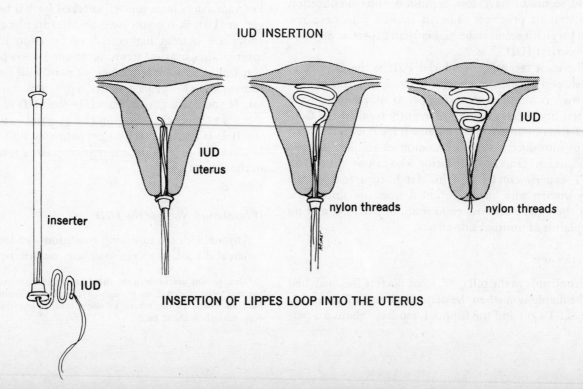

IUD INSERTION

inserter   IUD   IUD uterus   nylon threads   nylon threads   IUD

INSERTION OF LIPPES LOOP INTO THE UTERUS

Check with your doctor if it goes on for more than a couple of days.

The major drawback is the expulsion rate, which on the whole is about 8–10 percent. (Lower for women who have had babies, higher for never-pregnant women using the loop or coil, lower for the Dalkon Shield.) The IUD is usually expelled in the first three months of use, and usually during the menstrual flow. It often comes out without your knowing it or feeling it. So check your tampon or sanitary napkin every time, and be sure to feel for the strings at the entrance to your cervix a few times a month.

Heavier and more irregular periods and more intense or prolonged menstrual cramps are possible, usually for the first three to six months of using the IUD. This varies among women. Heavier periods are the result of a thicker uterine lining; cramping occurs as the uterus works to shed the thicker lining and, until it grows accustomed to it, the IUD.

Breakthrough bleeding may occur between periods, due to irritation of the uterine lining. If it continues more than a few months it can often be corrected by use of a differently shaped IUD.

Back pain is an occasional side effect. If it persists it can often be corrected by the use of a differently shaped IUD.

Advantages and Disadvantages of the IUD

ADVANTAGES

You don't have to fuss with birth control at the time of intercourse (unless you are using foam or condoms at mid-cycle for closer to 100 percent protection).

You don't even have to remember to take a pill. If you are forgetful, or if your life is too hectic for you to keep track of pills, the IUD is a better method for you than the pill.

Contrary to what some people think, you can use tampons with an IUD.

DISADVANTAGES

Heavier periods and more frequent cramps make some women give up the IUD.

Some people don't like the idea of wearing something inside them all the time.

Some men have said that they can feel the IUD during intercourse. One man told us that when he does, he just shifts position slightly. If the IUD is all the way in and if the strings are properly trimmed, the IUD should not bother or poke the man's penis, although he might be able to feel the strings at the entrance to the cervix.

Responsibility

The woman sees a doctor and experiences the insertion and any side effects. The man or woman must check the strings weekly.

Cost

An IUD can be expensive to get, but costs nothing afterwards except for a visit to the doctor once every six months to a year. The initial charge is $35–$50 by a private doctor in Boston, $50–$100 in New York. If there are private doctors who do it more cheaply, your local Planned Parenthood association will have their names. Many clinics charge as little as $10, and in some places there is no charge at all.

DIAPHRAGM AND SPERMICIDAL JELLY OR CREAM

A lot of people make a face when a diaphragm is mentioned. "It's messy. . . . It's a hassle. . . . It fails all the time." This current disdain is a little ironic, because in 1880 when it was invented the diaphragm was a major breakthrough in the liberation of women from unwanted pregnancies. Until the 1960s, when the pill and the IUD started to remove birth control from the scene of intercourse, the diaphragm was the safest precaution women had—at one time one-third of American couples practicing birth control used the diaphragm.* Many of our mothers used it for thirty years without a slip. Whether our mothers *enjoyed* using it is a different question. Today our more positive feelings about our sexuality, and our increasing ability to communicate openly with the men we sleep with, make us more able to use the diaphragm happily. If you are just starting to have intercourse you may not want to add a diaphragm to your sex life immediately, but in a few months, when you are more easy about sex, you may be glad to get off the pill or the IUD for a method that is effective if you use it well and that has no side effects at all.

Description

A diaphragm, which must always be used with spermicidal cream or jelly, is made of soft rubber in the shape of a shallow cup. It has a flexible metal spring rim. When properly fitted and inserted, it fits snugly over

*J. Peel and M. Potts, *Textbook of Contraceptive Practice*, p. 63.

DIAPHRAGM AND CONTRACEPTIVE CREAM

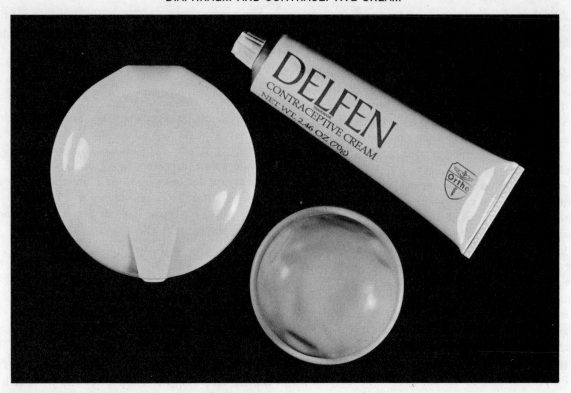

your cervix, locked in place behind the pubic bone and reaching back into the posterior fornix of your vagina. It comes in a variety of sizes measured in millimeters (mm), ranging from 50 to 105 mm, or 2 to 4 inches, depending on the size of your upper vagina.

How It Works

When the diaphragm is in place, holding spermicidal jelly or cream up to your cervix, the sperm cannot make it into your cervical canal. The sperm that swim up around the rim of the diaphragm run into the cream or jelly, which kills them. The sperm that remain in the vagina die in eight hours, as the vagina is a hostile environment to sperm. Some people smear jelly on the outside of the diaphragm to help kill sperm remaining in the vagina.

Effectiveness

The diaphragm is from 90–98 percent effective, depending on: the effectiveness of the cream or jelly (some are stronger spermicidal agents than others—see list under "Brands of Jelly and Cream"); proper fit and proper

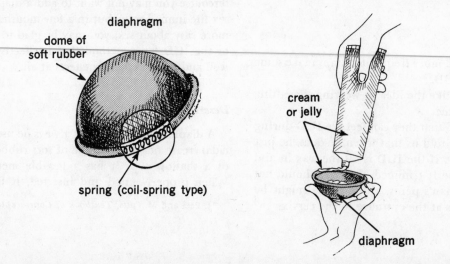

diaphragm
dome of
soft rubber

spring (coil-spring type)

cream
or jelly

diaphragm

care; and consistent and careful use. The main points in using a diaphragm are to use it every time and always to use a cream or jelly with it. Failures do occur about 2 percent of the time even when the diaphragm is properly used. Masters and Johnson found that the vagina expands during intercourse, so that the diaphragm moves around a bit (see chapter on "Sexuality"). The McGill *Birth Control Handbook* lists other reasons for slippage: cream on the rim, frequent insertion of the penis, and lovemaking positions in which the woman is on top (p. 28).

Reversibility

The diaphragm doesn't affect your fertility at all. Simply don't use it if you want to become pregnant.

Safety

The diaphragm is perfectly safe. The only risk you run is that of getting pregnant—and if you use it well, that risk is low. Some of us at some time felt scared that the diaphragm would slide up inside us and disappear, but as we got to know our anatomy better we have realized that the vagina stops about an inch beyond the cervix, and the diaphragm (or tampon) has no place to disappear into.

Who Shouldn't Use the Diaphragm

A woman with a severely displaced uterus (severe prolapse, for instance) cannot use a diaphragm. If your uterus is tipped forward or backward slightly, the doctor can choose one of the three kinds of metal spring rim (arcing, coiled, or flat) that would fit your particular anatomy.

A virgin, since her diaphragm size will change with first intercourse, should use a different method (foam and condom) the first few times and then go to be fitted.

A woman who doesn't like to touch her genitals and doesn't think she can get used to it, should not use a diaphragm, because she will dislike putting it in and taking it out so much that she probably won't put it in at all. You may feel very squeamish and embarrassed the first time you put your finger into your vagina, but as you get used to it and realize that your body is yours to touch, you should get over any uneasiness about inserting the diaphragm. You can also buy a diaphragm inserter.

How to Get a Diaphragm

The size of diaphragm you should use depends on the size and contour of your vagina. In this country it is usu-

ally a doctor who measures you ("fits" you) for a diaphragm. But this is not a hard thing to learn and could be one of the tasks that doctors start to share with nurses, midwives, or paramedical assistants. You should have a full gynecological examination at the time you get fitted for a diaphragm if you have not had one in the past year.

Very important: When you have been measured and fitted, you should practice putting the diaphragm in right there in the doctor's office, so the doctor can tell you if you have put it in right. You can reach in and feel what it feels like when it is in right, and the doctor can help you if you have problems, so that when you get home you won't be "experimenting." Some doctors neglect this important step. The doctor will probably give you a prescription for the proper size of diaphragm, and if your local drugstore requires one, a prescription for a good spermicidal cream or jelly.

How to Use a Diaphragm

Somebody said once that if someone handed you a toothbrush with no instructions and you had never seen one before, you might not use it very well for a while. The diaphragm is also a tool, and like any tool, it is simple to use once you've practiced with it. Putting it in the first time might feel awkward, but it will become easier and quicker with every insertion.

Who should put it in: There's a part of all of us that feels that we should go off into the bathroom, insert the diaphragm, and appear like a diaphanous angel ready for spontaneous sex. But there's also a part of us all that resents that role. It seems that many of the people who are happiest with the diaphragm insert it as part of sexual foreplay—the man and the woman do it together. This sharing seems to work best in a long-term relationship. One woman told us she prefers to put it in in the bathroom because she wants to be able to wash the cream off her hands. And if you are a couple that gets carried away with sexual intensity, it's probably best to put the diaphragm in in advance. But for most women putting it in together with the man is a much less burdensome and more enjoyable way of using the diaphragm.

When to put it in: The diaphragm can be inserted up to two hours before intercourse, since the creams and jellies hold their spermicidal potency in the body for about that long. The closer to the time of intercourse, the better: one-half hour is safer than two hours.

Preparation and insertion: Put about one teaspoonful of cream or jelly (three-quarters of an inch if it comes in a tube) into the shallow cup, or on the dome side, whichever side the doctor has told you to put up against your cervix. Spread the cream around. (Some books say to put the cream on the rim also; others say that cream

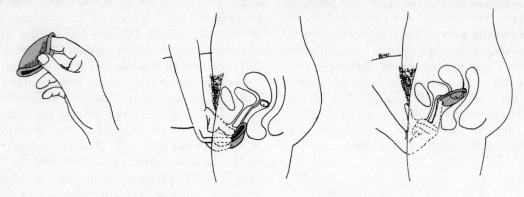

INSERTION OF DIAPHRAGM

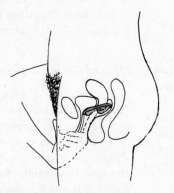

CHECKING OF DIAPHRAGM

on the rim makes the diaphragm slip; an effective compromise might be to put cream around the inside of the rim, not on the top of the rim.) Then squeeze the cup together by pressing the rim firmly between your thumb and third finger. You can buy a plastic inserter if you have trouble doing this with your fingers. Squat, sit on the toilet bowl, stand with one foot raised, or lie down. With your free hand spread apart the lips of your vagina, and insert the diaphragm up to the upper third of your vagina. If you have not used tampons or reached into your vagina before, remember that it angles toward your back. Push the lower rim with your finger until you feel the diaphragm lock into place. You should then reach in to make sure you can feel the outline of your cervix through the soft rubber cup. For more protection, insert a little extra cream or jelly with an applicator when the diaphragm is in place. When it's in right and fits properly, you should not be able feel the diaphragm at all, nor should the man. (Some men notice that the tip of their penis is touching soft rubber instead of cervical and vaginal tissue, but this not painful or bothersome.)

Leave the diaphragm in for at least six to eight hours after intercourse, as it takes the spermicide that long to kill all the sperm. You can leave it in for twenty-four hours or more if you want to. Douching is unnecessary, but if you want to douche, you must wait until the end of the six to eight hours.

Subsequent intercourse: If you have intercourse again within the six hours, you must add more cream or jelly with an applicator. Add it to the outside of the diaphragm, leaving the diaphragm in place.

Care: Wash the diaphragm with mild soap and warm water, rinse and dry it carefully, dust it with cornstarch, and put it in a container (away from light). Don't boil it. *Check it for holes* every so often by holding it up to the light or filling it with water and looking for leaks.

Possible Side Effects

A particular cream or jelly might irritate your vagina or the man's penis. Check the brand list on p. 127 for different ones to try. Some women are allergic to the rubber and need to use a plastic diaphragm.

Life of Product

Get your diaphragm size rechecked every year at your annual gynecological examination. You will need a new size if you gain or lose ten pounds and after a pregnancy. The diaphragm will last a couple of years with proper care.

Brands of Jelly and Cream

In choosing one brand over another, you should consider factors of effectiveness, smell and taste (oral-genital play), and any allergic reaction on your part or the man's. If you don't like the brand you're using, feel free to change. Some spermicides are made for use with a diaphragm, some for use alone; since the ones intended to be used alone are a little more effective, it makes sense to use one of those with your diaphragm. The *Consumer's Union Report on Family Planning* (New York, 1966) lists the following creams and jellies for use alone, in descending order of spermicidal effectiveness: Delfen Vaginal Cream, Koromex-A Vaginal Jelly, Preceptin Vaginal Gel. Some of the brands listed for use alone or with a diaphragm are: Certane Vaginal Creme, Contra Creme, Creemoz Vaginal Creme, and Lactikol Vaginal Jelly.*

Cost

A diaphragm costs about $4.50. The medical examination for this is about $15 at private offices, less at most clinics. Jellies and creams vary in price, costing about $2–$3 for a 2–3-ounce tube (there are about 12 applications in a 2½-ounce tube).

Advantages and Disadvantages of the Diaphragm

ADVANTAGES

A good method if you have infrequent intercourse. (Also good with a regular sex partner who is cooperative and helpful about using it.)

No side effects or dangers.

Very effective if well used.

The diaphragm is helpful if you want to have intercourse during your period and don't want your menstrual flow to make a mess. It will hold up to 12 hours of menstrual discharge.

Using the diaphragm can be a good kind of body education. If you are unfamiliar with what your vagina feels like, using a diaphragm will teach you! And in the long run the more familiar you are with your body, the more you will enjoy sex.

DISADVANTAGES

Closely related to sex act. If either you or your partner feels that sex must be absolutely spontaneous, with

*The following contraceptive jellies and creams are effective in helping to prevent VD (see "Venereal Disease" chapter for more details): Certane Vaginal Jelly, Cooper Cream, Koromex A Vaginal Jelly, Milex Crescent Jelly, Ortho Creme, Ortho Gynol Jelly, Preception Gel. Foam, not for use with a diaphragm, is also effective.

no interruptions, putting in the diaphragm will seem like a hassle.

You must remember to use it every time, be sure not to run out of cream or jelly, be sure to have it with you when you need it.

The discharge of cream or jelly can be a nuisance. Try different brands, and if necessary, use a tampon, pad, or Kleenex for leakage after intercourse.

Some women have mentioned that they experience a cutdown of cervical stimulation during intercourse when they use a diaphragm. Some of them like this, others don't. Since many people are not aware of cervical stimulation anyway, this will not be a factor for everyone.

Responsibility

The woman goes to the doctor to be fitted. After that the responsibility can be shared, although a lot of women do the whole thing themselves.

CERVICAL CAP (NO LONGER MUCH USED)

This product hasn't been used much since 1950, when diaphragms were generally substituted. It is like a diaphragm only smaller, made to fit securely over your cervix, where it mechanically blocks sperm. It is convenient because it can be left on for days or weeks; it must be removed only during menstruation. Spermicidal foam, cream, or jelly can be inserted at the time of intercourse for additional protection. Unless the woman puts it in every time she has intercourse, there is no chemical protection on the inside of the cap, as spermicides are effective for three hours at most. For this reason, and because the cap is harder to put on than a diaphragm, and because it can slip off during intercourse, the cervical cap is not as safe as the diaphragm.

CONDOM

(Rubber, Prophylactic, "Safe")

Description

A sheath, usually made of thin, strong latex rubber, designed to fit over an erect penis to keep the semen from getting into the woman's vagina. A condom usually comes rolled up, unrolls to about 7½ inches; the open end has a 1⅜" diameter rubber ring around it to help keep the condom on the penis, and the closed end is

PLAIN-ENDED CONDOM

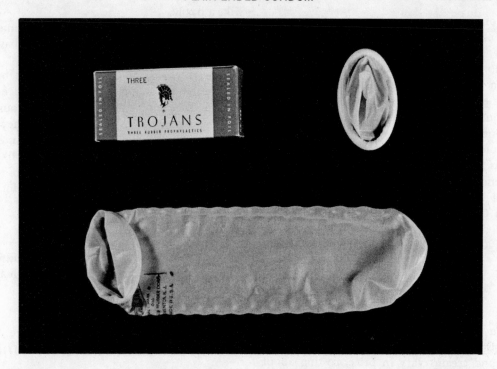

either plain or tipped with a little nipple that catches the semen and helps to keep the condom from bursting. "Skin" condoms (made of lamb membrane) are more expensive but tend to cut down less on sensation. Lubricated rubber condoms are available for couples who need extra lubrication, but these tend to slip off the penis more easily and have to be used extra carefully.

Effectiveness

Used alone, a good-quality condom is 85–95 percent effective, depending on how carefully it is used. The method of combining condoms with a spermicidal foam, cream, or jelly is highly effective. If you have forgotten two pills, lost your IUD, or have no other available means of birth control, use foam and condoms together for nearly 100 percent protection!

Reversibility

Perfectly reversible. To get pregnant, just don't use condoms.

How to Use

The man or woman unrolls the condom onto the erect penis before intercourse—*not* just before ejaculation, since the first few drops of the male discharge often contain enough sperm for pregnancy to occur.

CAUTIONS

Leave room at the end of the plain-ended condom for the semen: a half inch of space left between the end of the penis and the condom will keep the ejaculate, which comes out fast, from bursting the condom.

Unroll the condom carefully to avoid catching air in the end.

Use a lubricant to prevent tearing—spermicidal foam, cream, jelly, K-Y Jelly, or saliva, but *not* vaseline. Apply the lubricant after the condom is on the penis.

The man must hold the rim when he withdraws his no-longer-erect penis after ejaculation; otherwise the condom might slip off, and sperm will get into the vagina.

In case of accident, use cream or jelly or foam as quickly as possible. Also see the section, "The Morning-After Pill," p. 135.

Responsibility

This is the only effective temporary means of birth control that the man can use. As with the methods that are primarily up to the woman, it makes use of the condom much more enjoyable if both partners join in putting it on as part of the sexual foreplay. With a couple who sleep together more than a few times, condoms are a good way for the man to share the burden of birth control. In a shorter-term relationship, in which you may not know whether you'll be having intercourse or not, condoms can be very convenient. But if you just expect that the man will have a condom in his pocket, you may be disappointed. If you don't know the man well enough to trust that he'll have a condom with him, it makes sense for you to have something with you to protect yourself. Ideally, you could take a package of condoms with you, but for many of us, at least today, it would be hard to pull out a rubber and suggest that the man use it.

Advantages and Disadvantages of the Condom

ADVANTAGES

It is cheap, easily available, easy to use.

It is a method of birth control that gives some protection against VD. It helps to prevent the spread of gonorrhea and syphilis through penis-to-vagina contact. It also protects partners from infecting and reinfecting each other with an infection like trichomonas.

If the man tends to ejaculate too quickly, a condom can decrease the stimulation of his penis enough to help him delay ejaculation and prolong intercourse.

A condom catches the semen, so if the woman wants to go somewhere right after intercourse, she won't feel drippy.

DISADVANTAGES

The condom has to be used right at the time of intercourse. For some couples this ruins the spontaneity of sex, unless the woman puts it on the man and makes it part of sex play.

It often cuts down on the man's sensation, as his penis is not directly touching the vaginal walls. Many men resist using condoms for this reason, forgetting the effects that women's birth-control methods can have on a woman's enjoyment of sex. Pills can decrease her desire for sex, an IUD may make her bleed and have cramps for more days of the month than is normal for her, a diaphragm if not put in by both partners can make her lose interest, and so on.

The condom eliminates one source of lubrication for intercourse (the drops of fluid that come out when the man gets an erection), so it can irritate a woman, especially during the entrance of the penis into her vagina. Use of the lubricants mentioned above can help eliminate this problem.

How to Get Condoms

Since cheap condoms sold in vending machines in men's rooms, etc., are more likely to be defective, condoms should be obtained only in drugstores or at family-planning agencies. Many men say they were embarrassed the first time they bought condoms, particularly if the druggist asked, "What size?" and the man didn't know he was referring to the size of the package. Condoms are made in a standard size, they come in packages of three or 12, and they cost about $1.25 for three rubber ones and $1.50 for three lubricated rubber ones. Some high-quality condoms are: Ramses Rubber Prophylactics, Trojans Rubber Prophylactics, Trojan-Enz Rubber Prophylactics. A wide variety of good-quality condoms can be obtained at reasonable prices (in unmarked envelopes!) from Population Services, Inc., 105 N. Columbia Street, Chapel Hill, North Carolina 27514 (919-929-7195).

Life of Product

Condoms have a shelf life of two years. A condom kept in a wallet or a pocket for very long will deteriorate. A high-quality condom can be used five or six times if properly cared for. Put it in a bedside glass of water temporarily, then wash it, dust with cornstarch, and reroll.

"THE FOAM"—AEROSOL VAGINAL SPERMICIDE

Description

Foam is a white aerated cream having the consistency of shaving cream, which contains an effective sperm-killing chemical. It comes in a can with a plunger-type plastic applicator.

How Foam Works

Deposited just outside the entrance to your cervix at the top of your vagina, foam blocks the sperm and kills them as well.

Effectiveness

Foam is not as effective as a diaphragm used with cream or jelly, or as a condom. Because it spreads more even through the vagina, it is more effective than cream or jelly used alone. It is best used in combination with a condom, as an extra precaution with an IUD, or as a supplement for the first month of pills. If it must be used alone, two full applicators should be inserted, as close to the time of intercourse as possible. If you absolutely don't want to get pregnant, don't count on foam alone.

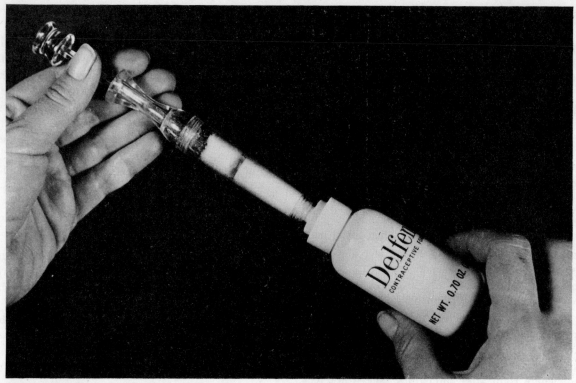

FOAM APPLICATOR BEING FILLED

How to Use Foam

Use no more than fifteen minutes before intercourse. Shake the can very well, about twenty times—the more bubbles the foam has, the better it blocks the sperm. Put the applicator on top. When the applicator is tilted (Delfen) or pushed down (Emko), the pressure triggers the release valve and the foam is forced into the applicator, pushing the plunger up. Lying down or standing with one foot raised, use your free hand to spread the lips of your vagina, insert the applicator about three to four inches, and push the plunger. If you have never used tampons you may want to practice inserting the applicator. You'll find that your vagina angles up and toward your back, and does not go straight up in your body. Your aim is to deposit the foam at the entrance to your cervix, not beyond. Use two applicators full. Wash the applicator with mild soap and water before putting it away. (You don't have to wash it immediately.)

CAUTIONS

Put in more foam every time you have intercourse again, no matter how soon.

Leave the foam in for 6-8 hours. If you want to douche, you must wait.

Keep an extra can on hand, as Delfen comes out of the can more slowly but doesn't otherwise indicate when you're running out.

HOW TO INSERT SPERM-KILLING FOAM, CREAM, OR JELLY

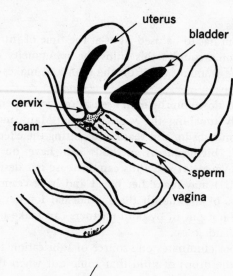

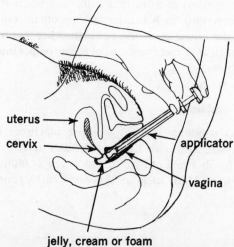

jelly, cream or foam

Side Effects

Foam irritates some vaginas and some penises. Delfen, which is most effective, also tends to be most irritating.

Responsibility

Basically the responsibility is the woman's. But either you or the man can put it in.

Advantages and Disadvantages of Foam

ADVANTAGES

It is an easily available stopgap method until you can get to a doctor to be examined for a more effective means of birth control.

It is quick, taking about 30 seconds to use.

It is less drippy than cream or jelly.

Foam is effective in helping to prevent VD (see chapter on "Venereal Disease").

DISADVANTAGES

It is not effective enough to depend on.

Using it can be a (brief) interruption of sex if the couple does not treat it as part of the sex play.

How to Get Foam

Foam can be bought in a drugstore without a prescription. If one druggist gives you trouble or refuses to sell it to you because you are "too young," try another. Better yet order it from the Population Services, Inc. (see p. 129 under "How to Get Condoms" for their address), and at the same time order some condoms to be used with the foam. Even though you don't have to see a doctor to get the foam, it makes sense to have a checkup yearly (more often if there's a chance that you've been exposed to VD).

Cost

Foam costs about $3.25 for a medium-sized can (with an applicator), which contains enough for use about 20 times.

Brands

Delfen Foam is widely considered to be the best, much more effective than Emko, the other well-known brand. If Delfen irritates you or the man, you can try Emko, but remember that it is less effective.

JELLIES AND CREAMS FOR USE ALONE (WITHOUT A DIAPHRAGM)

How They Work

Spermicidal cream or jelly comes in a tube with a plastic applicator. When deposited outside the cervix just before intercourse, cream or jelly (1) forms a film or coating over the cervix which blocks the sperm from entering the cervical canal, and (2) kills the sperm by chemical action.

Effectiveness

Creams and jellies are not as effective as foam, so unless foam irritates your tissues, don't use creams or jellies alone. Cream or jelly used with a diaphragm is more effective than foam, because the diaphragm holds it right up to the cervix, where it should be. If you must use cream or jelly alone, get your partner to use a condom.

How to Use Them

As near as possible (under 15 minutes) to the time of intercourse, fill the applicator and insert into your vagina and push the plunger. (See "Foam" section, p. 130, for insertion details.) Do this twice. Use an additional full applicator for each additional act of intercourse. Leave the jelly or cream in for 6–8 hours; if you want to douche, you must wait.

Possible Side Effects

The stronger, more effective creams and jellies tend to be more irritating to the vagina and penis than the others.

Reversibility

Just don't use it if you want to get pregnant.

Responsibility

Responsibility is primarily the woman's, but you both can put it in.

Advantages and Disadvantages of Cream or Jelly

ADVANTAGES

The only advantage is that they can be bought at a drugstore without a prescription and no medical examination is necessary, so you can get them on short notice.

As foam is more effective and just as easy to obtain, try it first. Certain brands are effective in helping to prevent VD (see footnote in section on the diaphragm).

DISADVANTAGES

There can be problems of leakage, allergy, or reaction to the smell or taste. Jelly tends to be gooier than cream.

Purchase, Cost, and Brands

Creams and jellies are available at all drugstores. See section on foam for purchase hints and mail-order source. See section on the diaphragm for prices, and names of effective brands.

BIRTH-CONTROL METHODS THAT DON'T WORK VERY WELL

WITHDRAWAL (COITUS INTERRUPTUS, OR "TAKING CARE," OR "PULLING OUT")

Description

Withdrawal of the penis far away from the vagina just before ejaculation ("coming"), so that the semen is deposited outside the vagina and away from the lips of the vagina as well.

Who Uses Withdrawal

Worldwide, this is the most universally used of all methods, a folk method that is practiced without medical initiative and is passed on from one generation to the next. It is not so widely used in the United States in general, but is depended on by quite a number of United States couples who don't have access to good birth-control information and care—many teen-agers, some college students, people who can't afford medical fees.

Effectiveness

Withdrawal is not highly effective because the drops of fluid that come out of the penis right after it becomes erect can contain some sperm, enough to cause a pregnancy. Also, withdrawing at the last minute can be difficult, and the man cannot always get out in time to avoid contact not only with the vagina but also with the vaginal lips (sperm have been known to swim all the way from the vaginal lips up into the fallopian tubes).

Responsibility

The man is responsible for withdrawal. The woman is completely dependent on his control over his ejacula-

tion, and must trust him greatly in order to be free of anxiety.

Disadvantages of Withdrawal

Withdrawal is the only last-minute method other than abstinence, but it has a number of drawbacks in addition to its high failure rate. The man must keep in control and therefore cannot relax and lose his self-consciousness. When used over a long period, it can lead to premature ejaculation by the male. Withdrawal can also be hard on the woman: the man might have to withdraw before she reaches orgasm, completely interrupting the flow of her sexual response; also, a part of her consciousness is wondering whether he's going to make it out on time, so that she, too, cannot entirely relax into her sexual feelings. Some couples who have used withdrawal for a long time have been able to work out these problems.

RHYTHM METHOD (SAFE PERIOD)

This is the only birth-control method approved by the Catholic Church. We mention it in such detail because some Catholic couples are trying to use rhythm without the assistance of a doctor or clinic, and because too many teen-agers and college students, unable to get good contraceptive advice and care, try to avoid pregnancy by timing their intercourse according to some vague idea that there is a "dangerous" time around mid-cycle. *You can get pregnant at any time during your cycle,* because in any cycle you might ovulate early or late.

How to Practice Rhythm

Rhythm is based on the fact that a woman usually releases only one egg each menstrual cycle. The egg has an active life of 12 hours; sperm about 4–5 days. Therefore, there are 5–6 days each month on which intercourse could lead to pregnancy: 4–5 days before ovulation (egg release) and the half day after. A woman normally ovulates 12–16 days before her menstrual period. The rhythm formula follows:

1. Keep a written record of your menstrual cycle for 12 consecutive months. Count the first day of menstruation as day one of the cycle, and the day before the next period as the last day of the cycle. At the end of 12 months figure the number of days in the shortest and longest cycles.

2. Subtract 18 from the shortest cycle's number; this determines the first fertile, or unsafe day.

3. Subtract 11 from the number of days of the longest cycle; this determines the last fertile day, or the day on which the unsafe period ends.

THE RHYTHM METHOD
How to Figure the "Safe" and "Unsafe" Days

Length of Shortest Menstrual Cycle	First Unsafe Day After Start of Any Period	Length of Longest Menstrual Cycle	Last Unsafe Day After Start of Any Period
21 days	3rd day	21 days	10th day
22 days	4th day	22 days	11th day
23 days	5th day	23 days	12th day
24 days	6th day	24 days	13th day
25 days	7th day	25 days	14th day
26 days	8th day	26 days	15th day
27 days	9th day	27 days	16th day
28 days	10th day	28 days	17th day
29 days	11th day	29 days	18th day
30 days	12th day	30 days	19th day
31 days	13th day	31 days	20th day
32 days	14th day	32 days	21st day
33 days	15th day	33 days	22nd day
34 days	16th day	34 days	23rd day
35 days	17th day	35 days	24th day
36 days	18th day	36 days	25th day
37 days	19th day	37 days	26th day
38 days	20th day	38 days	27th day

4. Each month bring the last of 12 cycles up to date by adding the cycle just counted to the bottom of the list and crossing off the oldest cycle on top.

A daily record of basal body temperature (measured on a special thermometer, which only registers a few degrees, from 96 to 100 degrees, in 1/10 degree gradations, which are wide apart and easily read) is used in combination with the chart of cycles. The basis of this is that whatever a woman's so-called normal temperature may be, there are characteristic (though slight) daily variations within each month caused by ovulation. The cycle runs like this: After each menstrual period the temperature on awakening is low. It may be still lower on the day associated with ovulation, which is assumed to occur just before or just after the lowest morning-temperature reading. After ovulation, because of the action of newly formed hormones, progesterones, the temperature rises several tenths of a degree and remains up until a day or two before menstruation begins. If pregnancy occurs, the temperature remains consistently high for several months, since progesterone continues to be formed. Suspect pregnancy if BBT (basal body temperature) is high for more than 18 days.

Effectiveness

This depends on the regularity of your menstrual cy-

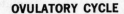

OVULATORY CYCLE

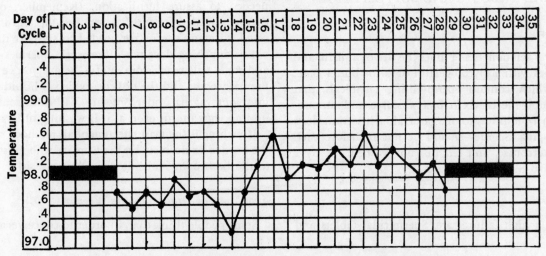

TEMPERATURE VARIATION DURING MENSTRUAL CYCLE

cles. If there is a variance of more than 10 days between the longest and shortest cycles, the rhythm method is not effective, because the safe period is too brief (true for about 15 percent of women). The method requires a lot of self-control and cooperation between partners. It has about a 20 percent pregnancy rate, which is lower if you diligently use a thermometer and calendar and always abstain if there is a chance of ovulation. The method is not good after pregnancy; several months are needed to recalculate the safe period.

CAUTION: For the rhythm method to work at all, it must be practiced under the guidance of a doctor, nurse, or clinic. If you are using rhythm vaguely, avoiding what you think are unsafe days, read the rest of this chapter and choose a birth-control method you can depend on.

Reversibility of Rhythm

Since the mid-cycle unsafe days are days when you are most likely to get pregnant, knowing which days they are will help you to get pregnant when you want to—just have intercourse on those days!

Responsibility for Rhythm

This method must have the cooperation of both sex partners, as rhythm takes a lot of self-control.

Disadvantages of Rhythm

It is complicated to practice rhythm properly, taking your temperature every morning for a year and watching the calendar carefully. The high failure rate increases the anxiety about pregnancy. It can be hard on your sex life: there are only certain days when it is all right to have intercourse, and a partner who isn't in the mood for it then feels guilty, while a partner who wants it during an unsafe time feels guilty and frustrated.

VAGINAL TABLETS AND SUPPOSITORIES

Description

Drugstores sell tablets 2–3 times the size of aspirin, and suppositories with a glycerogelatin or cocoa-butter base, both of which contain sperm-killing chemicals that spread around the cervix (tablets dissolve and suppositories melt) 15 minutes to one hour after insertion deep into the vagina. So they should be put in before each time of intercourse, and left in (not washed out by a douche) for 6–8 hours afterward.

Effectiveness

There is a high failure rate. Spermicidal tablets and suppositories are not as effective as creams or jellies, and much less effective than foam, because the spermicide does not get evenly distributed through the vagina.

Brands

There are many tablets and suppositories. Here are the ones listed by the *Consumer's Union Report on Family Planning:* Durafoam Vaginal Foaming Tablet (12 for $1.00), Zeptabs Vaginal Tablets Effervescent (6 for 90 cents), Lorophyn Suppositories (12 for $1.47).

Why People Use Them

Some women probably use them because they are cheap, can be bought in a drugstore with no trips to the doctor involved, and because they seem less messy than foam or jelly or cream. (The high pregnancy rate of tablets and suppositories should outweigh these conveniences.) Also, many women use these products because this is the only method they know about. Magazines and other publications rarely advertise pills, IUDs, or diaphragms (such advertisements are illegal in many places), but the tablets and suppositories are widely advertised as a "solution to your most intimate marital problems." What is most confusing is that these same magazines carry ads for such feminine-hygiene products as Norforms; the ads are worded in the same suggestive way, leaving many people with the impression that the hygiene products *also* prevent pregnancy.

NONMETHODS

Douching

Some women try to flush out their vagina with water or other special solutions immediately after intercourse—trying to remove semen before sperm enter the uterus. The idea is to keep the sperm level below the number needed to assure fertilization. (Remember, only one sperm is needed for fertilization, but the trip is complicated, so many sperm are needed to support the odds.)

But douching does not often work. Sperm swim fast, and some will reach your uterus before you've reached the bathroom; and the douche, which is liquid squirted into your vagina under pressure, will push some sperm up into your uterus even as it is washing others away.

Douching is the least effective of all methods, and puts the burden exclusively on the woman, who must hop up to the bathroom immediately. Don't use it!

Avoidance of Orgasm by the Woman

Some people think that, in order to conceive, a woman

must have an orgasm; one theory says that at the time of orgasm a woman's uterus or vagina releases a liquid similar to the man's seminal fluid, which helps the sperm up toward the egg. This is all false. One of the major differences between men and women in the field of reproduction is that a man must have an erection to cause a pregnancy, whereas a woman can conceive without any sexual arousal at all. Avoiding orgasm won't keep you from getting pregnant!

Avoiding Actual Intercourse

Some couples who follow sex play just to the point of intercourse and then stop, run the risk of pregnancy if the man ejaculates right at the entrance to the woman's vagina. If the woman's vaginal lips are well lubricated, some of the 300 million sperm will start to swim up into her vagina, and some might reach her uterus, where they can live for 4–5 days. Pregnancies do happen this way.

Note: *mutual masturbation* (partners stimulate each other manually or orally until they reach orgasm) can be a pleasurable experience and a good means of birth control as long as you are both careful that no semen gets on the lips of your vagina.

Norforms and Other Feminine-Hygiene Products

Remember, these are not birth-control methods.

AFTER UNPROTECTED INTERCOURSE— "THE MORNING-AFTER PILL"

Some college health services, some clinics, and some doctors will give you a series of high-dosage estrogen pills if you come in *fewer than three days* after unprotected intercourse in the middle of your menstrual cycle. A lot of estrogen at that point in your cycle will usually affect the uterine lining so as to make it impossible for a fertilized egg to implant. Check the "Birth-Control Pills" section, p. 117), for the side effects of estrogen, and you will see why this is not a method to be used often. The dosage used at Yale is 50 mg of diethylstilbestrol (two 25-mg tablets) to be taken together once a day for 5 days. You might want to get antinausea pills at the same time. Your local or regional Planned Parenthood group can tell you where to get "morning-after" medication.

WHEN YOU ARE ALL DONE—STERILIZATION

Sterilization is a 100 percent effective, usually final form of birth control, available for men and for women.

It is legal in all states, although many hospitals are conservative about it and require that the person be a certain age, with a certain number of children, and so on, and that he or she have the spouse's signed consent. (Other hospitals, notably in ghetto areas, tend to do too many, and not entirely voluntary, sterilizations. Black women in the South are all too familiar with the "Mississippi Appendectomy," in which their fallopian tubes are tied or their uterus is removed without their knowing it.)

Increasing numbers of doctors in the United States are willing to perform a sterilization operation on anyone who is fully aware that the operation is in most cases irreversible. If you or your sex partner want to be sterilized, and the hospitals and doctors in your community won't do it, you can call your local or regional Planned Parenthood association, Zero Population Growth office, or write to the Association for Voluntary Sterilization (addresses at end of chapter under "Helpful Organizations").

Choosing to get sterilized is a big decision. If you have no children or only one child, you will run up against shocked and adverse reactions from many closed-minded people. You will also have to deal with your own deeply internalized feelings that someone who is infertile is inferior. Even after three or four children the decision can be difficult, because so many of us have been encouraged to think of childbearing as our only accomplishment.

For either a man or a woman making this decision, which goes against many of our society's norms, it helps to talk with other people who have been sterilized. A woman who was sterilized a year after her only child was born, wrote to us and shared with us her experience of intense pre-operation fear that she would be regretful, followed by, after the operation, a beautiful sense of relief and joy that she was free to proceed with her life. Remember: sterilization means that you can no longer produce your own children; you are always free to adopt a child if you feel you want to be a parent.

In the traditional sterilization operation for a woman, the woman is put to sleep with a general anesthesia, a fairly large abdominal incision is made, a piece of each fallopian tube is cut out, and the two ends are tied off and folded back into the surrounding tissue. Some doctors, particularly at the time of an abortion, tie the tubes through a small incision at the back of the woman's upper vagina. A more recent development is the *laparoscopy technique*, in which, a tube with mirrors and lights is inserted through a small incision in the (unconscious) woman's abdomen, and the tubes are visually located and then cauterized (burned) with a small instrument entered through another incision. The traditional tubal ligation is major surgery, requires a 4–5-day hospital stay, and is accordingly very expensive—at least

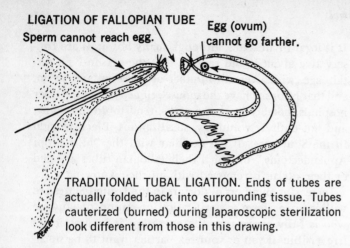

LIGATION OF FALLOPIAN TUBE
Sperm cannot reach egg.

Egg (ovum) cannot go farther.

TRADITIONAL TUBAL LIGATION. Ends of tubes are actually folded back into surrounding tissue. Tubes cauterized (burned) during laparoscopic sterilization look different from those in this drawing.

$300 in most places. The laparoscopic technique and the vaginal-incision technique require a shorter hospital stay, sometimes only one day, and in some places are being done on an out-patient basis. They are, accordingly, much cheaper, and require less time for recovery. Sterilization does not affect a woman's hormone secretions, ovaries, uterus, or vagina. Her menstrual cycle continues. An egg ripens in and bursts out of an ovary every month, but stops part way down the tube, disintegrates, and is absorbed by the body. Her sexual response, which depends on her hormones, clitoris, and vagina, is not lessened at all, and in fact usually improves as soon as she no longer fears pregnancy.

Sterilization for the man, called a vasectomy, is usually done in a doctor's office or in a clinic. The whole procedure requires about three visits—a preliminary visit (which often includes the wife), the operation, and a follow-up visit weeks later for a test of the sperm count. The operation takes about half an hour. The doctor applies a local anesthetic, locates the two vas deferens (tubes that carry sperm from testes to penis), removes a piece of each, and ties off the ends. Experimental operations have been made in which a piece of plastic is put into the tube to plug it up temporarily so that if the man later wanted to have a child he could have the plug taken out. This technique has not yet been successful, but when it has been perfected it will be an excellent means of birth control.

Vasectomy leaves the man's genital system basically unchanged. Sperm are made, his sexual hormones remain operative, and there is no noticeable difference in his ejaculate, because sperm make up only a tiny part of the semen. Some men, even knowing these facts, are still anxious about what a vasectomy will do to their sexual performance. These men should not have vasectomies, because worrying about sexual performance is likely to impair a man's ability to have an erection, even though the production of sperm and male hormones continues.

FUTURE METHODS OF BIRTH CONTROL

Male Contraceptive Research

A few years ago a birth-control pill was developed for men, but it drained a man's ability to have an erection as well as acting as an antidote to the potency of the sperm-producing cells. Now researchers are working on a sperm-capacitation pill in Sweden and California. This will stop the sperm's ability to penetrate the egg. It may be available in two to three years. As yet no compound has reached serious clinical trial.

Many women have been talking recently about pushing for research into effective birth-control methods for men. Since men play a role equal to women's in creating pregnancy, it makes sense for them to share the burden of preventing it. It makes women angry to see so relatively little research being done on methods for males. Women suspect that male research scientists would be unwilling to offer men a contraceptive that exposed them to as many side effects and potential risks as the pill or even the IUD does to women.

But what if there were a pill or a shot for men? Except for women in certain very trusting long-term relationships with just one man, how many women are in situations in which they can absolutely trust their sex partners to keep them from getting pregnant? As part of the active-passive, pursuer-pursued, predator-prey, male-female stereotypes that we act out in sex, men say many persuasive things to women to try to get them into bed. Why would a man not say he was taking birth-control pills if he wanted to persuade a woman to sleep with him? If he was lying, the woman and not he would get pregnant.

Even in a marriage the financial burden of a child would probably not scare a man into remembering his pill, as the threat of unwanted pregnancy and total responsibility for child care make a woman remember hers. Therefore, getting men to share the burdens of birth control involves a lot more than finding methods for them to use! For now, many of us prefer to keep the control in our own hands.

Female Contraceptive Research

Prevention of ovulation, implantation, or sperm entrance into uterus by use of hormones. These experimental methods are just variations on birth-control pills in that they introduce synthetic hormones into the woman's body:

The minipill—a continuous low dosage of progesterone that is supposed to keep the cervical mucus too thick for sperm to penetrate, and to hinder uterine lining development. Much breakthrough bleeding and other drawbacks make this method not as promising as it seemed at first.

Subdermal implants of capsules containing progesterone that would leak into the blood a little every day, accomplishing the same effects as the minipill.

Progesterone-coated IUD would add contraceptive effects of progesterone to effects of IUD.

Progesterone-coated vaginal ring that would fit like the rim of a diaphragm. The ring releases enough progesterone every day to suppress ovulation. The ring is removed for 7 days once a month to allow cyclic bleeding to take place.

An injection of 50 mg of medroxyprogesterone acetate (Depo Provera) every three months suppresses ovulation. Side effects are irregular bleeding, no real menstrual period, and most important, a 12–21-month delay in ovulation if the woman decides she wants to become pregnant. Some women who want no (or no more) children are using this method already.

New IUD designs. See the IUD section for a discussion of the Copper-T, now in experimental use.

A promising development—the prostaglandins. Prostaglandins are hormonelike chemical substances that have been found in male semen (hence their name, from "prostate," the gland in which seminal fluid is made) and in many body tissues. They have been discovered to cause uterine contractions, and are being experimentally used to induce labor and to cause abortion. As a birth-control method, prostaglandins would be put into a vaginal suppository or an injection which a woman would use if her period was late or perhaps not until after a pregnancy test had proved to be positive. The prostaglandins would make her uterus contract, causing a period whether she was pregnant or not. (Someone who believes that "life" starts at the moment of fertilization would call this a mini-abortion.) Current side effects of prostaglandin injections include nausea, cramping, and diarrhea. These side effects would have to be minimized before prostaglandins were generally used. Since a normally fertile woman using no birth control would tend to conceive only once every 3–4 months, a woman using prostaglandins for birth control would have to use them only a few times a year. The rest of the time her body would be free of birth-control devices or medications. It seems that several more years of research are necessary before prostaglandins can be widely used.

Helpful Organizations

Association for Voluntary Sterilization, Inc., 14 W. 40 Street, New York, N. Y. 10018 (212-524-2344).
　　Will provide information on sterilization, speakers to interested groups, and referrals to doctors all over the country.

Planned Parenthood-World Population: National Headquarters, 810 Seventh Avenue, New York, N. Y. 10019.
　　Clinics and offices throughout the United States. Clinics provide birth-control (and some of them vasectomy) services for anyone. Offices provide information and local or national referral for birth-control, sterilization, and abortion services.

Zero Population Growth, Inc., Los Altos, Cal. 94022.
　　Whether or not you agree with ZPG that overpopulation is the world's major problem, you can get birth-control, sterilization, and (in some cases) abortion information from your local or regional ZPG chapter. Some ZPG chapters are trying to establish or have already set up vasectomy clinics.

FURTHER READINGS

(All are paperbacks except Demarest and Sciarra.)

Calderone, Mary, ed. *Manual of Family Planning and Contraceptive Practice.* Baltimore: Williams and Wilkins Co., 1970.
　　Long, careful, detailed.

Demarest, Robert, and John Sciarra. *Conception, Birth and Contraception.* New York: McGraw-Hill, 1969.
　　Clear, informative text and beautiful drawings on all pertinent subjects, including male anatomy. An excellent book for a school, library, or clinic.

Gray, Marian and Roger. *How to Take the Worry out of Being Close.* 32 pp. Oakland, Cal., 1971.
　　A lively and clear description of birth-control methods, abortion, venereal disease, and "itchy infections and infestations." Order from Marian Gray, P.O. Box 2822, Oakland, Cal. 94618 (25 cents, lower in bulk).

Kistner, Robert W., M.D. *The Pill.* 329 pp. New York: Dell Pub. Co., 1969.
　　Dr. Kistner is a great believer in the pill, and tends somewhat to de-emphasize risks and side effects. So take what he says with a grain of salt, but read his book if you want to know in detail how the pill works and what it does.

McGill University Student Society. *Birth Control Handbook.* Montreal, Can., 1971.
　　A detailed, complete, simple, and unbiased description of birth-control methods. The McGill authors did more research and go into more detail than this chapter has been able to do. Highly recommended.
　　Send 25 cents for mailing to New England Free Press, 791 Tremont Street, Boston, Mass. 02118, or to *Birth Control Handbook,* P.O. Box 1000, Station G, Montreal 130, Quebec, Can. Bulk orders $45 per 1,000 copies. Send check or purchase order in advance.

Neubardt, Selig. *Contraception.* 157 pp. New York: Pocket Books, 1968.
　　Amusing, perceptive, and clear.

Peel, J., and D. Potts. *Textbook of Contraceptive Practice.* Cambridge, England: Cambridge University Press, 1969.
　　Quite technical and thorough; includes sociological and legal aspects. Under 300 pp.

Seaman, Barbara. *The Doctors' Case Against the Pill.* New York: Peter H. Wyden, Inc., 1969. 273 pp.
　　Ms. Seaman is alarmed by the dangers of the pill, and cites numerous case histories to show that the pill can "cripple and kill." A good antidote to the pro-pill, "almost-anyone-can-take-the-pill" attitude in such books as Robert Kistner's *The Pill.* You should read both sides. (Also available in paperback [Avon Books]).

Yale University Student Committee on Human Sexuality. *The Student Guide to Sex on Campus.* New York: New American Library, 1971.
　　Clear, complete, informative. Not as detailed on birth-control methods as the McGill booklet. Approx. 150 pp.

11
Abortion

INTRODUCTION

ABORTION is our right—our right as women to control our bodies. In almost every community in this country a woman with an unwanted pregnancy is frustrated and obstructed by laws, hospitals, doctors, by high prices and poor communications. The same public whose sex-filled media urge her to be sexy turns on her with moralistic disapproval that isolates her and forces her to deal with her problem in secret. Some strong and concerned people have changed a few state laws and started some good abortion-referral services and humane clinics, but for too many American women legal abortions are hard to get, hard to pay for, and once gotten, are alienating and lonely experiences.

Why do unwanted pregnancies occur? Some of us become pregnant without thinking about it because we have been forced to believe that we are acceptable only as sex objects or as mothers. Or we are taught that sex is not quite right (even though we are taught to be sexy and flirt) so we're scared to ask those who may know where to get birth control and which birth-control methods are most effective. Or even when we do ask, many of us can't get birth control—it's not easy for teen-agers anywhere, and it's hard for any of us who can't afford the medical fees and drug prices. And even if we can get the most effective method for pregnancy prevention, it may not be the best method for all of us (e.g., we may have a family history of breast cancer and should not take the pill). And every method except the pill fails to work 2 percent of the time or more. Birth control is better than nothing, but there is no such thing as an ideal method, that is, one that is safe, simple, cheap and 100 percent effective. Birth control fails us because the methods are imperfect, not because we are irresponsible. Nevertheless the consequences fall on us.

In places where legal abortions are hard to get, the risks are great. Although the risk of death for an abortion done under proper medical supervision during the first 12 weeks is less than for a full-term pregnancy, not all women who want abortions can get them legally. And of those who can, many have spent so long securing information about getting an abortion and then getting an appointment that they go beyond 12 weeks after their last menstrual period, when the procedure gets more difficult and more dangerous.

Until recently illegal abortion has been one of the most common causes of maternal death in this country. The casualties are difficult to count, since many women who came into emergency wards and died of acute peritonitis (infection spread through the abdomen) were victims of botched or dirty abortions but wouldn't say so because they were afraid of arrest. Many women who recovered from such infection found that they were sterile. The risks to our mental health were enormous, too, when legal abortions were very hard to get. We had to deal with the fear and trauma of getting a "criminal" abortion, or we had to place ourselves at the mercy of hospital boards which in most states decide whether a case "deserves" a legal "therapeutic" abortion. We had to wait anxiously and to act in secret. But now, in the places where women have access to legal abortions, the devastating effects of the botched illegal abortion are rarely seen. One of the earliest and greatest triumphs of the awakening Women's Movement in this country has been the widespread change in attitudes toward abortion which is just beginning to be felt nationwide.

When legal abortions are hard to get, poor nonwhite women suffer most. In 1969: 75 percent of women who died from abortions (mostly illegal) were nonwhite; 90 percent of all legal abortions were given to white private patients. If you do not live in or near New York State, or in Alaska, Hawaii, or Washington State, these figures probably hold for your area.

138

tercourse too soon after the abortion, thereby allowing germs to enter the uterus through the vaginal canal before the uterus has had a chance to completely heal. Nausea, vomiting, heavy cramping, or a temperature of 100.5 degrees Fahrenheit or over are all signs that warn of possible infection.

Incomplete abortion. This results when a doctor fails to remove all fetal material in the uterus. The abortion may then have to be completed by a dilation and curettage of the uterus. The danger signs to watch for are a foul-smelling vaginal discharge, cramping, nausea, vomiting, or hemorrhage as described above.

Before you go for your abortion it is important that you have the address and phone number of a doctor or clinic that you can go to if any complications should occur, because if complications do occur, it's a crisis, and that's not the time to have to search out a doctor who will see you.

Aftercare

Although a woman can usually get up and resume her normal activities a few hours after a vacuum suction abortion, it is a good idea for her to be on the lookout for the above danger signs, and observe these directions carefully after the abortion: No douching, tampax, tub baths, or intercourse for four weeks after the abortion. This will cut down the chances of getting an infection. The idea behind this is that infectious germs entering the vaginal canal might cause infection in the uterus at this time. Thus exterior masturbation or oral intercourse are not prohibited.

Because of this chance of infection some doctors prescribe an antibiotic, such as tetracycline. But this is controversial, because others feel that an antibiotic will mask the symptoms of infection. Ergotrate is another drug that is sometimes given. It helps the uterus contract to its normal size, thereby diminishing the chances of infection or possible hemorrhage. If an antibiotic has been prescribed, you should not drink any alcoholic beverages for seven to ten days after the abortion, since the effect of the alcohol might work against the antibiotic.

Birth Control After an Abortion

Some women say after their abortion, "I'm never going to have sex again, so I don't need birth control." If you're feeling this way you've got to be honest with yourself about the chance of your having intercourse again. At the time of your abortion someone at the hospital or clinic may talk with you about birth control. This may seem like a hassle when you are so concerned

with what's happening to you right then. Clinics do this because many women got pregnant because birth-control information was just not available to them where they live. This is a good time to ask for this information of any of the counselors, who (in the New York clinics at least) are very sympathetic and well informed.

Some clinics will insert an IUD at the time of your abortion. Check this if you are interested. (See chapter on "Birth Control" for information on IUDs.)

If you plan to take the pill as a method of birth control, it is a good idea to start taking it right after the abortion even though you can't have intercourse for four weeks, because it is not until the second month of taking the pill that you can be positive that it has stopped ovulation (see chapter on "Birth Control") and is therefore working as an effective method of birth control.

You should plan to have a postabortion checkup four to six weeks after your abortion. This is another time when you could discuss birth control. If you plan to use a diaphragm, you could have your size checked or be refitted at this time.

Your period will start about four weeks after the abortion. But, remember, it is important *not* to have intercourse the first month after the abortion: you are fertile and you are open to infection.

Abortion Counseling

Probably the most important person you would come in contact with during an abortion would be the abortion counselor. Since this is such a new and challenging field, we've asked abortion counselors to tell us about their work, their working conditions, and any important psychological effects of their job.

Most counselors agree that an important factor in their work is the number of cases they handle a day. They feel that there should be enough counselors so that patients can be treated considerately and effectively. If a counselor is obliged to see too many patients in a day, both she and the patient can begin to feel like impersonal, mechanical parts of the "big business" of the clinic.

Some counselors have reported feeling greatly frustrated at not being able to have more decision-making power in the clinics in which they work—helping decide on procedures, what literature should be available for the patients, and so on. But groups of counselors are getting together in workshops to help each other learn how they can be more effective.

Some of the things women want to talk about in these workshops are how they *feel* working as abortion counselors. On the one hand, it's an extremely rewarding feeling. Many women report that as abortion counselors they feel for the first time that they have a meaningful job where they really sense they're helping other women.

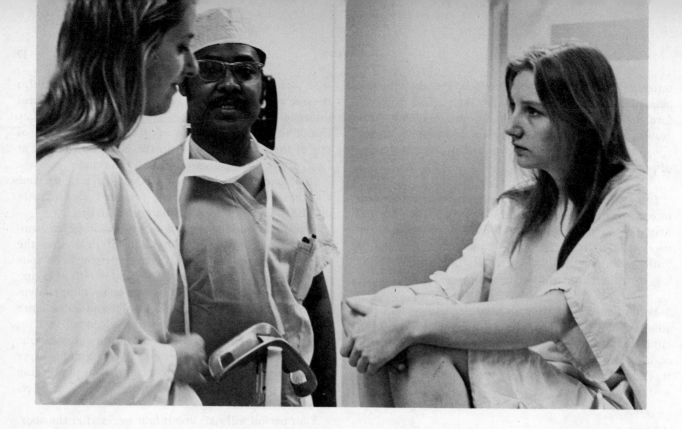

"Just knowing that I can help another person to relax in her time of crisis is important to me. Some women come to an abortion thinking that it's the most hideous crisis in their lives—but hopefully in a time of crisis you can learn something about yourself. Through counseling, women can get down to those real feelings. They look at their relationships with men; they see who their friends are; they learn about their bodies and birth control, reflect on their sexuality, get support. . . ."

Inevitably there is also the less positive side. "Many [of us] counselors have abortion nightmares. I've had a few. But of course, when I was a student I had student nightmares, and when I taught I had teaching dreams." Like all other jobs in which there is a great deal of human contact, it is not a job that just any person can handle. It calls for strength and warmth and control and a kind of responsiveness to each individual woman.

Nurses also have reported strong feelings about assisting at abortions (see article in *The New York Times,* February 1, 1972, p. 32). Some nurses who were used to working in the delivery room trying desperately to save even the smallest babies found that sometimes they were salting out babies larger than the ones they had tried to save. This, understandably, was very difficult to accept. The nurses most deeply disturbed ask to be transferred to different sections of the hospitals. Others are helped by ventilating their feelings in counseling sessions.

Other nurses felt degraded by being assigned to an abortion section without any proper psychological training. They also felt they could not do a good professional job if they could not develop some kind of personal relationships with these women they were serving.

However, most nurses who continue to work in the abortion units have a positive attitude toward the work and feel that it is the personal right of a woman to control her own body and to have an abortion if she wants one.

ILLEGAL ABORTION

The Doctor-Performed Illegal Abortion

When legal resources fail her and she cannot get to New York, the woman with an unwanted pregnancy starts asking friends of friends, nurses, and taxi drivers in a frightened and hysterical nosing around, which ends her up on a doctor's table if she is lucky, in the hands of some semimedical quack if she is less lucky, at the mercy of her own mutilating hands if she is desperate, and in the emergency ward of a hospital if serious complications develop.

It is important for a woman to know the whole range of abortion methods, so that she will know what she is talking about with her doctor, and more important, so she can judge the methods of an illegal abortionist and find the courage to walk out if her life is in danger. (Don't pay in advance if you can help it.)

Many illegal abortions up to 12 weeks are performed by doctors who give D & Cs or vacuum aspiration abortions in hidden offices. Many do it for profit but some do it because they believe abortions should be done but are scared to court arrest by doing them in the open. The cost ranges from an occasional humane hundred or so, to the usual $600–$1,000. Except for a more hasty departure afterward, and the exclusive use of a local anesthetic, the abortion performed by a skilled and conscientious illegal abortionist who keeps his tools clean is just as safe and comfortable as a hospital abortion. While on the whole the rural woman has a harder time than the city woman in finding an illegal abortion, Lawrence Lader describes the abortion practice of small-town doctors who have some kind of understanding with the local police. Lader also tells of the woman whose unsympathetic gynecologist told her to go elsewhere and then at the end of her long and panicked search turned out behind face mask and gown to be her illegal abortionist (Lader, *Abortion,* pp. 42–51).

Methods of the Unskilled Abortionist

The dirty D & C. The D & C in the hands of hurried incompetents, with no anesthetics, no antiseptics, and dirty tools is frightening and dangerous.

The catheter method. Catheters are narrow tubes sold at drugstores for drawing off urine. The catheter is inserted into the uterus through the cervix, a dangerous procedure when attempted by an amateur. Germs introduced into the uterus by the catheter cause an infection. The uterus contracts, thereby "spontaneously" aborting the fetus.

The high douche. Forced douche or injection under pressure of such over-the-counter chemical agents as soap, turpentine, Lysol, vinegar, or lye will produce an abortion if the solution reaches the fetus or sufficiently irritates the uterus. Extremely dangerous.

Both the catheter method and the high douche work on the theory that an infection or dangerous substance will kill the fetus before it kills the woman. They can result in permanent disability or death.

Air pumped into the uterus. This method causes air embolism (air into the bloodstream) *and* sudden and violent death.

Self-induced Abortion

The most unskilled abortionist of all is the woman herself.

External means. Women try extremely hot baths, severe or prolonged exercise, violence to the lower abdomen, and various long sharp tools for self-mutilation. Some of these attempts are very dangerous. None of them work.

Drugstore abortifacients. The woman can also get from her "friendly" druggist a number of abortifacients which, all expensive, endanger her life to varying degrees and almost never work.

1. Soap-base pastes and douche solutions are among the most dangerous. Soap goes directly to the uterine veins to cause blood-vessel blockage, *shock,* and *death.*

2. Desperate women douche with almost any liquid they can think of, running the risk of severe burning of tissues, hemorrhage, shock, and death.

3. Suppository tablets of potassium permanganate, a caustic tissue-destroying agent that damages the vagina walls and can cause massive hemorrhaging, ulcers, and infection, are sold despite an FDA prohibition.

4. Among the useless folk remedies sold are quinine pills and Humphrey's Eleven pills, which women take in massive, expensive doses (literally hundreds of pills) because once a woman who thought she was pregnant took some around the time when her period was due, and, lo and behold, her period came.

5. Women also take quantities of birth-control pills, which actually support the pregnancy if anything, and when used in this way, are suspected of causing genital deformity in the fetus.

6. Castor oil and other strong purgatives are used to no abortive effect.

Of the many thousand women in the United States who yearly get illegal abortions or try to abort themselves, between two and five thousand actually die. Thousands more spend time in the hospital with septic abortions, peritonitis, gangrene, air embolism, and other acute repercussions. Unknown numbers of them find themselves infertile later on when they want to plan a pregnancy. (At a 1969 abortion conference in Boston, sponsored by the Unitarian Universalist Women's Federation, it was disclosed that 10–20 percent of a local infertility clinic's patients had had previous septic abortions.) And many thousands of women escape from the frightening experience physically whole but with a new cynicism, and rarely acquire any better contraceptive techniques than they were using when they got pregnant.

FUTURE PROSPECTS

If we look to the future it seems that the technical aspects of the abortion procedure will probably be simplified very soon. In some places a medical instrument known as the Karman cannula is being used on an experimental basis. It is a narrow piece of flexible tubing which can be inserted into the undilated cervix before the fifth week after conception. Attached to the tube is a syringe that sucks out the contents of the uterus including the fertilized egg. This procedure has to be done just about as soon as a woman misses a period and by someone carefully trained in the proper use of this technique. It is relatively simple to do, takes only about a minute and the woman feels only minor cramping.* Prostaglandins are also being used on an experimental basis to terminate pregnancy. We should follow the progress of the research in this field and try to keep well informed about the various ramifications for women of these different methods.

Even as abortions become more readily available around the country, there are still some things to look out for. Decent working conditions should prevail in the clinics; good abortion counseling and birth-control instruction should be available; health-insurance programs and welfare should cover abortions for married and single women; costs should be kept down by elimination of profit-making referral agencies and the scaling down of doctors' fees.

Women's groups—there is so much that we can do. We should be pressuring legislatures and hospitals to provide abortions locally. We should be starting abortion counsel-

*Newsweek, July 24, 1972, p. 62.

ing and referral services where there are none. If there is a service in your area, make sure the women are getting supportive counseling and not just referrals. Do what you can to help the women who need to deal with postabortion feelings. Start a fund to lend money to women who can't afford the abortion prices and travel costs, particularly teen-agers.

We should put pressure on drug companies to invest in research to develop the kinds of products that help us to take better care of ourselves—for example, do-it-yourself kits to determine if you are pregnant or if you may have VD, or even a do-it-yourself Pap kit. Schools should be urged to give courses in health care, taught by sympathetic persons in an atmosphere of frank and open discussion. Surveys should be made of public health facilities to see what services they offer and if these services are meeting the needs of the public.

And the key demand for us to organize around is the demand that would enable us to eliminate this whole chapter: we must press for the development of really good forms of birth control and demand their wide dissemination. Abortion is by no means a good method of birth control. It should be used only when a birth-control method fails. Besides the psychological and physical discomfort, it seems that forced dilation of the cervix may weaken the muscles and lead to a small risk of miscarriage or premature birth in subsequent pregnancies. Women should not be coerced into making the choice of whether or not to have an abortion—a choice that for some is so traumatic and painful. The key to what we

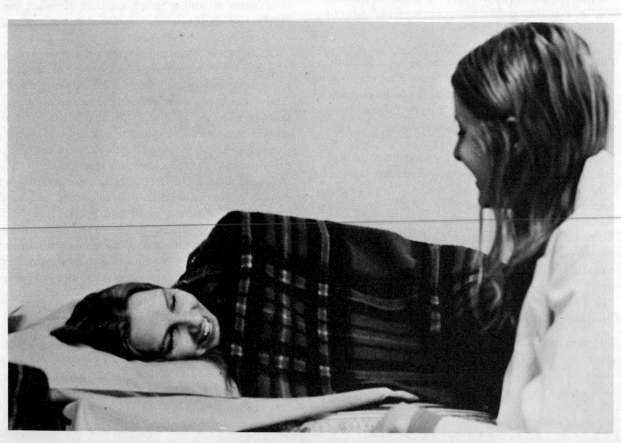

want for ourselves is not to be "allowed" to have abortions, but to have real control of our bodies through safe and foolproof methods of birth control.

TWO PERSONAL EXPERIENCES

1969

Probably the most insidious untruth about abortion is the so-called postabortion guilt feelings on the part of the woman. In fact, many women have been taught to expect and in some perverse way, may welcome, the "cleansing effect" that anticipated postabortion guilt offers them —as though they have to atone for their crime. For, as long as this society fails to recognize and refuses to sanction the right of a woman to have an abortion whenever she chooses to do so, the fear of postabortion self-recriminations represses her as surely and as effectively as any prohibitive law is capable of doing. The problem, then, is how to get women to face the reality of postabortion *feelings* while shaking off the shackles of superimposed guilt feelings. Ironically, guilt, the psychologists tell us, grows out of anger—anger at ourselves for feeling inadequate and unwomanly, but also anger at a society that reveres us as mothers and child raisers, but despises our rights to make the decision not to have a child. Perhaps, then, sharing my personal experience might in some way show my sisters that guilt and its attendant emotions need not follow an abortion.

"I'm sorry," the voice said to me over the phone, "the test was positive." From that moment on I was a changed woman. I was going to become a mother. But was I really, in the true sense of the word? Any woman who has ever conceived understands the mixed emotions I was feeling. Understand, then, the thrill I felt in knowing that life was beginning. My body is constructed to bear children, and it was fulfilling that purpose. But then I was forced to ask myself: Is that *my* purpose as a rational as well as a biological human being, and am I not reacting to a societal stimulus as well as a biological one in feeling good about being pregnant?

For me the answers to these questions resulted in my decision to abort my pregnancy. For I realized that these vague biological stirrings inside of me could never justify giving birth to a child I did not want and was not prepared to raise. Neither was I willing to subject myself to the ordeal of pregnancy and waiting, only to relinquish the child at the end of it all. It's all crystal clear to me now in telling about it. At the time, my decision was not so well thought out, but rather grew out of the conviction that I could not under my circumstances continue

with an unwanted pregnancy. For me the fetus represented an undesirable growth that had to be expelled and with it also any guilt feelings about what I intended to do. Not once did I ever think of the fetus as a human being, but rather as an entity that contained some of the properties and carried the potential for human life in much the same way that a fertilized egg contains the properties and potential for life. If, then, the destruction of a fertilized egg is within our power, why not a fetus?

Finding an illegal abortionist was not easy. The few legal avenues that are open did not even occur to me (I had my abortion in 1967), although I'm sure I would not have qualified for a so-called therapeutic abortion. Like millions of desperate women before me, I went underground. My search led to a registered nurse (I was told) who did illegal abortions. My contact was a woman who had recently undergone an abortion by the R.N. and seemingly had suffered no physical ill effects from it. The negotiating was done entirely through my intermediary, and after settling on the price ($400), the date was fixed. All the while I was not able to pry out of my contact many details about the procedure, which really panicked me. There was no one else to ask, so I went into the thing "cold turkey," and all of my dreaded fears about the physical pain were realized.

The woman came to my apartment on Friday, spread me out on the kitchen table, and inserted a catheter tube up my vagina into my uterus. This, I was told, would in time start the contractions in the uterus that would lead to the expulsion of the fetus. When I questioned the abortionist further, she put me off as though I were undeserving of anything more than what she had just done for me for $400. I had to be content with her vague instructions about what to do when the bleeding began while trying to stifle my anxiety about complications. The entire procedure took about 15 minutes, and her attitude was one of "do the abortion and run." It was apparent that with the exception of two friends who remained with me (who were as ignorant of the process as I was) I was strictly on my own.

And so began a 48-hour ordeal of pain and anguished waiting for it to be over. At that point I had little regard for myself as a worthwhile human being, I was someone to be scorned and avoided—I was a walking, bleeding catheter tube. On Sunday the contractions began, and by the middle of the afternoon it was over. The force of the uterine contractions had dislodged the catheter tube and it slipped out easily and along with it the fetus. Looking at the fetus was an experience I will never forget. I had been approximately two months pregnant, and at that stage the fetus had acquired some of the characteristics of a human being as we know it. It was about an inch long, and I am unable to remember its color. I do remember staring at it in a curious, somewhat detached way; it looked so strange, and indeed it was. Its appearance did not shock or repel me, partially because of the fact that by that time I had shut myself down emotionally and was feeling only relief that it was over.

It was only much later that I was able to internalize how I felt and continue to feel, and then to verbalize, as I have tried to do here. Even now my total emotional reaction to it escapes me, except in one vitally important way. At no time, even in the shadow of societal taboos, did I believe that I was doing something wrong or committing some offense against nature—since, in fact, it is my nature and my right to determine my destiny as a woman. Since that time my confidence in the rightness about my decision has grown and along with it a sense of dignity and self-determination about myself as a woman.

1972

It has become very important for me to write about my abortion, yet it is difficult to know where the beginning is. I am at a place in time where my life, by my own efforts, is beginning to change. After having two children (ages six and seven and a half) reach a point of some adjustment in school I began to feel I needed and wanted more from life. I decided to return to school, to a plan that had been interrupted by my marriage and children. As many women who have gone or will go back to school know, that is a process of awakening within ourselves that is incredibly exciting. After one marvelous year (with at least one to go) I found myself pregnant. I couldn't believe it. It seemed somewhat like a very bad dream that I would wake up from at any time. The idea of a third pregnancy was suffocating. I just couldn't go through another five or six years of intensive child rearing.

I couldn't—didn't want to—talk to anyone about my pregnancy, and I felt really alone. The burden of every anxiety and fear of childbirth, unwanted babies, guilt about abortion, death, life—everything I could possibly lay on myself, I did. I tried to accept the fact that I was pregnant so that I could make plans for my life that included a baby, but all the while I kept hoping for a miscarriage. The idea of abortion—the word—came in and out of my head, and was quickly dismissed. I felt strongly that abortion was not a choice for me. I, as a person I thought I had begun to know, did not have the freedom to make that choice. I had believed abortion was every woman's right, but those were hollow, liberal thoughts for me. It's so easy to be a liberal when you're comfortable. For me abortion was a whole life-death question that I could not bear to settle.

I simply couldn't make a choice. I neither wanted to bear another child nor did I feel I could allow myself the alternative of an abortion, which I believed so strongly was a destructive, violent act. It's important to say that my husband was adamantly opposed to a third child, which didn't help me at all in making a decision. We argued bitterly—I defending anything he was against. We really turned our backs completely on each other, and the support we had so often given to each other was gone. The situation was hopelessly deadening. It's so hard to describe those feelings. I really just wished I could die.

I went to bed at night hoping to wake up to a miscarriage, and I guess it was at this point—when I was down very low—that I realized that I was actually considering an abortion. I saw that my problem was not so much that I was having difficulty adjusting to the idea of a third child but that somewhere in the back of my mind I understood I could make a choice—and that realization was really mind-blowing.

I tried to be really honest with myself; and it seemed that to hope for a miscarriage was about the same as wanting a guilt-free abortion. That's really the way I looked at it. If nature would only expel this fetus, everything would be all right.

I began to talk to other women about myself—my feelings, my life, everything. They were really supportive. I started thinking about myself and what I really wanted. I tried to sort out my feelings—what was real, what were the influences of my Catholic upbringing, society, my husband, myself. I couldn't stop thinking about a fetus as a child—as my six- or seven-year-old playing in the yard. I kept getting very entangled in the sanctity of life: this fetus was growing within me whether I was awake or asleep, all the time. When does one have the right to destroy life, potential or real? When is life real? I wanted to just stop and search a bit for an identity that I thought I had found but that had become confused by the realization that I could consider aborting a fetus. Fetus—to me a child.

I was completely muddled—and I had nowhere to go. But friends kept helping and supporting—women supporting no decision, just me as I was. At about the point when I felt completely spent and done in, I began to think about the responsibility of making a decision. It became clear to me that my confusion was a result of my unconscious desire to avoid making a real decision. I couldn't come around to the reality of the situation. I had to take on the responsibility of saying "I want to have this child and I will accept that" or "I do not want another child and I must accept the responsibility of aborting this fetus." I had to say that I was real, that my life was real and mine and important. Those feelings were very hard to come to. I don't think I believe in them fully even now, but I did begin to think of myself in a direct way, and I began to feel more sure of myself. There was a certain strength in knowing that I could make a choice that was mine alone and be entirely responsible to myself. It became very clear to me that this was not the way to have a child, that in thinking about the sanctity of life I had to think about the outcome of my pregnancy, which would be a human being/child that was not wanted. On the strength that I had begun to feel as a woman I made the decision to have an abortion. There was no decision of right or wrong or morality —it simply seemed the most responsible choice to make. It is still upsetting to me—the logic of it all—but somewhere within me it is still very clear, and I'm still very sure of that decision.

In writing about this now it all seems so simple, but a two-month process that involved a whole spectrum of emotions is incredibly difficult to go back over. The feelings all are still within me but very hard to express verbally.

After I made my decision to have the abortion I had a great deal of support from some beautiful women who helped me over a lot of bumps. That support became very crucial to me—I'll never forget it.

My feelings the day of the abortion were in some ways very much numbed and at the same time quite clear. I was very sure of my decision that day, much more than at any other time, but my emotions were somewhat shut down. Perhaps it was in self-defense; I had questioned my decision so many times that I just had to stop. I remember thinking the next day that what had happened to me had nothing to do with my concept of the word "abortion" and all the images that word brings into one's head. What in reality had happened was that I had become a person I control—someone who is able to say, "This is the way my life must go." I was fully awake during my abortion, and although it was difficult to go through, it was especially important, because I felt in control of the situation. I had made my decision and was able to carry it through without losing touch with what was happening to my body. (Also, being awake and aware alleviates some of those fantasies about what has happened to you, what a fetus may look like, and so on.) I also had a woman friend with me throughout the abortion, which was a really beautiful thing. Mentioning her in one sentence can give no indication of the feelings we shared, but because of her and because of two very loving friends who accompanied me to New York, I remember that day as one of strength.

In retrospect, my feelings are very contrary and complex—some high, some low. I do not feel guilt—almost rather guilty over my astonishing (to me) lack of guilt. I have felt at many times very strong and sure in my identity as a woman—a very real person.

In this beginning (again) to try and know myself, it has become very clear to me that it is essential for women to be open with one another; that the sharing of experiences, anxieties, fears, and laughter makes us feel we are not alone but one in a unity shared by all women. Before I had my abortion I wondered how I would feel about the women I would meet at the clinic. It all seems so strange now, but I felt that I had made my decision —could I accept theirs as well? What actually happened when I walked in the waiting room was that I became all those women and they were me, and the experience we shared together as women will never be forgotten— it is rather a very sustaining remembrance.

FURTHER READINGS

Caillouette, James C., and Thomas Callister. "Practical Management of Septic Abortion," *Hospital Medicine*, Vol. 6, No. 1, January 1, 1970.

Cherniak, Donna, and Allan Feingold, eds. *Birth Control Handbook.*
Production by the workers of Journal Offset, Inc., Montreal, Can., 1971.

Committee on Psychiatry and Law. *The Right to Abortion: A Psychiatric View.* New York: Charles Scribner's Sons, 1970.

Ebon, Martin, ed. *Abortion.* New York: Pocket Books, 1971.

Lader, Lawrence, *Abortion.* Boston: Beacon Press, 1967.

Nemy, Enid. "Even Now, Helping with Abortions Is Traumatic Shock for Some Nurses," *The New York Times*, February 1, 1973, p. 32.

"On Abortion and Having Children," *Women's Health and Abortion Project Newsletter*, Vol. 1, No. 10 (November-December 1971). 36 W. 22 Street, New York, N.Y. 10010.

Schulder, Diane, and Florynce Kennedy. *Abortion Rap.* New York: McGraw-Hill, 1971.

"Who Shall Live," *Man's Control over Birth and Death.* Report prepared for the American Friends Service Committee. New York: Hill and Wang, 1970.

Women's Health and Abortion Project Pamphlets, 36 W. 22 Street, New York, N.Y. 10010: *Abortion in New York City, 1970–71, Vacuum Aspiration Abortion, Saline Abortion,* and others.

12
Deciding Whether to Have Children

BOTH WE and our children fare better when conception is chosen freely out of a desire for a child to love and care for, and not as a means to fulfill other needs—for identity, security, and social approval. But those of us who have no children, many of us who are pregnant, and those of us who have children—whether we are living with men, other women, or in a group, or living alone and raising our children alone—all experience a lot of confusion about motherhood.

Those of us who have children, often don't fully understand the reasons why we had them. Many of us have a sense that biological and social pressures pushed us into motherhood before we had had a chance to develop into whole human beings. Motherhood and the living situations in which we are being mothers make us feel restricted. We need time and space to grow, ourselves, but these are hard to find. If we don't have children yet, it is legitimate and good to wait until we feel ready, or to choose not to have children at all. Yet our society doesn't give much moral support for such decisions.

What are some of the social pressures for motherhood? We grow up in a society that leads us to believe that we will find our ultimate fulfillment as women-people by living out our reproductive function. There is a widespread idea that because women have the special biological ability to bear children, that is what all normal women should do, regardless of our individual talents. Our parents, our institutions and their mouthpieces, the media and advertising, persuade us from birth that we must be pretty to attract men so that we can get married and have homes and children. At the same time, we are discouraged from trying to express ourselves in the world of work. Our society makes use of us in our homes as free domestic labor and in the work force doing the boring and dead-end jobs.

This same society neglects to make legally and economically accessible the tools for our control of pregnancy—birth control and abortion; so when we are quite young we are surprised by intense sexual feelings, which

we had not been told about, and then trapped by the biological efficiency of the reproductive process. Many of the mechanisms by which our society encourages/coerces women to have children are hangovers from a time when population growth was nationally desirable. Population growth is no longer a national goal, but promotherhood influences are still strong.

Societal pressures, internalized, become psychological pressures. Because our opportunities, hence our motivations, are limited, we ourselves often begin to believe that in motherhood we will find greater satisfaction than as students, workers, artists, political activists, or doctors. Many of us become pregnant because there is little else that we feel we can do well. Motherhood is the course of least resistance. Tired of looking for jobs and trying to decide who we are, we look forward to pregnancy and motherhood as a time when we can put our identity crises on the shelf and relax, secure in the "legitimacy" of our maternal role. Yet our essential selves don't give up. The confusion and unhappiness that many of us feel at least some of the time when faced with motherhood can be positive indications to us that our total selves, not just our mother-selves, are struggling to make themselves heard.

We make the actual decision to have a child for many different reasons.

* * *

I had a gut desire to have a child. It took me so long to have a successful pregnancy. And all my friends had children.

* * *

I had this idea at the back of my mind, which I didn't come to terms with until pregnancy—I didn't want to get a job, I wanted to stay home with a baby.

* * *

Part of my reason for having a baby is that I'd been thinking a lot about death, and I wanted something that would assure my immortality.

* * *

I wanted a daughter, because I wanted to raise her differently than I'd been raised.

* * *

I was afraid I'd grow old without having done anything.

* * *

I was afraid our marriage would break up if we didn't have a baby to hold us together.

* * *

I needed to know that I wasn't sterile.

* * *

I was ready to be pregnant because I had nothing else to do, and I figured I'd have to have a baby sometime. My husband wasn't too enthusiastic, but I decided to anyway, and he went along with it because he figured that since it's a "woman's role" to raise kids, the decision should be mine.

* * *

My husband kept asking when we were going to have a baby. He wanted a child to carry on his name.

* * *

I had no one to love. I wanted someone who would love me and depend on me more than anyone else. (What I didn't know was that a baby couldn't provide me with other kinds of love I needed just as much—self-love, and love of a peer and companion.)

* * *

I was alone in the apartment while my husband worked all day. I was lonely.

* * *

I had a baby before I was ready to take on the job of it, partly because no one ever really told me what a big and total job it is. I had never spent much time with children or infants, so I had no idea what a life change was involved.

* * *

Most of us who spoke above felt that whether or not we have now come to terms with our motherhood, we got pregnant for the wrong reasons. But we also have a strong sense that there are *good* reasons why some—not all—of us may want to have children. We may want to live through the total experience of childbearing and child rearing; we may want to learn from our children how to experience life directly; we may believe in and love ourselves so much that we want to extend our spirits and our ways into the future—being careful, however, to let our children be themselves: we may simply want to share our love with and to enjoy our children.

* * *

I've learned to stop and watch my kids. All the energy I've put into getting in touch with the child in me I use now to stop and just listen to all the messages my children are giving me. . . . I feel like it's taken me a good part of both my kids' lives to learn to enjoy them. It's as

if one day I woke up and said, "Hey, there are two people here." The more I've treated them more like people, the more they've become separate from me. I feel like I don't have to be doing all the giving; they have been giving me a lot of attention all the time, but I haven't been seeing that. That giving and receiving between parent and child is different from that with my friends.

* * *

How to make the choice clearly? A good general rule is to try to see clearly whether we are expecting our children to make up for serious lacks in ourselves and in our lives. Can we fill these lacks in other ways? If we can, and we still want children, then our reasons are probably good. It makes sense to find out if we like being with kids; we should test ourselves by caring for friends' children or helping in a play or preschool group. Occasional baby-sitting isn't a fair trial; we should try to get into a situation where we really take responsibility for someone else's kids, and then take a lot of time to examine our feelings about being with children. We should talk with friends who have borne children and friends who have adopted them and friends who have none.

Still another important thing to consider is the living situation in which we'll be raising the child. So far in this country the monogamous nuclear family, husband and wife, is the only socially sanctioned and socially affirmed place/home/environment in which to bring up children. But motherhood in the splendid isolation of the autonomous nuclear household can be lonely and difficult. If the father has a full-time job, total responsibility for child care falls on the mother; even if the father is at home some of the time there is, for many of us, continual arguing and maneuvering over who should take care of the children at certain times and whose responsibility it really is. If we plan to have children in a nuclear family, we should look into possibilities of sharing child care and other domestic work with neighbors. And we should be sure to talk with our husband or the father-to-be *before* we become pregnant, to see if we can work out some basic agreements about sharing the care as well as the pleasure of our child.

Some of us, wary of marital-nuclear family life or separated or divorced from a bad marriage experience, choose to be or find ourselves to be single mothers. Right now the life of a single mother with children is terribly difficult unless she has many helpful and supportive friends and unless the father of the children spends time with them and helps to support them. For too many of us, feeling lonely and vulnerable, the choice is to try to squeeze by on welfare. Or we take a job that means we'll pick up our children at five, arrive home tired, clean the house, feed the children, find time and energy to play with them and really *be with* them . . . and what's left for us? And we constantly run up against the social stigma attached to mothers and babies without husbands and fathers. It's even harder for those of us who are lesbians or who identify primarily with women.

For both married couples with children and single women with children, communes are an alternative place to live in, so that the whole burden of child rearing doesn't fall on the mother or on the mother and father.

* * *

Lisa has become such a warm, open, self-sufficient girl. She doesn't cling to me as she used to. She seeks attention from other adults almost as much as from me. She has her own world with the other children here. . . . And then there's me. I have more time for myself. It's a new freedom I still have trouble getting used to although we've been here over a year. I sometimes forget that I don't have to run to meet Lisa's needs; she can and will turn to others here. My time with her has been much "better quality" time.

* * *

Communal child rearing challenges our ability to move out of some old restrictive ways of looking at parenthood. How do we begin to share the responsibility for raising our children? How do we trust other adults to do right by them? How do we encourage our children to turn to and respond to others? And whether we do or do not have children of our own, what do we risk by becoming very close to another's child? How will we or the child feel if the commune breaks up and we must separate? How do we deal with feelings of "interfering" and begin to share in a whole new responsibility for raising a child we didn't give birth to? There are no easy answers, but some of us feel that our lives and the lives of our children will be better if we accept the challenge of communal living.

Many of the factors that will influence our childbearing decision are beyond our individual control. We must join together and work, therefore, to make some changes in our society so that the decision of whether and when to have children will be a free and clear one for all of us. No one should have to make the choice that many of us must make today between commitment to motherhood and to serious work, or between earning enough money to support our children and seeing them enough to really feel like their mother. We need child care at our jobs and twenty-four-hour community-controlled child care in our neighborhoods; we need paternity leaves for fathers, as in Sweden; we need to have half-time jobs accepted as the norm, so both parents can live fully human lives. We would like to see guaranteed income for all individuals, so that a woman who wants to have children is not forced to be financially dependent on a man.

Some of us will decide that we want to wait to have children.

* * *

I want to have children when I can appreciate them and love them for what they are: separate people who will develop their own ways. . . . I'm afraid I would not be able to relate to them without imposing my neurotic needs on them. . . . I want to be strong, so that my daughter will see that a woman can be strong. Being strong means working out my feelings of passivity and masochism. It means being able to be alone without fear. It means separating my sexual powers from my total life energy, so that I don't use my sexuality in an aggressive way toward my child. . . . I know that I'm not strong enough now to fulfill infant needs for love, nourishment, protection, and limits and guidance.

* * *

Some of us have decided not to have children, and we need a lot of support in this decision.

* * *

The fact of being an only child makes it hard for me to choose not to have children. My parents have been very understanding, but in many ways they let me see how much they would like a grandchild. I would like to make them happy, but I do not want that to be a prime reason for bearing a child. . . . I see my decision as very much my own to make, because mothers have so much of the responsibility for care of the young in this society, and are required to give so much of their emotional lives to their children. Women have been programmed to put other peoples' needs before their own. I have always had trouble doing this—I have always seen my life as my own. . . .

When I lived with three other family units in a commune for a year I became very upset by the quality and emotional content of much of the parent-child interaction. I saw the high levels of anxiety that these parents had, and their inability to deal with their own emotions openly with the children. I think I got a glimpse of the nightmare that some women experience when they have to cope with meeting the emotional needs of several children. . . .

After I made the decision not to have children I felt an enormous sense of control over my life. . . . I could pursue my life goals as a stronger person because I had come to terms with myself. I got from the women's movement a lot of strength and a sense that women must be free to determine their own life patterns and their own destinies without suffering lifelong guilt for not having lived up to society's or their family's expectations.

* * *

13
Childbearing

INTRODUCTION

WE WANT to understand our childbearing experience. We literally have been kept in the dark about what we can expect physically and emotionally when we conceive and give birth to our children.

We have needs that are not being met. One great need we have is to experience our childbearing year as a continuum. This continuum begins with conception and our decision to carry our child to term. It includes pregnancy, labor, and delivery, the period immediately after our child is born and the postpartum period. (Adjustments may last up to a year or more after birth.) We have a great need for knowledgeable medical care, which begins early in pregnancy and sometimes continues for several months after our child is born. And we need personal support, one or more people to be with us and support us throughout the whole cycle.

The present medical system doesn't provide for these needs. Pretending to help us, it tends to interfere with natural processes. For instance, doctors and hospitals have set what to us are artificial boundaries. Each period of childbearing is handled by a different set of "experts." During our pregnancy we see one private doctor or a series of doctors or nurses in a clinic. We might deliver our baby with someone we know or with someone we've never seen before. After the birth we're cared for by a new set of attendants and nurses, while our baby will have his or her own doctor. When we come home we don't have a doctor anymore, and we care for ourselves or depend on family or friends. So an experience that could be a unified one is all broken up. We begin to rely on one person or set of people, then we are shunted to another set.

In this country we are denied control over our own very personal childbearing experience. Childbirth, which could be as much a part of our everyday lives as pregnancy and child care, is removed to an unfamiliar place for sick people.* There we are separated at a crucial time from family and friends. We and our present children suffer from this sudden removal; to our children it's a mysterious absence. In the hospital we are depersonalized; usually our clothes and personal effects, down to glasses and hairpins, are taken away. We lose our identity. We are expected to be passive and acquiescent and to make no trouble. (Passivity is considered a sign of maturity.) We are expected to depend not on ourselves but on doctors. Most often for the doctor's convenience, we are given drugs to "ease" our labor. (We have let ourselves be convinced by doctors who have never experienced labor and by our unprepared frightened forebears that our labor will be too painful to bear.) After our baby is born s/he is taken away for an hour, for a day, or longer. We pay a lot of money for our hospital space, sometimes more than we can afford.

Our obstetricians are trained mainly to deal with complications of childbirth. "Well," we say, "you never know. Something might happen. We need our doctor." We are afraid on many levels. We have been taught to have very little confidence in ourselves, our bodies, in other women's experience. In fact, 95 percent of our deliveries are normal. Most of us could very easily give birth with the experience and help of a trained midwife, either in a hospital, a special maternity house, or at home among family and friends. However, emergency equipment must be present or ready.

We want to improve maternity care for ourselves and all women by calling into question the present care we receive. This care interferes with the rhythm of our lives. It turns us into objects. We want to be able to choose where and how we have our babies. We want adequate flexible medical institutions that correspond to our needs.

*Lester Hazell states: "Pregnancy, labor and delivery are states unto themselves but they are by no means illnesses" (*Commonsense Childbirth*, p. xxxiv.) In France women go to special maternity houses—not hospitals—to have their babies.

In addition to the medical context of our child-bearing year, our society's attitudes toward pregnancy and motherhood, internalized by us, can color and distort our experience of pregnancy, delivery, and postpartum. There is a huge gap between the reality of pregnancy and motherhood—often exciting, but also often hard and often depressing—and the glorious myths that have shaped our expectations.

Voicing some of the most common and pernicious myths, here are some paragraphs from a booklet—written by a man—which is handed out by doctors to pregnant women:

A woman is likely to glow and look more beautiful during this period while her body is fulfilling its ultimate physical function. For each woman pregnancy has its own unique mystery, emotional response and contentment. Yet, while every mother-to-be differs in these respects, there are innumerable experiences which are common to all. They bind every woman into that exclusive sorority called Motherhood.

. . . .

Doctors who devote their practice to the care of pregnant women report again and again how amazing it is to observe a girl become a woman physically and emotionally in nine months. For many, the prospect of motherhood makes them mature. They become poised, proud, confident and beautiful. Nature, in her own mysterious manner, seems to have devised an intricate balance that prepares the body for a baby and the mind for acceptance of motherhood. A conscientious woman responds to these responsibilities. She uses them to become a better person and a contributor to the growth of society.*

We take issue with several of these myths and mistruths.

1. "A woman is likely to glow and look more beautiful during this period . . ." Such a glorification of a pregnant woman's looks leaves no room for the times when we feel ugly, for feelings like "I'm so fat and cumbersome," or "My husband looks at other women because my belly is so big."

2. ". . . her body is fulfilling its ultimate physical function." In other words, at some point in our lives we are supposed to become pregnant. Society puts great pressure on us to have babies, and smiles approvingly when we become pregnant. If we've become pregnant accidentally, if we have negative feelings about being mothers, if we don't feel ready, society doesn't answer us except with its continuous congratulatory smile. We are forced to smile in answer, covering up our more complicated feelings, and we tend to deny ourselves our legiti-

mate anxieties; then sometimes they appear after our child is born in forms we're not prepared to handle.

3. "For each woman pregnancy has its own unique mystery." It's true that for each of us pregnancy will mean something different. We'll experience it on many levels, from a deep sense of creativity and an awareness of process and unity to having to pee more often than we did before. However, we have to beware of society's tendency to mystify what is happening to us. For one thing, people tend to fall back on words like "mystery," "ultimate," "beautiful experience"; or they push it really far and refer to "that exclusive sorority called Motherhood." Mystifying words and attitudes keep us ignorant, immobile, and passive at a time when we most need to know specific details about what to expect and what to do. Why such mystification? Women, who menstruate bloodily, carry children in their wombs as animals do, give birth with obvious effort and some discomfort, are close to nature. But our male-dominated culture is threatened by this physicality and creates pretty myths about us which we come to believe.

4. "For many, the prospect of motherhood makes them mature." Propaganda. We don't grow up by being pregnant. We have a lot of the child still in us. Both pregnancy and childbearing bring out in us long-buried childhood feelings.

5. "Nature, in her own mysterious manner, seems to have devised an intricate balance that prepares the body for a baby and the mind for acceptance of motherhood." Propaganda again. Nature doesn't whisper to us the things we need to know. Unlike animals, for instance, we have to learn what kinds of food to eat so that we will remain healthy and the baby will grow optimally. It's by our own effort and striving in our heads and hearts that we prepare ourselves for motherhood. No mystery about it. For too many years we have been confused, because we've been expected to know instinctively what to do both before and after our child is born.

6. "A conscientious woman responds to these responsibilities. She uses them to become a better person and a contributor to the growth of society." These days, in this world, lots of new babies aren't needed. But this man is saying to us: "Your maturity consists in understanding what your role is. [Because you are biologically able to bear children.] You are to be mothers and wives and stay at home, and be proud of making your contribution to society in that way." This is another form of the "biology is destiny" argument. There's a you'd-better-toe-the-line-or-else tone to this last sentence.

All of these myths provide us with socially backed "positive" attitudes toward pregnancy and motherhood which blur our thinking and feeling about ourselves. It has been important to us to help each other to name and

*William Birch, *A Doctor Discusses Pregnancy*. Budlong Publishing Company, Chicago, Illinois, 1966.

reject such myths about childbearing, in order to connect with the real experiences of our pregnancies and to accept our often mixed feelings about being pregnant and about being mothers.

There are many steps we can take as we move to become more active, conscious, and critical participants in our childbearing experience. We have to learn as much as we can about pregnancy, childbirth, and mother and child care (care of ourselves and our children after birth). We have to educate ourselves, arming ourselves with all kinds of knowledge so we can make our own choices. Too often in a critical situation we're not aware we have choices. We need to prepare ourselves by getting a lot of how-to information to cope with specific situations during each phase of childbearing. With our own knowledge we can actually prevent certain complications from ever arising.

We must assume more control over what happens to us in and out of hospitals during our time of childbearing. We must work from the inside to make hospitals more humane places in which to have our babies. We desperately need more good, humane doctors, and especially more women doctors. And we must work from the outside in for the development and legalization of midwife services, neighborhood clinics—which will give us decentralized and more personal services—and efficient mobile medical units, which could operate within each neighborhood so that we could have our babies more naturally and cheaply and safely at home. We must also work on and along with doctors and nurses to demystify, to deprofessionalize medicine, so that we become more at one with what happens to us. (At the end of the "Childbearing" chapter, "Some Proposals for Change," p. 218, see the list of demands and suggestions for change that we have put together over the past three years.)

In this unit we divide our discussion into three parts, pregnancy, childbirth and postpartum care, because there are specific things we need to know and do during each period. It's crucial to remember that each phase is interconnected with the others.

SECTION ONE: PREGNANCY

A PREVENTIVE PROGRAM: WHAT YOU CAN DO TO PREPARE YOURSELF

Taking Care of Yourself:
Choice, Commitment, Preparation, Feelings, Emotional Needs

Some of you decide to have a child and soon afterward become pregnant. Clearly you have chosen before conceiving to become pregnant.

* * *

We wanted to be pregnant for a lot of reasons. We had made love for two years without birth control. We weren't sure we could have a baby. I was really happy when we finally were trying to have a baby.

* * *

I had a gut desire to have a child. It took me so long to have a successful pregnancy. I was living alone. I was lonely. A desire for a life-style change.

* * *

Some of you become pregnant unexpectedly, without feeling ready, without being ready. You haven't chosen to conceive.

In either case pregnancy begins physiologically at the moment of conception.

If you have planned your pregnancy, when you find you are pregnant you know you have already chosen to keep your baby. If you haven't planned your pregnancy, when you find you are pregnant you have to decide whether or not you will continue your pregnancy. When you decide to continue it you have made your first crucial choice—to be pregnant. Sometimes it takes a few months to make this choice. Some women let time decide.

* * *

After three months I knew my pregnancy was irrevocable, I wasn't going to end it. I felt it was taken out of my hands.

* * *

I didn't want to have another abortion, I really was amused by the idea of having a kid; I wanted a kid. I didn't feel I could ever consciously decide to have a kid, I didn't know what grounds to base that decision on.

* * *

The pregnancy is established now in each case. You have chosen to let the pregnancy run its course.

You make a second kind of choice when you think of how you want to be pregnant, when you decide to deal with all the kinds of changes that childbearing involves. This commitment can come at any point—at the beginning, middle, or even toward the end of your pregnancy. If your pregnancy was unexpected you might be so confused and so hassled that for a long time you drift along not being able to think clearly. It's not uncommon during pregnancy to feel often out of control. It's to your advantage that you take on/assume/choose your pregnancy as early as possible, for the more you know about the process (what's happening in and to your body) and about your feelings, the more you can be in control of what happens during pregnancy, childbirth, and the postpartum time.

The first step in planning to have your first child begins with planning for a fundamental change in your life. It's not easy to experience beforehand what that change will mean. Your body and mind will change during your pregnancy, your life will change with the birth of your child. A new being will enter your home, someone unknown, whose temperament may be totally unlike yours, and whose needs and demands remain constant day in and day out.

Think of these changes and then take advantage of every tool and every scrap of information available. Use what used to be thought of as a time of "waiting," of simple passivity, to prepare for the changes ahead.

For many of us it has been important to spend time with sympathetic people during our pregnancy—to be in contact, talking, sharing work, checking feelings and questions. But in this society it can be hard to move out of isolation. In our middle-class-oriented industrial culture we usually marry and move away from our families and friends. We are often isolated in our nuclear cells—apartments and houses. In our isolation it's hard to find other pregnant women to talk to. It's frustrating, because we have lots to talk about.

It can be hard to bring up our questions and anxieties, because our bodily functions are often treated as taboo subjects. And if we save these questions for doctors or nurses, most often they can't answer us satisfactorily. Usually they don't know the things we need to know, aren't aware of feelings we may be having, or can't really take the time to speak with us. So we have to make an effort to talk among ourselves. (One thing to be a little careful about as we turn to each other for information and support is that some people who offer information and advice can misinform us or frighten us needlessly with stories of their own pregnancies and births, which they themselves didn't understand.)

During pregnancy we need to depend on someone.

* * *

You have to know how to ask for help. It's all right to ask, even for a cup of tea. Most of the time I had a lot of energy and was able to do things for myself, but there were times when I was really tired and I really didn't want to do physical things. The thing to aim for is instead of denying that the pregnancy makes a difference, just admit it. It made me aware of my own physical limitations.

* * *

At the beginning I felt independent. But toward the fifth month, when we came back from vacation, Dick went to work, and I felt very isolated from the "real" world.

Then I had no one. I needed to be able to talk to people, and I wasn't talking to people.

* * *

You need to make a continuity for yourself. If you can, find one or more supportive women or men to share your whole experience with, to lean on at times of need and stress, to whom you can easily say, "I need you."

* * *

I depended on my mother and two friends. One friend had factual information that I trusted.

* * *

Often it's hard to ask your man for this kind of support. He might be too busy, not able to cope too helpfully with your problems—and then, he's not a woman. But it's still good to have him involved as much as possible in your pregnancy, as he will be living with all the joys and problems of your childbearing and he'll need preparation too.

Some of you will be isolated on farms, in mountains, in suburbs. Maybe you feel more isolated than you need to feel. Maybe close by there are people to talk to. Some your seeking out other people or groups. If you do have only your doctor or your clinic to depend on, try to find out as much as possible about all that is happening to you.

This emphasis on preparation may begin to sound repetitious. But one thing we don't concentrate on enough —our society doesn't teach us to do so intelligently—is the fact that establishing a new human being, especially during the early weeks and months of its life, is an extremely complicated, demanding piece of work. So keeping your health and sanity is vitally important.

It's also important to realize that no matter how well prepared and ready you feel at each step, something unexpected will usually happen. At least the knowledge you have will help you be more open, more flexible, more able to meet new situations with confidence.

And, finally, don't knock yourself out as you learn about yourself. There will be enough time. Take it easy.

Taking Care of Your Physical Needs

There are three crucial ways for you to take care of your physical needs during pregnancy (thus helping you feel better emotionally). First you must see a doctor as early in your pregnancy as possible so that he/she can give you a complete physical checkup. Most serious complications can be prevented by a combination of your knowledge and his/hers. Those of us who work all day or who live far from hospitals or who can't find or afford baby-sitters have a hard time getting prenatal health care. But given the present health-care system in this country, we know that it is up to us to seek and find the care we need. For guidelines to this search see the section

"Choosing and Using Medical Care" in the chapter on "Women and Health Care" (p. 242). Prenatal care is a form of preventive medicine, for when we are pregnant we are not sick. Our goal in seeing our doctor is to prevent sickness.

Second, it is good to exercise to develop and strengthen your body.

Third, you must eat well throughout your pregnancy. This is what we're going to discuss next.

Nutrition

Eating well as an example of prevention. You are pregnant now. You have to eat nutritious food. By eating well you'll help prevent some minor discomforts and help guard against some major illnesses in yourself and your baby. Studies in progress and studies made over the past forty years show that eating well is vitally important to ensure the health of your growing body. In this section we'll talk about (1) good nutrition (some facts and figures); (2) a good diet for your pregnancy; (3) why these foods are important; (4) controversy about nutrition; (5) gaining weight; (6) toxemia; (7) edema; (8) diuretics; (9) diet pills; (10) salt; (11) the effects of drugs on pregnancy; and (12) nutrition as a political issue.

Good nutrition—some facts and figures. In general, doctors and obstetricians know very little about the role of nutrition in pregnancy. (In the ob/gyn examinations medical students have to take before becoming doctors there is no question relating to nutrition.) And often they may seriously misinform us about our diets and about medication.

There is strong evidence that if we eat well, we bear strong, large, lively babies. During World War II in Great Britain pregnant women were given priority in food-rationing programs, and even under adverse conditions the stillbirth rate fell from 38 per 1,000 live births to 28—a decrease of about 25 percent.

If women eat well during pregnancy and gain weight, there's much more chance that the baby's weight will be adequate. It should be obvious that if the baby's birth weight is adequate, the baby is less apt to die or get sick after birth. Women and babies from poor homes are most vulnerable to disease and complications, never having had adequate medical care or adequate diet. The incidence of low-birth-weight infants is affected by (a) the socioeconomic status of the mother; (b) biologic immaturity—if a girl is under seventeen years of age her baby will more likely weigh less than it should; (c) low weight gain during pregnancy; (d) poor nutrition; (e) infections, and (f) chronic disease.* Good nutrition, then, helps prevent stillbirth, low birth weight, and prematurity from low birth weight. It also helps prevent infections, anemia in mothers, and brain damage and retardation in babies.

A good diet for your pregnancy. Every day you must eat: (a) one quart (four glasses) of milk—low-fat, whole, or buttermilk (equivalents such as cottage cheese and yogurt are fine; skim milk is less good); (b) two eggs; (c) one or two servings of fish, liver, chicken, lean beef, lamb, pork, or cheese (alternatives are dried beans, peas, or nuts); (d) one or two servings of fresh green leafy vegetables—mustard, collard, or turnip greens, spinach, lettuce, or cabbage, or fresh-frozen vegetables; (e) two or three slices of whole-wheat bread; (f) a piece of citrus fruit or glass of lemon, lime, orange, or grapefruit juice; and (g) one pat of margarine, vitamin-enriched. Also (a) four times a week a serving of whole-grain cereal—Wheatena, farina, or oatmeal; (b) five times a week a yellow or orange-colored vegetable; (c) liver once a week; and (d) three times a week a baked potato.

Why these foods are important. All these foods together contain combinations of proteins, vitamins, and minerals that are crucial to your health and must remain in a certain balance in order for your body to function well and for you to provide good materials for the growth of your baby.

PROTEIN (meat, fish, eggs, milk, beans, and cheese). You've got to eat high-protein foods. Protein contributes to build tissue, a solid placenta, and a strong uterus. It keeps the blood sugar, the immediate source of body energy, at a high level. It furnishes amino acids. You'll need about 80–100 grams of protein a day.

VITAMIN A (vegetables, whole milk, fortified milk) builds up resistance to infection, strengthens mucous membranes, and has a vital function in your vision. Vegetables are good laxatives.

VITAMIN B (bread, whole grains, liver, brewer's yeast, wheat germ) is said to help to prevent nervousness, skin problems, lack of energy, constipation, and changes of pigmentation in your skin.

VITAMIN C (citrus fruits) detoxifies the junk foods you eat, takes care of poisons produced by bacteria and viruses, keeps capillary and cell walls strong, and builds a strong placenta. It helps absorb iron from the gut and acidifies urine.

VITAMIN D (sunshine, vitamin D-fortified milk, or fish-liver oil) works with calcium to strengthen bones and tissues, helping the calcium to be absorbed from the blood into tissue and bone cells.

VITAMIN E (whole grains, corn, peanuts, eggs) governs the amount of oxygen your body uses. You use more oxygen than you need to if you lack vitamin E. It promotes healing and influences the metabolism of vitamin A.

---

* "Maternal Nutrition and the Course of Pregnancy," p. 4.

VITAMIN K is necessary to the clotting mechanism. Vitamin K is synthesized by gut bacteria and doesn't come directly from food.

FOLIC ACID (leafy green vegetables). Symptoms of folic-acid deficiency are anemia and fatigue. Excessive folic-acid deficiency can lead to nerve damage. Orally administered folic acid can remedy the deficiency. Essential for protein synthesis in early pregnancy; also essential for blood formation.

IRON (liver, raisins, dark molasses, fish, egg yolks, meat). You need vitamin B to use properly the iron you get. Iron is a main component of hemoglobin, and the blood hemoglobin, composed of complex molecules of protein and iron, carries oxygen to your baby and your cells. The baby also draws on your iron reserve to store iron in its liver to last for the duration of her/his milk diet after birth. Also during labor you'll need a lot of oxygen (supplied by hemoglobin) for your uterus; the baby's brain cells need oxygen too. Your own iron stores are seldom large enough to meet the requirements of pregnancy, and many young women are already iron-deficient before pregnancy. Food rarely provides enough iron. Most doctors prescribe ferrous sulfate as an iron supplement.

CALCIUM (milk, stone-ground grain). Sleeplessness, irritability, muscle cramps, nerve pains, and uterine ligament pains can be signs of lack of calcium. You can take extra pills—calcium gluconate or calcium lactate. They should be taken on an empty stomach with sour milk or yogurt. Vitamin C (acid fruit or juice) helps in the absorption of calcium and iron. *All of us must insist that our doctors give us iron, calcium, and folic-acid supplements in the form of pills.* By taking them we are sure to prevent serious deficiencies.

ZINC AND COBALT (seafoods) are trace minerals, which are necessary to the building of certain enzymes that speed chemical reactions.

CALORIES. You need calories to carry on your life and your pregnancy. You can't get good nutrition without calories, but it's calories without nutrition that you need to avoid, like sweets (candies and cakes). Severe caloric restriction is potentially harmful. Women under seventeen especially need a lot of calories as they are still growing. And toward the end of pregnancy everyone needs more calories.

FLUIDS. Drink six to eight glasses daily. Water aids the circulation of blood and body fluids. It helps the distribution of mineral salts and stimulates the digestion and assimilation of foods.

It's important to know that the nearer most foods are to their native state, the higher their food value. (See chapter on "Nutrition," p. 75).

Controversy about nutrition. Our doctors don't agree with one another about the role of nutrition in pregnancy. While all doctors do agree that we should eat milk, eggs, leafy green vegetables, and fruit, they will disagree about our intake of salt, our weight gain, the number of calories we need, the value or harmfulness of diet pills. Up till now we have accepted our doctors' words as truth. For example, many of us who had children recently were advised not to gain much weight and were put on low-salt, low-calorie diets. We accepted these restrictions without question. We didn't question our doctors intelligently because we didn't have enough information. Now we're learning about a large and growing body of research that criticizes the traditional pregnancy diets we had. We must become acquainted with the findings of this research.

Gaining weight. Now you are eating well, and you find you are gaining weight. As your pregnancy advances you might feel voracious. There has been much controversy over whether or not it's O.K. to gain much weight beyond the weight of the uterus, placenta, fetus, and amniotic fluid. Some studies show that as long as your diet is well balanced you may gain extra weight. Again, there is a positive correlation between weight gained during pregnancy by the mother and high weight of the newborn baby. The pattern of your weight gain is more important than the total amount; that is, some women might gain one pound every week, other women two pounds every week. If the pattern remains fairly regular, everything is all right. A sudden large gain after the twentieth to twenty-fourth week, especially if you haven't been eating well, might mean excessive water retention (edema). Be attentive: check your own weight weekly. Weight loss or no gain should be checked by a doctor too.

The main thing to remember is to balance your diet over the whole course of your pregnancy. Even if your doctor has limited you to a twenty-pound weight gain for the entire pregnancy, and you have already gained twenty pounds by the time you're in your seventh month, it's important that you continue to eat well rather than to restrict your diet radically. You'll need vitamins, minerals, proteins, and other nutrients even more toward the end of your pregnancy.

There are two important objections against gaining *a lot* of extra weight. One is that excessive weight gain can put too great a strain on your circulation and your heart. The other is that many women find it very hard to get rid of all that extra weight after the baby is born; and sometimes not being as light as you want can be depressing after all those months of heaviness.

Toxemia. (See also "Toxemia," p. 169.) Many of us are cautioned by our doctors not to gain much weight during pregnancy so that we won't swell up and get toxemia. Most of us have never known exactly what toxemia is.

* * *

During my pregnancy I thought that if my hands or ankles started to swell, something would happen—I would suddenly be in some kind of danger, a danger that I didn't understand.

* * *

[From a description of a clinic] Women . . . were threatened with frightening stories about deaths from toxemia.

* * *

What is toxemia? Metabolic toxemia of late pregnancy (MTLP) is a condition that has several stages: The first stage is characterized by edema (swelling due to water retention), high blood pressure, and protein in the urine. It usually happens after the twentieth to twenty-fourth week of pregnancy. Pre-eclampsia (the first stage) may be mild or severe. In the second stage a woman might have trouble with her vision, or severe headaches. In the most severe state, the eclamptic stage, she might have convulsions and go into a coma. Usually women don't advance into the eclamptic stage if they are receiving medical care.

Whereas the large body of doctors is unsure of the causes of toxemia (in one major obstetrics textbook* there's a long chapter on the subject of eclampsia that contains at least eighteen theories about how the illness is caused, and a related bibliography of one hundred and eighty articles, only three of which deal with nutrition). Dr. Thomas Brewer, who runs a clinic for poor women in California, is convinced after twenty years of study and clinic work that toxemia of pregnancy is caused mainly by malnutrition. When women in his clinic were placed on good diets, the incidence of toxemia dropped radically. M. Bertha Brandt states that "Toxemia may be associated with undernutrition and low total serum proteins" (p. 75).†

"Maternal Nutrition and the Course of Pregnancy" points out that the lower a state's per capita income, the higher the incidence of toxemia and the higher the maternal mortality from toxemia. Mississippi and South Carolina rank fifty-first and fiftieth in low per capita income. Whereas the rate of mothers dying from toxemia per 100,000 live births is 6.2 nationwide, in Mississippi it is 30.2, and in South Carolina 20.3. The author of the above-mentioned textbook, Nicholson J. Eastman, has written a letter to Brewer admitting that malnutrition plays an important and possibly *the* most important part in causing toxemia.

We don't have the medical expertise to evaluate Dr. Brewer's findings, but the facts seem to establish the

credibility of his argument. We also cannot say too strongly that if toxemia has already been systematically prevented by good nutrition, then it's clear that all pregnant women should be well nourished at the very least. Whatever symptoms and sicknesses remain, one known cause of this sickness would be eliminated. Perhaps toxemia itself will disappear, one of those "diseases" that need never be, one of the diseases of an unequal society.

Edema. (See also "Edema," p. 169.) Associated with weight gain during pregnancy is a condition called edema. In edema your body tissues retain water, and this retention causes face, hands, legs, or feet to swell. Doctors in the past and present immediately connect weight gain with toxemia. However, they must make distinctions. They must not confuse accumulation of fat with weight gained as a result of edema. And studies have been made indicating that there are at least two kinds of edema. Physiological edema—which is not serious if your diet is well balanced—involves swelling of the legs, arms, and hands usually at the end of the day. There is also a condition called pathological edema, similar to "hunger swelling," which occurs if you have been deprived of protein, vitamins, minerals, and salt. A doctor must first correctly distinguish between these two kinds of edema by analyzing your nutritional intake and by applying various other methods of diagnosis.

Diuretics. Too often doctors will automatically give you diuretics (water pills) if you have edema. These diuretics may be harmful. They can cause many undesirable side effects in mother and fetus. The immediate effect of these pills is to cause your body to eliminate water excessively. You urinate more. They are dehydrating. Among other things they cause nausea, vomiting, diarrhea, jaundice, muscle spasm, dizziness, headache, and loss of appetite. These diuretics appeared in 1958 and have been pushed by the drug industry, regardless of their effects. However, when wisely used, they can be helpful. Occasionally they are essential.

Diet pills. Diet pills are "speed" (amphetamines). They are drugs. Women who gain weight are sometimes given these pills. They go straight through the placenta to the fetus. They are given to you to kill your appetite, to make you feel good for the moment even when your diet isn't as good as it should be. They only serve to mask problems of poor nutrition. You shouldn't be taking these pills. And if you are eating adequately, you won't need to take them. There are other ways to stop eating too much if you find you are indeed eating too many of the wrong kinds of food. Don't ask your doctor for diet pills.

*N. J. Eastman and L. M. Hellman, *Williams Obstetrics*, 13th edition, Appleton-Century-Crofts.
†Nancy A. Lytle, ed., *Maternal Health Nursing*, 1967, p. 75.

Salt. When you are pregnant you need a certain amount of salt. Salt is stored in fluids outside your cells, and it leaves your body as you perspire. So you need to replenish it. For instance, if you happen to lose some blood and you have adequate salt in your system, then extra salt and water can move into your bloodstream and you don't readily go into shock. Also, if you are preparing to nurse, salt and water mean less dehydration, which is better for milk production. Margaret Robinson did a study in which she found that women on low-salt diets developed leg cramps, and increased salt intake relieved them. You should not avoid salt in ordinary amounts, though it's necessary to avoid oversalted foods, since too much salt can lead to excessive fluid retention. In cases of toxemia, salt can be harmful. It increases hypertension and blood pressure, fluid retention and edema.

Effect of medication. Your decision about whether to use a drug must be a compromise between possible good effects (to you) and possible bad effects (to you, to your baby). It is very important to know that any drug you take gets through the placental barrier to your fetus. Some drugs produce malformations of the fetus (they have teratogenic effects). Some drugs alter the level of hormones in the maternal/fetal circulation and thus alter the function of the placenta. This is a very limited list of drugs and their possible effects:

Narcotics—possible prenatal habit (addiction) formed in fetus.
Some antihistamines (check with your doctor)—may produce malformations (are teratogenic).
General anesthetics—may produce malformations (are teratogenic) at high concentrations.
Cortisone—reaches fetus and placenta and may cause alterations.
Antithyroid—may cause goiter in infants.
Tetracycline—may cause deformities in babies' bones and stain their teeth.

In general, if you are affected by a drug it will get through to your baby.* Try as hard as you can to know what drugs you're taking, and what effects they might have, and take no drugs unless you are convinced they are absolutely needed. This also includes simple over-the-counter "drugs" like aspirin and sleeping preparations.

Nutrition—a political issue. All of us, rich and poor, have to struggle separately and together against ignorance, our own and our doctors'. Our struggle is much greater if we don't have enough money to buy needed foods, if good fresh foods aren't available, if we aren't getting good continuous medical care. We all quickly have to learn what we need and why.

We asked Dr. Brewer how the women he works with manage to get enough of the right foods. He answers:

The women I work with manage because out here in California there is a "welfare system"; vicious as it is, it does provide something . . . as differentiated from many parts of the rural Deep South. Once a woman learns the life-and-death importance of eating enough, she usually manages. The fact that women in my clinic have healthy babies is the best evidence that they do manage. There are exceptions . . . such as a young woman with twins who fell behind in her protein intake and got sick because of it.

We have to fight for an economic system which provides all of us cheaply with essential foods. We have to fight for a medical system which educates its doctors toward providing *preventive* services, and which educates doctors who deal with women about their real needs.

THE PREGNANCY ITSELF

Introduction

During your pregnancy there are two kinds of development: (1) the physical and emotional changes you are going through, and (2) the growth of the fetus within you—two stories going on at once.

Though your pregnancy will have much in common with other women's, it is yours and unique. (And each pregnancy you go through will differ from the others.) In talking to women who have been pregnant and who are pregnant at the same time you are, you will discover that there's no one, right way to be pregnant. Also realize that when we talk about experiencing changes and emotions, there are many exceptions and many combinations.

For instance, many changes will take place in your body as the fetus develops in you. Some of these changes are just changes, some can lead to discomfort. For though we are adapted to bearing children, discomforts can arise, and complications too.* You'll all have changes to deal with. You might feel many discomforts, few, or none at all. You'll want to know what the changes will be, why they occur, when they occur, and any discomforts you

---

*" . . . fresh examples keep accumulating of congenital malformations which follow drug administration in early pregnancy and which presumably are caused by these drugs" ("Cause, Prevention and Treatment," reprinted in Nancy A. Lytle, ed., *Maternal Health Nursing,* p. 193).

*"Regardless of the fact that from a biological point of view childbearing is considered a normal reproductive process, the borderline between health and illness is less distinctly marked during this time because of the numerous physiologic changes that occur in the mother's body during the course of parturition" (Elise Fitzpatrick, *Maternity Nursing,* p. 443).

might feel. Some minor discomforts, if neglected, can lead to major complications.

As for your feelings, they will vary tremendously according to who you are; how you feel about having children; how you feel about your own childhood, your parents, or the people who reared you; whether or not you are with a man—and if you are, how you feel about your man. At each stage you will feel conflicts as well as harmonies. Sometimes you'll feel positive, sometimes negative. You'll have doubts and fears. It's important to know that these doubts and fears occur during a "good" pregnancy too, for in a very real sense your body has been taken over by a process out of your control. You can come to terms with that takeover actively and consciously by knowing what's happening to your body, by identifying your specific feelings (especially the negative ones, because they are the most difficult to deal with), and also by learning what the fetus looks like as it grows. Its growth is dramatic and exciting.

The length of a normal pregnancy can vary from 240 to 300 days. We'll divide our discussion into trimesters (approximately three three-month periods). This division will be relevant for some of you and not for others. Your feelings will ebb and flow and not always follow predictable courses. But since we have so many changes and feelings to talk about, it's more convenient to talk within the framework of trimesters.

The female ovum can be fertilized 12 to 24 hours after leaving the ovary. The fertilized egg takes about 4 to 5 days to reach the uterus. Implantation (attachment to the uterine wall) occurs between 5½ to 7 days.

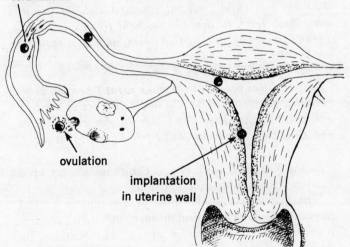

fertilization

ovulation

implantation
in uterine wall

First Trimester

Physical changes. You might have none, some, or many of the following early signs of pregnancy. If you have had regular periods, you will probably miss a period (amenorrhea). However, some women do bleed for the

first two or three months even when they are pregnant, but these periods are usually short and there's scant blood. Also, about seven days or so after conception, the tiny group of cells-to-become-the-embryo, the blastocyst, attaches itself to the uterine wall, and you might have slight vaginal spotting called implantation bleeding, for new blood vessels are being formed.

You might have to urinate more often because of increased hormonal changes; pituitary hormones affect the adrenals, which change the water balance in your body, and you retain more body water. Also, your growing uterus presses against your bladder.

Your breasts will probably swell. They might tingle, throb, or hurt. Your milk glands begin to develop. Because of an increased blood supply to your breasts, veins become more prominent. Your nipples and the area around them (areola) may darken and become broader.

You might feel nauseated, mildly or enough to vomit, partly because your system is changing. One theory is that the higher level of estrogen accumulates even in the cells of the stomach and causes irritation as acids tend

WOMAN IN 6TH WEEK
OF PREGNANCY

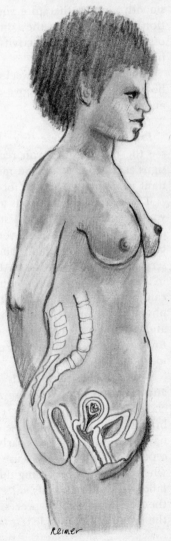

Reimer

to accumulate. The rapid expansion of the uterus may be involved. If you feel nauseated, eat lightly throughout the day rather than taking large meals. Munching crackers or dry toast slowly before you get up in the morning can really help. Avoid greasy, spiced food. Avoid fasting. Apricot nectar helps.

You might feel constantly tired.

You might have increased vaginal secretions, either clear and nonirritating or white, yellow, foamy, or itchy. The chemical makeup as well as the amount of your vaginal fluids is changing. If you are uncomfortable for any reason or if you have questions, see your doctor. (See also the section on "Vaginal Diseases," p. 260.)

The joints between your pelvic bones widen and are made movable about the tenth or eleventh week. Occasionally the separating bones come together and pinch the sciatic nerve, which runs from your buttocks down through the back of your legs.

Your bowel movements might become irregular, both because of the pressure of your growing uterus and again because the heightened amount of progesterone relaxes smooth muscle; therefore your bowels might not function as efficiently as they did. Also, if you are resting often, your decreased activity might cause some constipation.

During the first ten weeks you'll feel relatively few body changes. All the above are fairly common, not too annoying.

Procedures for detecting pregnancy. TESTS. You will see the doctor when you recognize some of the above signs as pregnancy; or you might discover you are pregnant while being checked for something else.

There are pregnancy tests to determine whether or not you are pregnant. These tests might be given by your doctor or by the nurses at your clinic. Or you might go first to a pregnancy lab. Some labs charge $8 for their services. Some charge less. At some you can get results in a few hours, at others you have to wait overnight. You can look up pregnancy labs in the Yellow Pages of your phone book, and perhaps check their prices, promptness, and accuracy through local women's groups. In some towns you can only have pregnancy tests made through local doctors or hospitals.

There are two main kinds of pregnancy tests, biologic and immunologic. Both use a hormone (HCG—human chorionic gonadotropin) secreted by the developing embryo and found in the urine of pregnant women. Pregnancy can be detected as early as three weeks after conception. Both kind of tests use urine. In the biologic tests, when the urine containing this hormone is injected into laboratory animals—rats, mice, rabbits, or frogs—it causes them to ovulate. This process takes a few days, whereas the fastest immunologic test takes only a few seconds. In the latter test, a drop of urine is mixed on a slide with a drop of serum sensitized to it and two drops of another substance; if the hormone HCG from the placenta is present, the mixture won't coagulate.

These tests are 95–98 percent accurate, but can be false if they are performed too early (before there's enough hormone in the urine), if there are technical errors in handling or storing the urine, or if the test animal doesn't respond as it should. Sometimes even if you are pregnant, your first or second tests will be negative. Keep testing. Some women don't show positive signs at all in tests. There are also rare occasions when a pregnancy test can be falsely positive. Usually a diagnosis of pregnancy can be made without these tests. If the test is positive, if you want to keep your baby, and you haven't yet seen a doctor, it's a good idea to see one or go to a clinic as soon as you find out. It's a good preventive measure.

PELVIC EXAM. If you are pregnant (1) the doctor can feel that the tip of the cervix has become softened, (2) he can see that the cervix has changed from a pale pink to a bluish hue because of increased venous blood circulation, (3) the uterus feels softer, and (4) the shape of the uterus changes: where the embryo attaches itself to the inside of the uterus it makes a bulge, which can sometimes be felt on the outside of the uterus.

SOME WOMEN JUST KNOW THEY ARE PREGNANT. Some of us feel we know the moment we become pregnant. Or from one sign—a missed period, tender breasts—we become tuned into the fact that our bodies feel different. Or we find out at the doctor's.

* * *

With my first child I missed a period and my breasts hurt. With Jesse, I knew the moment I conceived him. There's no way of pinning that down, no way of explaining how I felt. I just knew.

* * *

I realized I was pregnant the same night I became pregnant. I lay there all night. I'd had a very active sex life, and it was the first time I had ever felt this way. I wasn't expecting to get pregnant, but I felt different that night.

EXAM SCHEDULE. Doctors and clinics usually set up a fairly routine examination schedule.

The first visit should consist of a complete general physical exam: (1) Medical history; menstrual history; previous babies, pregnancies, operations, abortions, illnesses, drugs taken. (2) General physical exam. It's important that you either bring any previous records that you have, or try to be complete in your description of what's happened to you physically. (3) Exam for pregnancy, which includes (a) examination of your breasts to see if there are changes in the glands; (b) a pelvic examination, as described above, which shows the position and consistency of the uterus, condition of ovaries and fallopian tubes, consistency and color of the cervix; (c) taking a blood sample to determine its type and Rh factor (see Appendix, p. 179) and provide blood for a blood count, hemoglobin analysis, syphilis checkup, and a hematocrit to see if you're anemic or not (right proportion of cells to fluid); (d) urinalysis;* (e) weight and blood pressure checked.

Insist that your doctor give you supplemental vitamin and mineral (calcium and iron) pills. Also insist on a Pap smear, a check to see if you have had German measles (rubella), and a blood-sugar test.

Your next visits will be monthly and much shorter. The heartbeat and position of your fetus will be checked, as well as your urine, weight, and blood pressure.

At the beginning of your eighth month you'll see the doctor every two weeks.

During the ninth month you'll see him or her once a week. S/he will take internal measurements (if s/he hasn't already) to see if your pelvis is large enough for the baby to come through; s/he will check the thinning of the cervix wall (effacement), the width of the opening of the cervix (dilation), and the position of the baby. S/he will keep checking the heartbeat.

If you can, try to find a pediatrician early, and try to check his or her competence.

We describe the schedule above as an ideal schedule, ideal only in the context of our present system, and not really ideal at all, because it stops with childbirth and doesn't deal with your emotions. At the other extreme of exam scheduling, many women from poor areas never see a doctor until it's time for them to deliver. Or conditions in some hospitals and clinics are so bad that it's very difficult for women to feel motivated to come regularly for appointments.

Your feelings about yourself and your pregnancy. At the beginning of a first pregnancy, of any pregnancy, there are so many variations in feeling, from delirious joy to deep depression.

SOME POSITIVE FEELINGS. You might feel an increased sensuality, a kind of sexual opening out toward the world, heightened perceptions, like being in love. A lot of new energy. A feeling of being really special, fer-

*If you are pregnant, you become more susceptible to urinary tract infections. Five percent of women have latent urinary tract infections. Because the hormone progesterone relaxes smooth (involuntary) muscle, the collecting area in the kidneys and the tube connecting kidneys to bladder becomes larger. Urine tends to stagnate there, aggravating any latent infection. Signs of infection are increased urination, hurting or burning, backache. In the first trimester of pregnancy your infection should be treated with sulfa drugs.

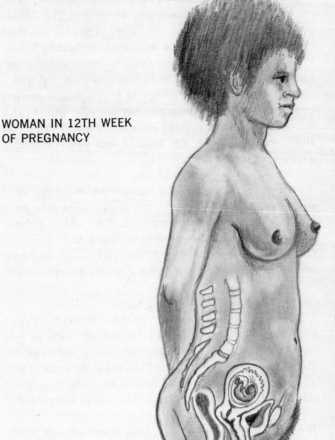

WOMAN IN 12TH WEEK OF PREGNANCY

tile, potent, creative. Expectation. Great excitement. Impatience.

* * *

Being pregnant meant I was a woman. I was enthralled with my belly growing. I went out right away and got maternity clothes.

* * *

It gave me a sense that I was actually a woman. I had never felt sexy before. I went through a lot of changes. It was a very sexual thing. I felt very voluptuous.

* * *

It meant I could get pregnant finally after a lot of trying, that I could do something I wanted to do. It meant going into a new stage of life. I felt filled up.

SOME QUESTIONS. What's going to happen to me? How will being pregnant change me? Will I be able to cope well? How long can I keep my job? Who am I? What image can I form of who I want to be? What is my baby going to be like? What about my man?

SOME NEGATIVE FEELINGS. (These are all relevant, natural, to be dealt with, not avoided or ignored. The deeper you go into these feelings, the better prepared you'll be to handle them close to the birth and afterward.) Shock. I'm losing my individuality. I'm not the same anymore. I'm a pregnant woman; I'm in this new category, and I don't want to be. I don't want to be a vessel, a carrier. I won't matter to people now, only my baby will. I can't feel anything for this thing growing in me. I can't feel any love. I'm scared. I'm tired. I feel sick.* I wish I weren't pregnant. I'm not ready.

* * *

Sometimes it seemed like I had gotten pregnant on a whim—and it was a hell of a responsibility to take on a whim. Sometimes I was overwhelmed by what I'd done. A lot of that came from realizing that I had chosen to have the baby without the support of a man. I was scared up until the third trimester that I wasn't going to make it.

* * *

Some of you will be too busy to think often about your pregnancy. Others will have more leisure. Some of you will be interested in your pregnancies in different degrees, your awareness switched inward at different times. You might be interested and involved in pregnancy without coming to terms with what it means to have a baby.

* * *

When I first felt her move, I knew there was life inside me. But I didn't realize I was having a baby until my doctors literally pulled her out of me upside down and she sneezed, and then she lay next to me, and I felt her tiny breath on my fingers.

* * *

Maybe the last three weeks I started looking at other babies.

* * *

At the beginning of pregnancy it's sometimes a relief not to think about it, and you can even forget it if you want to. At some point during pregnancy you might want to escape from the inevitability of what is happening to you.

* * *

If pregnancy meant anything, it meant being married. I no longer felt it was easy to get out. It was like a seal on the marriage.

* * *

Growth of the fetus. You can't feel the changes going on inside you. Both the placental systems and the complicated systems of your fetus are developing on a miniature scale. This is fantastically exciting to learn about. Knowing what's going on inside our bodies at each stage makes pregnancy a much less alienating and frightening experience than it has often been in the past.

We regret that we don't have enough space to describe the step-by-step development of the fetus. But there are several good books on the subject. We especially recommend Geraldine Lux Flanagan's *The First Nine Months of Life* and Anthony Smith's *The Body*, which are available in paperback (see bibliography).

Second Trimester (Thirteenth to Twenty-sixth Week)

Physical changes. At about the fourth month the fetus begins its bulkier growth. Your waist becomes thicker, your clothes no longer fit you, your womb starts to swell below your waist, and beginning with the fourth or fifth month you can begin to feel light movements. The fetus has been moving for months, but it's only now that you can feel it. Often you will feel it first just before you fall asleep.

You are probably gaining weight now. Eat as well as you can. (See section on "Nutrition.")

Your circulatory system has been changing, your total blood volume increasing, as your bone marrow produces more blood corpuscles and you drink and retain more liquid. Because of the increase in blood production, you need more iron. Your heart is changing position and increasing slightly in size.

In some women the area around the nipple, the areola, becomes very dark. The line from the navel to the pubic region gets dark too, and sometimes pigment in the face becomes dark, making a kind of mask. The mask goes away after pregnancy, but usually the increased color around your nipples and in the line on your abdomen doesn't go away.

Some women salivate more. You might sweat more, which is helpful in eliminating waste material from your body. Sometimes you'll get cramps in your legs and feet when you wake up, perhaps because of disturbed circulation. It's believed that calcium relieves these cramps. Just relax—the cramps will go away. Or rub them if you want to, or keep your feet elevated and warm.

Your uterus is changing too. It's growing. Its weight increases twenty times, and the greater part of this weight is gained before the twentieth week.

As your abdomen grows larger the skin over it will stretch, and lines may appear, pink or reddish streaks. Your skin may become very dry; add oil to your bath and rub your skin with oil.

By mid-pregnancy your breasts, stimulated by hormones, are functionally complete for nursing purposes. After about the nineteenth week a thin amber or yellow

---

*And there are many theories about the nausea that accompanies pregnancy: That it is peculiar to Western culture; that on some deep level, though we are raised in a society that adulates motherhood, we are disgusted by the animal fact that we have conceived and are now pregnant; that by vomiting we are trying to get rid of the fetus in a symbolic way; that nausea is a result of anxiety and tension, of the many pressures we feel.

substance called colostrum may come out of your nipples; there's no milk yet. Your breasts are probably larger and heavier than before. If you are planning to breast-feed, some experts feel it's a good idea to begin gently massaging your nipples. If your nipples are inverted (turned in), pull them out gently several times a day by putting your thumbs on each side of your nipples, pressing down into the breasts and away from the nipple. You should wash your breasts daily with mild soap or clean water. It's also a good idea to support them by wearing a good supportive bra, as they can begin to feel very heavy.

Your bowels and your entire digestive system might move more slowly. Indigestion and constipation can occur. You might have heartburn because of too much acid in your stomach. Again, a good diet eases these situations. Eat frequent small meals if possible. Avoid greasy foods. Dried fruit helps constipation, also fresh fruits and vegetables. Drink a lot of fluids. Avoid choosing

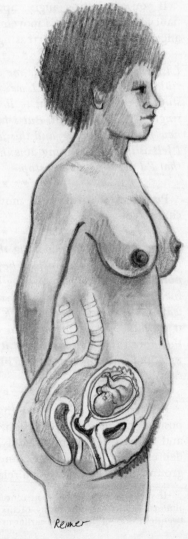

WOMAN IN 16TH WEEK
OF PREGNANCY

Reimer

medicines yourself and taking strong oily laxatives. Avoid laxatives containing sodium.

Also as a result of pressure, veins in your rectum (hemorrhoidal veins) may become dilated and sometimes painful. Lie down, with your rectum high, and apply ice packs. "Tucks pads" and "Preparation H" are O.K. Or take warm baths and apply vaseline. Varicose veins are veins in your legs that have become enlarged and can hurt. Again because of pressure by pelvic organs, the veins and blood vessels that carry blood from your legs to your heart aren't working as smoothly as before. A tendency to varicose veins can be hereditary. Many women find it very helpful to wear support stockings a half size larger than their ordinary stockings. And lots of rest, with legs elevated, is good.

Many women have nosebleeds because of the increased volume of blood, also perhaps because of increased hormone levels. (It's also possible to have sympathetic nosebleeds during periods.) Put a little vaseline in each nostril, and that will stop the bleeding.

We want to speak of edema here again (we discussed it in the section on nutrition). Edema is swelling of the face, hands, ankles, wrists, or feet as a result of retention of water by the body tissues. Some edema during pregnancy is normal. If you are uncomfortable, try to lie down, with your feet raised, several times a day. Cut down on carbohydrates for a while, and get more physical rest. See if this helps. If edema persists, check with your doctor.

Toxemia (see section on "Nutrition"). After the twenty-fourth week of pregnancy you might develop high blood pressure, edema, or protein in your urine.* You might have mild pre-eclampsia, with the symptoms mentioned above. You should check with your doctor. Your blood pressure should be observed on at least two occasions at least six hours apart, and the amount of albumin (a protein) in your urine must be checked at least two times. Or, toward the third trimester of pregnancy you might have severe pre-eclampsia, indicated by very high blood pressure, a large amount of protein in your urine with a decrease in the amount of urine, blurred vision, a severe continuous headache, or swelling of your face and fingers. Pre-eclamptic conditions can develop in a few hours. Unless these pre-eclamptic stages are checked immediately, eclampsia—convulsions and coma—might occur. (These must be treated in the hospital; your life and your baby's are at stake.) There is disagreement about the treatment of pre-eclampsia, with various claims made for the reduction of weight gain, curtailment of

*Toxemia develops mainly in very young (under sixteen) women, older women, and women with their first pregnancy. Women with diabetes, high blood pressure, and chronic kidney disease are most susceptible, as are women who carry twins, or have too much fluid in their uteri.

salt, hormonal treatments, and the use of diuretics. *It's essential to repeat that all medical people agree that toxemia of pregnancy is preventable by constant prenatal care, good diet, and supervision.*

What about smoking tobacco? The 1971 Surgeon General's report, "The Health Consequences of Smoking," analyzes over 100,000 births showing that the infants of smoking mothers weigh an average of 6.1 ounces less than infants born to nonsmoking mothers. Low birthweight newborns have more survival difficulties than fatter babies do. In the area of premature births, more than fifteen different studies have shown a significantly higher number of premature births in smoking versus nonsmoking mothers.

Caffeine is not destructive, but don't drink lots of coffee. It crosses the placenta, but is relatively harmless in moderation. You may feel less fatigue if you cut it out for a clear interval—like six weeks.

Alcohol (a depressant drug). If you drink, drink a limited amount. It contains a lot of carbohydrates. It crosses the placenta, but doesn't harm the fetus. Occasional wine is good for relaxation, but only on a good diet.

Your clothes should be loose and comfortable, warm in winter and cool in summer. Many women modify their own pants by piecing in an elastic stretch panel in the front. Simple unbelted smocks are useful as dresses. Large men's shirts are useful too. Maternity clothes in stores are so often ugly and expensive. Ask your friends for any clothes they might have.

Get as much rest as you possibly can.

Your feelings about yourself. How will you feel about your changing changed body?

* * *

I was excited and delighted. I really got into eating well, caring for myself, getting enough sleep. I liked walking through the streets and having people notice my pregnancy.

* * *

But many of us watch ourselves growing outward so quickly (when we hadn't grown for years too much in any direction) with mixed emotions. Our confusion is legitimate. We have been brought up to be mothers eventually. During pregnancy we change from the slim wraiths we were (supposed to be) to large-bellied women. We are making a visible transition from one role to another, moving from one myth to another. Some women try to hide their pregnancies from the world and even from themselves either by continuing for a time to wear the same clothes as before even when they no longer fit, or by wearing clothes so baggy that no one can see what is happening underneath.

You've got to find yourselves beyond and in spite of

these myths. It's possible to feel comfortable and happy with the changes you are going through.

Your feelings about your baby. If you are feeling really good, or ambivalent, or even bad, the first movements you feel your baby make can be very beautiful and very moving.

* * *

I was lying on my stomach and felt—something, like someone lightly touching my deep insides. Then I just sat very still and for an alive moment felt the hugeness of having something living growing in me. Then I said no, it's not possible, it's too early yet, and then I started to cry. . . . That one moment was my first body awareness of another living thing inside me.

* * *

And after the first movement—in the fourth or fifth month—you might wait days for another sign of quickening.* Then the movements will become frequent and familiar. The baby begins to feel real. You can feel from the outside the hard shape of your uterus.

If you are feeling angry, upset, threatened by pregnancy, then your baby's movements serve to focus your anger. You might feel increasingly taken over.

* * *

Last night its kicking made me dizzy and gave me a terrible feeling of solitude. I wanted to tell it stop, stop, stop, let me alone. I want to lie still and whole and all single, catch my breath. But I have no control over this new part of my being, and this lack of control scares me. I felt as if I were rushing downhill at such a great speed that I'd never be able to stop.

* * *

Perhaps feeling the baby move for the first time will change you.

* * *

Sitting on a rock overlooking the domesite, trees growing right out of the rock. They cling and flourish on nothing. Images of the growing life inside me, also coming from nothing, getting nutrition from my body the way the tree does from the rock. . . . Occasionally I give it warmth, mostly when it moves. The more it moves, the more I like it. I also resent it an awful lot; I feel big, ugly and uncomfortable, and in spite of Len's protestations, I feel alone.

* * *

It's important again to say that even during the most positive pregnancies you might have moments, hours, and days of depression, anxiety, and confusion. These depressions are probably connected to all the underground anxieties you have in relation to your own moth-

---

*If you aren't sure when you conceived your baby, you can be almost certain that quickening occurs between the eighteenth to twentieth week of pregnancy, earlier in second pregnancies.

er and your childhood; doubts that come from our societal ignorance about pregnancy and childbirth; doubts you have about your own identity; economic problems; having too many children already; and problems in your relationship with your man.

* * *

It seems that my feelings about my pregnancy, my body, the coming of the baby, were inextricably wound into my feelings, problems, hopes, and fears for our relationship. . . . It's hard to separate which feelings were a result of my unhappiness about us (a lot of the bad feelings about my body arose because Bob showed very little interest in my enlarged, changing body), which ones were my own negative feelings about having a less functional body (I wanted to keep working and active, but my body was so cumbersome that I was always worn out and tired), and which ones were just moods caused by pregnancy.

* * *

We all have general fears too. Fear of the unknown, especially if it's a first pregnancy. No matter how much we do know about the physiological changes in our bodies, there's something incomprehensible about the beginnings of life. And by becoming pregnant we open ourselves to possible changes, complications, and events that are risks in a sense. We become much more vulnerable.

* * *

I remember feeling overwhelmed by sad things I saw, and was overwhelmed by things that could happen to innocence. I'd wake in the night and think people were going to come in and take things, take the baby from me. I was beginning to be out of control. I was terribly afraid of chance. I've always been afraid of irrationality, of fate.

* * *

For two nights now my falling asleep has given rise to that old childhood dream-image of falling down a deep, dark, square hole ever diminishing in size.

* * *

We fear that our babies will be deformed. Four percent of babies are born with diseases and one percent with physical malformations.* Some of us have dreams, fantasies, and nightmares about deformity. These are normal, universal, international.

* * *

When I was about six months pregnant, and Dick was starting school again, I was home alone, isolated for days at a time. My nightmares and daydreams started around then. Really terrible fears of the baby being deformed. All my life I've always been the good girl. I knew I wasn't really good. I knew I had bad thoughts, but I was never allowed to express them. So I thought that my

*See Appendix, p. 180, for the facts about diagnosis of birth defects in early pregnancy.

baby's deformities would be the living proof of the ugliness and badness in me.

* * *

We fear our own death, the child's death.

In fact, we do have to face the fact that some women miscarry, and some babies die. While it's difficult, threatening, and sad to think of, we know it happens. Though it's not usually useful, and is also very hard to prepare ourselves for death, it helps to know what has happened to some of us, so that if we or our friends experience such tragedy, we can in some way be acquainted with the event. This knowledge is a kind of preparation. It's vitally important to be able to reach out to friends when tragic things happen, and to help break down their feelings of isolation. It also helps us to know that we can and need to ask for help if such a thing happens to us.

* * *

I went into the hospital for the birth of my first child. . . . The child's lungs became infected and he died two days later. I never saw him. When I began to return to myself I found that despite all those times I had told myself that nothing could really happen, I had nothing but an empty belly. I don't know if we should be warned ahead of time to worry needlessly about something that happens to a very few women, but as one of those women, I definitely needed to feel some sense of sharing with others in the same position—not to cry over what had happened, but to work out how to face other people. That's the hardest part—nobody wants to deal with death, especially when your friends are at the childbearing age themselves and can't help being afraid of you for what you stand for. I found that my friends wanted me to pretend nothing had happened—that there had been no pregnancy even. I don't think it was just my particular friends—it's natural to want to avoid those things. And so my fantastic pregnancy, in which a lot of things went on in my head and body that helped me to change and get myself together, had to be buried. Even now, after a year, I can see their pain and fear for me as I start into my eighth month of pregnancy with my second child. I have to be the one who keeps them calm, and I especially must assure everyone that this one will be okay.

* * *

Denying that unpleasant things happen is to deny to ourselves and to our friends the reality and totality of our experience. Recognition of misfortune is an affirmation.

And then, we feel guilty about having fears. Don't they in some way suggest that as mothers we will be weak and inadequate? The myth is that we can't allow ourselves these depressions, because we are supposed to be strong, mature, maternal, accepting, loving all the time.

It's vital to us to realize that our feelings are legitimate. We should feel free and right in expressing them.

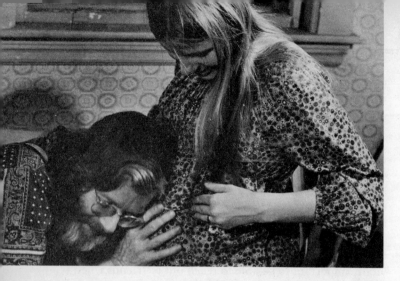

Men's feelings about you and your pregnancy. How will the man you are involved with feel about you? That depends on how you feel about yourself, on the relationship between you both, on how he feels about himself, and what he feels his part to be in your pregnancy. If he feels like getting involved, it's a very good idea to prepare with him and learn together, especially if he lives with you after your baby is born. He might feel attracted to you and close, and fascinated by your growing body. Or, for reasons having to do with his own background and upbringing, with his hang-ups, he might feel repelled, confused, and threatened by all your changes and your impending motherhood (his impending fatherhood). Or he might feel positive sometimes, negative sometimes. One man says:

* * *

Sometimes I thought you were very beautiful and your belly was beautiful. And sometimes you looked like a ridiculous pregnant insect. Your navel bulging out looked strange.

* * *

If you are having problems it's certainly best if you can talk together and realize that often your and his complex feelings are changeable. Talk can also lead to some deep, good questioning about the conventional ideas of beauty we are all brainwashed with. It's possible that he won't be able to talk about or to cope at all with the changes and responsibilities that your pregnancy implies. He might be jealous or resentful. Some men for many reasons seek out women other than the pregnant women they are living with, whether they're married or unmarried. Most men, while not actually leaving you, may withdraw from you emotionally at this crucial time.

If you are single and get involved with men during your pregnancy, these men will all have different kinds of attitudes toward you as a person, as a pregnant woman, and as a sexual being.

Intercourse. What about making love during pregnancy? There are two things to talk about: medical fact (and fiction), and your own feelings.

MEDICAL FACT AND FICTION. Traditionally, doctors have asked that we abstain from intercourse for four to six weeks before giving birth and up to six weeks after: altogether we were told to abstain for three months. According to a fairly recent Siecus study guide, this abstention was based on four unproven beliefs: (1) the thrusts of the penis against the cervix induce labor; (2) the uterine contractions of orgasm induce labor; (3) membranes may rupture, leading to infection; and (4) the sex act is physically uncomfortable.

It's tempting here to wonder how uncomfortable doctors are with the idea that we can be sexually active and potential mothers at the same time (don't mix sex with motherhood). These unscientific cautious abstention beliefs can deny us our sexuality and prevent us from maintaining a closeness to the man we're involved with when that closeness is much needed, before and after our child's birth.

What about the facts? Masters and Johnson have some evidence that the contractions of orgasm could set off labor, but the women in their study were close to term anyway. (In some cultures women ready to go into labor make love to induce labor.) The Siecus pamphlet concludes that intercourse toward the end of pregnancy is usually not dangerous. But you should not make love at any time during your pregnancy (1) if you have vaginal or abdominal pain, (2) if you have any uterine bleeding, (3) if your membranes have already ruptured (then there *is* danger of infection), or (4) if you have been warned or think that miscarriage might occur. If you have miscarried before, avoid intercourse the first three months during the time your period is due. That's important for you psychologically, so if a miscarriage should occur, you won't consider yourself responsible. And for the same reasons you shouldn't masturbate either, as orgasm could bring on miscarriage.* And throughout your pregnancy, be aware that during oral-genital contact, air blown into your vagina may be dangerous, causing air embolism.

All these remarks refer to unusual circumstances, and it's useful to be aware of them. For our main worries are that we will harm the baby in some (unknown) way. The truth is that intercourse during pregnancy is almost always harmless. (See section "Postpartum" for intercourse after pregnancy.)

Some of you will get strong uterine contractions when you make love or when you masturbate. These contractions are valuable and useful. They strengthen the uterine muscles. You know when they happen. Your uterus becomes harder. If you lie quietly and relax, they will

---

*Some recent studies are finding that a substance in a man's semen, called prostaglandin, and possibly a like substance created by a woman's orgasm, can induce labor a little earlier than it might ordinarily occur.

nearly always die down. Labor will start only if it's time.

Intercourse can be a good exercise for the muscles of the pelvic floor. Also note how completely you can relax after making love. It's useful to know how it feels to relax, because later, during labor contractions, that kind of complete relaxation can be useful.

Toward the end of pregnancy, when the baby's head has moved down, an erect penis can cause discomfort, for there's not a lot of room in there.

Later in your pregnancy the "traditional" position (man on top) can be uncomfortable. The pressure on your abdomen makes you feel that you're going to pop, and pressure on your breasts causes them to leak. Pillows under your back can make you more comfortable. But at no time should the man's whole weight rest on you, nor should great pressure be put upon your uterus. You can use other positions more happily: you can be on top, or he behind you. Sheila Kitzinger says men and women should make love "with emphasis upon a careful tenderness" (*The Experience of Childbirth,* Copyright © 1962, 1967, 1972 by Sheila Kitzinger. Published by Kaplinger Publishing Company, Inc., New York, p. 64).

YOUR FEELINGS ABOUT MAKING LOVE. You'll each have many and different feelings about making love.

* * *

I wanted to make love more than ever.

* * *

I remember feeling very sexy. We were trying all these different positions. Now that we were having a baby, I felt a lot looser, a lot freer. I used to feel uptight about sex for its own sake, but when I was pregnant I felt a lot freer.

* * *

I felt very ambivalent about making love. I had miscarried several times. I wanted to make love and I was scared to make love. As a single woman it was hard to find men who found me attractive with my belly so big. I had no sexual contact at all the last two months.

* * *

Some of you might have times when you really turn inward, when you won't want to or be able to "give" to a man. Pregnancy can be used as a good excuse not to make love if you want an excuse. And often you might be feeling very tired.

Masters and Johnson report an increase in sexual desire during the second trimester and a decrease during the third.

If you are living with a group of people. It's a good idea to think about how you want them to relate to your child. In an ideal situation most everyone wants to help care for it and feels commitment to it. Some communities exist that are themselves large extended families. But many groups are composed of people who will have very different commitments to your child. Often people don't want to have anything much to do with taking care of children. They either don't want to or don't feel ready to. Try to figure out just what you are expecting of each person and whether your expectations are realistic. Talk to each person if you can and find out how he/she feels about your coming child. Do it early.

* * *

You can't assume that people will automatically help on their own and know you need help. Also, with people who don't have children, you have to be explicit and tell them what to do. I don't think it's a good thing to have a lot of people take care of the baby at first, but I was glad that people helped me out. Also find out how they feel about you. Having chosen these people as your new family, you might expect to be cared for and nurtured, and you might find that people won't be able to meet your increased needs.

* * *

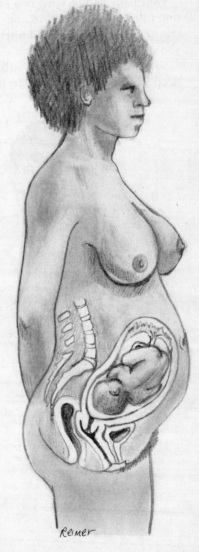

WOMAN IN 24TH WEEK
OF PREGNANCY

Reimer

Third Trimester (Twenty-seventh to Thirty-eighth Week)

Physical changes. Your uterus is becoming very large. It feels hard when you touch it.

*   *   *

I remember my friends' surprise when they put their hands on my belly to feel it. They expected it to be soft and somehow jellylike, and were amazed at its hardness and bulk.

*   *   *

It's a strong muscular container. You can feel and see the movements of your fetus from the outside now, too, as it changes position, turns somersaults, hiccups. Sometimes it puts pressure on your bladder, which makes you feel that you need to urinate even when you don't, and which can hurt a little, sometimes a lot for very brief periods. Sometimes, toward the very end of pregnancy, it puts pressure on the nerves at the top of your legs, which can be painful too.

Your baby will be lying in a particular position, sometimes head down, back to your front, sometimes lying crossways. It moves around often. Your doctor can help you discover which position it's in.

Sometimes your baby lies still. It's known that babies sleep in utero. If you don't feel movement for three to four days, and you're wondering, call your doctor if you can and ask whether he thinks it's a good idea to check the fetal heartbeat. Usually these are periods of "rest" for the baby and can last several days.

It becomes increasingly uncomfortable for you to lie on your stomach. You might experience shortness of breath. There's pressure on your lungs from your uterus, and your diaphragm may be moved up as much as an inch. Even so, because your thoracic (chest) cage widens, you breathe in more air when you are pregnant than when you are not. Sometimes when you lie down you might not be able to breathe well for a moment. Prop yourself up with pillows, and the pressure on your diaphragm will be lessened.

The peak load on your heart occurs in about the thirtieth week. Then cardiac work tends to go down until delivery.

You are still gaining weight. If you have hemorrhoids or varicose veins, try to avoid standing up for long periods of time, and when you sit or lie down, be sure your feet are raised.

Your stomach is pushed up by your uterus and flattened. Indigestion is common. Eat small amounts. Take Gelusil or Maalox, very mild medication. Sucking on the tablets is better than swallowing them. Don't take mineral oil; it causes you to excrete necessary vitamins.

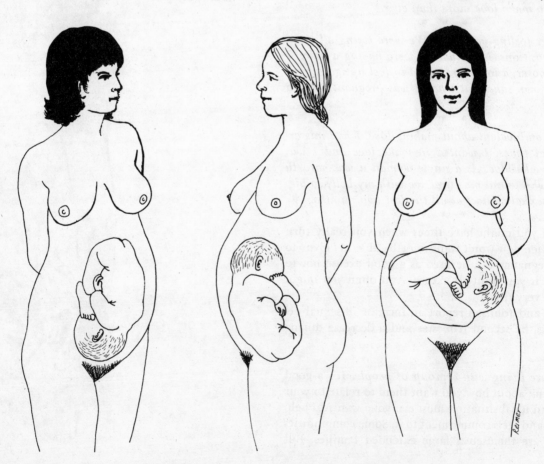

THREE POSITIONS A BABY MIGHT BE IN

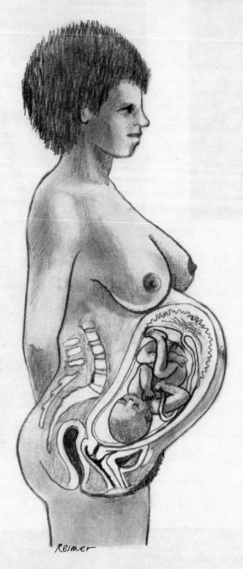

WOMAN IN
36TH WEEK
OF PREGNANCY

Your feelings about yourself and your pregnancy.

* * *

I had a feeling of waiting at the end, of nothing else being terrifically important.

* * *

I thought it would never end. I was enormous. I couldn't bend over and wash my feet. And it was incredibly hot.

* * *

At the end I started to feel it was too long. Dick took pictures of me during the eighth month. I saw my face as far away and sad.

* * *

I had insomnia. I couldn't get comfortable. I couldn't sleep, he'd kick so much.

* * *

I wonder what it looks like. How fantastic that it only has to travel one and a half feet down to get born.

* * *

My kid is dancing inside under my heart.

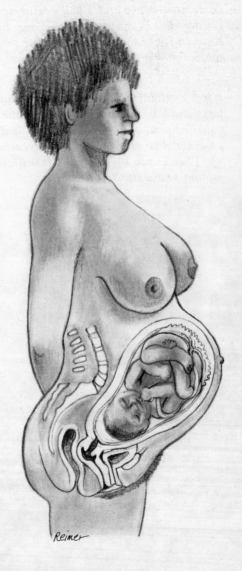

WOMAN IN
40TH WEEK
OF PREGNANCY

Avoid indigestion remedies that contain sodium.

Your navel will probably be pushed out.

Since your body has gotten heavier, you'll tend to walk differently for balance, often leaning back to counteract a heavier front. This can cause backaches, for which there are exercises. Your pelvic joints are also much more separated.

At about four to two weeks before birth, and sometimes as early as the seventh month, the baby's head settles into your pelvis. This is called "lightening," or "dropping" or "engagement." It takes pressure off your stomach. Some women do feel much lighter. And if you have been having trouble breathing, pressure is now off your diaphragm. This "dropping" can cause constipation; your bowels are more obstructed than they were.

As for water retention, an average pregnant woman retains from six and a half to thirteen pints of liquid, half of this in the last ten weeks. Ankle swelling is common.

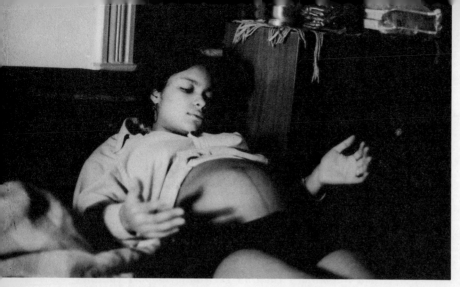

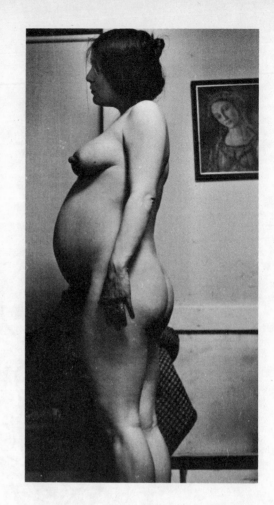

The relationship of mother carrying child is most beautiful and simplest.
I pity a baby who must come out of the womb.

* * *

Fairly confidently and calmly awaiting the baby—quite set on a home delivery. Doctor said Thursday I was already dilated two and a half centimeters, so it must be getting close. Getting a bit anxious, listening to every Braxton-Hicks contraction, awaiting with hope, and fear too, its change into the real thing.

* * *

I feel exultant and tired and rich inside. My belly is large and last night the baby beat around inside it like a wild tempest. I thought the time had come and was panicked and nauseated, then very excited. I woke Gene up. Then at five I fell asleep. Meanwhile I move in slow motion and wait.

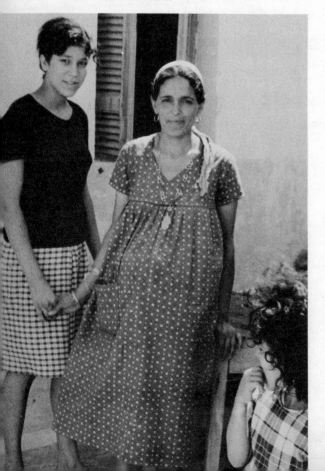

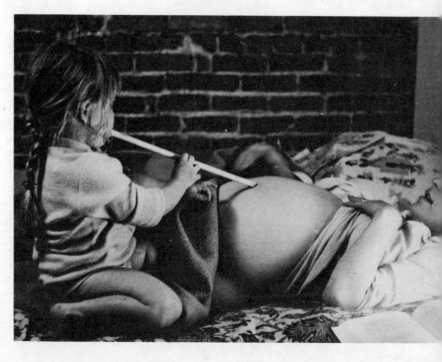

APPENDICES

Miscarriage (Natural Abortion)

Miscarriage is always an emotional event. There are different kinds of miscarriages at different times during pregnancy. If it happens early and the fetus is barely formed, you might be less affected than if it happens after the fourth or fifth month, once you have felt the fetus move within you and it has become real to you. But if you want a baby, even if it happens early, and especially if it has occurred once or several times before, it can be occasion for increased anguish and despair and can add to the tension involved in trying to conceive again. Many fears are increased, and you become more and more vulnerable and must work on building up defenses. If a miscarriage occurs in the fifth month or later, some women feel incredibly incomplete and find themselves waiting for something to happen; their time sense gets shaken up. This incompleteness can be felt even after an earlier miscarriage.

All of this is not to alarm, but to make women aware that miscarriage is a possibility during pregnancy (one in ten women miscarry) and can be very difficult to cope with. But anxieties can be lessened by your persistence both in learning reasons for your miscarriage and in being as much as possible aware and constantly in touch with your feelings and fears. It is also vitally helpful that you talk out these feelings, and very important that your friends not gloss over the event (because they feel so uncomfortable with it—and it can be hard to deal with), so that you are frustrated when you try to communicate your feelings. Often through talking both to the man involved and to empathetic friends you can sort out your own strong feelings and begin to know your anxieties.

If a woman is not fertile, the reasons for her infertility might be the reasons for miscarriage. (The man is less physiologically responsible for miscarriage than for infertility.) So, many of the tests performed for infertility are useful in determining why a woman will miscarry.

There are four general classes of causes for miscarriage: (1) defective egg or sperm; (2) faulty production of estrogen or progesterone; (3) anatomical illness or functional abnormalities, or general illness or infection; and (4) psychological reasons. Ten percent of women miscarry, and about 50 percent of the aborted fetuses are found to be abnormal. Some additional statistics: After a first miscarriage it's 85–90 percent sure that the next pregnancy will be all right; after a second there's a 50 percent chance; and after a third a 25 percent chance. A woman who has miscarried three times or more is sometimes called a habitual aborter. She should definitely have preventative (preconceptual) therapy and treatment.

Miscarriages are classified into stages or types. One miscarriage can pass through many stages.

Threatened abortion. There's a difference between bleeding and abortion bleeding. Some women when pregnant bleed slightly for a few months at about the time they are supposed to have their period. Sometimes as the blastocyst implants into the uterine lining there's slight bleeding. Sometimes the bleeding might be bright red. If this continues for several days, go to the doctor; he'll examine you for lesions. Early bleeding has no effect on fetal development. If bleeding does begin (slight brown staining, with little or no abdominal cramps), there is always uncertainty. The pregnancy might or might not continue. You will often be advised to go to bed until the bleeding has turned brown and then has stopped for twenty-four hours. Afterward you should not douche, be too active, or make love until the fourteenth week of pregnancy. Many women find the fact that there is no treatment hard to accept. And they find it extremely hard to accept the fact that if the bleeding continues for several days, it means almost definite miscarriage.

Inevitable. Severe cramps, cervical effacement, and dilation occur, with strong bleeding and clots. There is no way to stop it.

Complete. The uterus empties itself completely of the fetus, membranes, and the decidual lining of the uterus. During the first three weeks, spontaneous abortion is almost always complete. Sometimes then, and even later, it might feel like a really heavy period; sometimes you might not notice it at all, as it takes place around the time you expect your period. If the pregnancy is more advanced than three weeks, the doctor would very likely give you a D & C to be sure that every bit of membrane is out of the uterus. Unless it is completely emptied, the uterine muscles won't contract to compress the bleeding vessels and control the hemorrhage, and infection may occur.

Incomplete. Varying amounts of tissue remain in the uterus, either attached or free. Mild to severe cramps, perhaps pain in a specific place. Must have a D & C.

Missed. The fetus has died but remains in the uterus. Symptoms of pregnancy disappear, breasts get smaller, the uterus stops growing and gets smaller. Spontaneous abortion almost always occurs. There's a brown spotting. Doctors usually wait until it begins by itself and then give a D & C.

Sometimes a woman's cervix has been injured and can't hold in the fetus. A simple operation can be performed to prevent her from losing her baby, usually during the pregnancy.

In general, if you have a history of miscarriage, you should be fully examined along the lines of the infertility investigation. If you have miscarried only once, that usually means that the egg or sperm is defective and paradoxically, it's a healthy thing for your body to get rid of an embryo or fetus that isn't growing well.

The positive side of a miscarriage, for someone who has thought herself infertile, is that it means you can get pregnant.

Ectopic Pregnancy

If you're old enough to bear a child, have had intercourse, and feel abdominal pains you don't understand, it's possible you have an ectopic pregnancy, a pregnancy that is out of place (usually a tubal pregnancy). In ectopic pregnancy the fertilized egg implants itself, not in the wall of the uterus, but most often in the fallopian tube, or much more rarely, in the abdominal cavity, the ovary, or the cervix.

Tubal pregnancy. Fertilization of the egg by the sperm almost always occurs in the fallopian tube. If the function of the tube is impaired in any way—if the cilia (hairs) don't move as they should to propel the egg into the uterus; if the tube's structure has been changed by pelvic inflammatory disease so that there are "pockets" in it; if the tube is genetically malformed—then it's possible that the fertilized egg might attach itself to some part of the tube, instead of proceeding on into the uterus. The egg implants itself in the tubal lining. It establishes a beginning placenta and space for itself just as if it were in the womb. The fetus begins to grow. Because placenta and fetus are growing, both producing and using the usual pregnancy hormones, all the usual changes of a beginning normal pregnancy might occur.

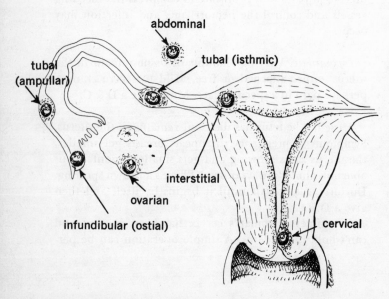

abdominal

tubal (isthmic)

tubal (ampullar)

interstitial

ovarian

infundibular (ostial)

cervical

So early symptoms of an ectopic pregnancy can be a missed period, breast tenderness, nausea, and fatigue. The uterus may also be slightly enlarged and softened because of the influence on it of placental hormones, as in a normal pregnancy. If you go to a doctor, s/he might diagnose a normal pregnancy after examining you internally and listening to your symptoms. It's difficult to discover an unruptured early tubal pregnancy.

As the pregnancy enlarges, the tube will stretch slightly. It's not made to expand indefinitely, and eventually, as the placenta burrows into the muscle wall of the tube, it bursts. This usually happens between the eighth and twelfth week.

Now the signs of ectopic pregnancy appear. Just before it bursts you might feel acute (sharp) stabbing pain at the site of implantation, or cramps, or a constant, dull abdominal pain, which is temporarily relieved by the rupture.* But then you'll bleed inside, and soon feel lower abdominal pain again. Or later you might feel aching pain in your diaphragm and sharp shoulder pain caused by blood flowing up to your diaphragm. If the bleeding is greater, you might be in shock, with low blood pressure and a high pulse rate. Symptoms of shock are hot and cold flashes, nausea, dizziness, fainting. If you experience any of these symptoms, see your doctor. Try to be aware especially that that first sharp abdominal pain might indicate a rupture, and go quickly to your doctor.

Sometimes, before or after the rupture, you might have a late period with mild, menstrual-type bleeding or fragments from your uterine lining, because the hormones secreted by the fetus are not strong enough to keep up the growth of the lining of your uterus, or the ovum has died and estrogen production has stopped. This bleeding can be misleading, as you and your doctor might think you have had an early "natural" abortion. If the lining of the uterus is passed, it should be examined microscopically, and if there's no evidence of trophoblastic tissue, ectopic pregnancy should be suspected.

Internal bleeding is of two kinds: a sudden acute bleeding, or much more common, a slow trickle of blood into the pelvic cavity. If there has been much bleeding, your abdomen will feel sore, breathing will be painful, and you might have pain in each shoulder.

A pelvic examination might show no findings at all or a number of findings: tenderness or mass in the fallopian tubes or ovaries; enlargement of the uterus; softening of the cervix; fullness behind the uterus. Blood tests might or might not be useful. Possibly the amount of chori-

---

*Dr. Edward Quilligan in his article "Ectopic Pregnancy" speaks of a dictum to the effect that if any woman of reproductive age feels abdominal pain, it has to be first investigated as a possible ectopic pregnancy.

onic gonadotropin (HCG) might be lower than normal for the age of the fetus.

Then your doctor might do a culdocentesis, inserting a needle vaginally into the space behind the uterus (pouch of Douglas). If nonclotting blood is found, ruptured ectopic pregnancy is a possibility, because the intraperitoneal blood doesn't readily clot. He or she might recommend operative diagnostic procedures like culdoscopy or laparoscopy.

The therapy—treatment—for tubal pregnancy is usually a salpingectomy, in which the entire tube is removed. This must be done under anesthesia in a hospital. There's disagreement over whether the ovary on that same side should be removed too.

It's likely that if a woman has had one tubal pregnancy, she'll conceive less readily than if she hadn't had it. (There's a 50–60 percent chance of not conceiving.) Chances of another tubal pregnancy are increased.

Abdominal pregnancies are very rare. Signs are (1) vague, persistent abdominal pain, (2) abnormal findings on pelvic exam, and (3) anemia.

Ovarian pregnancies are even rarer. Symptoms vary from none at all to those of a tubal ectopic pregnancy with intraperitoneal bleeding. The ovary is usually removed.

Cervical pregnancy may be associated with uncontrollable bleeding which may require hysterectomy. Fortunately it's also very rare.

Rh Factor in Blood

The Rh factor is a substance in the blood. At least 86 percent of us have this substance in our blood coating red blood cells: they are Rh-positive (Rh+). The people who don't have it are Rh-negative (Rh—).

If someone with Rh— blood receives transfusions of blood containing Rh+, the Rh— blood gradually builds up antibodies, which defend the blood from the hostile Rh+ factor, causing some red cells to be broken down and their products disseminated through the body, thus exerting a poisonous effect.

When you are pregnant there's a certain amount of blood transference between you and your fetus through the placenta, though each circulatory system remains fairly separate. Most of the exchange goes from the mother to the fetus. At birth, however, because of the separation of the placenta from the uterus, there can be a much larger spillover, and a quantity of the baby's blood can be absorbed by the mother. If you have Rh— blood and are pregnant for the first time and have not had a transfusion containing Rh+ blood, your first child will probably be all right. But at birth you can absorb your baby's Rh+ blood, and within the next seventy-two hours your own blood reacts and begins developing antibodies. These antibodies will be present in your blood during your next pregnancy, and will threaten the blood cells of your second growing fetus in varying degrees.

Thus every woman should have her Rh factor checked early in pregnancy. If you are Rh—, you should pay careful attention to the following: (1) The father's Rh factor should be checked. If he is Rh— too, your offspring will be Rh—, and there's nothing to worry about. If he's Rh+, it should be determined whether he has both Rh+ and Rh— genes, in which case the fetus, having some Rh— genes (like you), will be unaffected. If the man has only Rh+ genes, the fetus is much more vulnerable. (2) You should know whether you have had previous blood transfusions. Even matched blood types contain Rh— and Rh+ factors, so that it's possible (though hopefully rare now that people are aware of the Rh factor) for a woman with Rh— blood type B to have received Rh+ blood type B, and thus have already developed antibodies. (3) You should have your own blood tested for Rh sensitization (the presence of antibodies). (4) A fetal amniotic fluid sample can be taken through a needle to see whether the blood cells of the fetus are being altered. This test can be done throughout the pregnancy. If the bilirubin level in the fluid is high, it indicates that the fetus is affected and a blood transfusion may be given to the baby in utero. (5) You should ask your doctor about a new medicine called Rhogam, developed by the Ortho Pharmaceutical Company. Apparently if Rhogam is given to an Rh— woman within seventy-two hours after her Rh+ baby's birth, it prevents the build-up of antibodies and protects her next pregnancy. After each Rh+ pregnancy she should get an injection of Rhogam to protect the next pregnancy.

Ortho, the pharmaceutical company that distributes Rhogam, did a controlled experiment at an abortion clinic to try to see if Rh— women who had abortions developed antibodies after the abortion, and to see if Rhogam prevented these antibodies from developing. It was found that sensitization does occur but less than in pregnancies that go to term. Most physicians feel it's better to give some extra Rhogam and save some women from sensitization.

What can be done if the blood of the fetus is being invaded by maternal antibodies? There are techniques now for exchanging invaded fetal blood for good blood while the fetus is still in the uterus, and for exchanging the baby's blood after it is born. Check with your doctor about the benefits and risks of these techniques. Compel him or her to tell you everything you want to know. If s/he doesn't, don't pay him or her. Check with other doctors, if you can, to learn even more. Ask for names of other women with similar experiences, and find out from them what their experiences were.

Early Diagnosis of Birth Defects

A woman can now be tested early in her pregnancy for an increasing number of inherited disorders in order to determine whether or not the child will be affected by them.

The disorders that can be diagnosed in early pregnancy are (1) virtually all chromosomal abnormalities (such as Down's Syndrome—formerly called "mongolism"), (2) certain biochemical diseases (that is, some amino-acid disorders), and (3) sex-linked diseases, carried by females, but affecting males (hemophilia, muscular dystrophy).

These diagnoses can be made by studying the amniotic fluid and the cells in it which are from the fetus. About two tablespoonsful of amniotic fluid (the water surrounding the fetus) is withdrawn from the uterus by the procedure called amniocentesis.

Amniocentesis should be done between fourteen and sixteen weeks of pregnancy. There's a one percent risk of losing the baby if you choose this procedure early in pregnancy. Later the risk is greater. It generally takes about fourteen to eighteen days to do most of the laboratory work to make a prenatal diagnosis.

Who might want to have this done? (1) Mothers who have already had a child with one of certain hereditary biochemical diseases. (2) Women who are carriers of serious disorders that affect males only. (3) A mother who has had a child with a chromosomal abnormality and who may wish to have the test done because of increased risk or because she is anxious during this second pregnancy. (4) Sometimes women over forty who get pregnant, since the risk of having a child with a chromosomal abnormality increases as the woman gets older.

The amniocentesis can be done in a doctor's office either by your own obstetrician or an obstetrician connected with a prenatal genetics team.

Parents who are carriers of certain hereditary diseases can be diagnosed before the woman becomes pregnant by studying a blood or skin sample.

If you find that there might be a chance of your fetus having birth defects, it will be your decision, along with the advice of your physician, as to whether or not you will continue your pregnancy. One doctor suggests that if you would continue your pregnancy in either case, it would be wiser to omit the test.

Infertility

Many of us have difficulty becoming pregnant. Usually, if we have been trying to conceive over a long period of time, many tensions are built up. Trying to conceive on the mathematically right day, during ovulation, can become a self-conscious mechanical process that destroys good sex. Both you and your man might begin to resent each other, to hold unfounded grudges and suspicions, and above all, to feel inadequate.

How long should you wait before seeing a doctor? If you can't conceive a child after trying for two years, or for one year if you can't wait, or if you are past thirty (your fertility declines with increasing age), you should see a doctor interested in infertility who has had obstetrical and gynecological experience and knows about the physiology of reproduction. S/he should also be very knowledgeable about semen analysis. If s/he is a good doctor s/he will be aware of your tensions and hang-ups, and s/he will try to deal with the emotional and psychological conflicts you might have toward each other and maybe toward having a child. A doctor who runs through a series of tests without discussing your situation with you will be helping you less than s/he could.

Often you, the woman, will feel more guilty and responsible for not being able to have children than the man will. Studies show that 10–15 percent of the couples in the United States are infertile, and in more than 40 percent of these cases the man is responsible. It's possible that some men will resist (1) the idea that there's something amiss with them, and (2) going to the doctor with you. It's threatening for him as well as for you to consider himself impotent on some level, and even more upsetting to find out definitely that his sperm are not "powerful" or numerous enough. But if he's really interested in having a child and not threatened he'll consent to be examined first. It's usual to examine a man first, because it's a much simpler process. But now it's possible within the span of two menstrual cycles for a woman to get a series of diagnostic studies done in a carefully planned sequence; or she can, in two days in the hospital, have many tests done. Of course these tests cost money, and we should demand that they be made available to all women who need to have them, who want to have a child.

Before going into the specific factors the doctor will be looking for, it is important to mention the conditions on which our female fertility depends: (1) good general health, (2) desire to give birth to and rear a child, (3) no infection or inflammation in the reproductive tract—vagina, cervix, uterus, fallopian tubes, ovaries—and appropriate function of the anterior pituitary gland, and parts of the hypothalamus and cerebral cortex.

There are roughly twelve conditions that must exist in

order for an egg to be fertilized: (1) At a time properly related to the developmental stage of the endometrium (lining of the uterus), an egg must be discharged from the ovary. That presupposes that at least one ovary is intact, that it has "responsive" follicles, and that its activities are governed by a functioning endocrine apparatus. (2) Near the exact time of ovulation the hairs (fimbriae) of the fallopian tube must surround the lower half of the ovary and catch the ovum. (3) In the tube the egg must travel through the tube in four to seven days; otherwise the fertilized egg will not implant successfully. (4) Healthy sperm must be deposited in a healthy, intact vagina. (5) Once in the vagina, a sufficient number of sperm must go into the endocervical canal as a result of their efforts or because of "in-sucking" organic contractions of the uterus. (6) Once in the canal, there must be a good biochemical environment. The cervix must be in all ways intact. Its secretions must interact well (nontoxically) with the sperm. (7) From the canal the sperm must swim to the uterus. (8) Then into the fallopian tubes. (9) They must be able to swim against the push or with the help of the hairs to the farther third of the tube and there meet the egg during its time of viability. This depends on the vigor of the sperm, maybe on the chemical content of the tubal secretions. (10) Large numbers of sperm must affect the outer covering of the egg, so that it can finally engulf one. (11) As it is swept along the tube toward the uterus, the fertilized egg must undergo a series of maturational changes that make it into a blastocyst as it arrives in the uterus. It must be genetically and embryologically normal. (12) The endometrium must be ready to receive it; the secretory changes of the menstrual cycle must be adequately advanced, as controlled by the endocrine system.

Thus, if any of these things are prevented from coming about, the end result can be infertility.

If the doctor hasn't found anything wrong with you anatomically and if the man's semen is normal, then you return for the third step of the investigation, which consists of complete blood tests to check your normal endoctrine functioning and basic body health. You will have a complete blood count to check the number of red and white cells that you have; a hematocrit—a count of the percentage of red cells in a specimen of blood to determine anemia; a test to determine by checking white blood-cell count if there's any infection; and a differential—a check of the kinds of cells involved in the white blood-cell count. Your blood will be typed, for it's possible that incompatible blood types may be reflected in the sperm and in the egg. And as abnormal thyroid function may affect fertility, you'll have two or three tests to determine how efficiently the thyroid is working. You may have a two-hour postprandial (after-eating) blood glucose test to determine whether there's proper

functioning of glucose-control mechanisms—a test for diabetes. And, finally, you will have a urinalysis to check kidney function, hormones in the urine, and infections.

If everything described above gives no clues to what is wrong, the doctor will do a systematic investigation of the bodily systems of reproduction.

First s/he will want to find out whether your ovaries produce Graafian follicles, which upon ripening emit eggs. A few days before menstruation s/he will do an endometrial biopsy, which consists of taking a small sample of the uterine wall tissue to give information about whether ovulation takes place and how the endometrium develops. S/he may do a fern test twice, once during midcycle and once at the end of the cycle. When estrogen is present and highly concentrated during ovulation (midcycle), the cervical mucus under the microscope shows fernlike designs. At the end of the cycle the fern pattern will no longer be there, for the progesterone of a normally ovulating woman inhibits fern formation. Another way of determining ovulation is to record your basal body temperature rectally on a special thermometer. Your temperature is supposed to rise one degree Fahrenheit at ovulation and stay high during the life span of the corpus luteum. If there's no significant rise, progesterone isn't being provided in effective amounts. The basal body temperature is of greatest value with women who have regular menstrual cycles. All these tests of egg formation shouldn't be counted as conclusive. It might be that they'll have to be done a few times, for you might have an atypical cycle the first time. Any diagnosis of ovulation in order to be adequate should cover at least three cycles.

There are several kinds of menstrual disorders that indicate that something has gone wrong either with ovulation, hormonal levels, or some other facet of the menstrual cycle. Such conditions are: disfunctional uterine bleeding, possibly caused by persistent corpus luteum cysts, pelvic inflammations or infections, or anemia; dysmenorrhea (painful or difficult menstruation); amenorrhea (no menstruation); anovulatory bleeding (bleeding without ovulation). The doctor needs to follow a logical sequence of studies. A common cause for the absence of menstruation is the Stein-Levinthal syndrome: enlarged ovaries or ovaries with cysts. The cysts can be removed by a simple operation, or altered by hormones (Clomid).

If s/he must continue the search, the doctor will check the transportation of the cells by looking for tubal disorders (common if a woman has had gonorrhea). The fallopian tubes might be blocked, so that he will blow CO_2 through them (the Rubin test, CO_2 insufflation test). This test in itself might correct the blockage.

A hysterosalpingram may be taken of the uterus and tubes. A water-soluble radio-opaque medium is injected into the uterine cavity and tubes, and outlines structures so that any obstruction or malformation shows up clearly in an X ray.

Tubal disorders may be grouped under two categories: (1) mechanical obstruction by organic lesions, caused by pelvic inflammatory disease, ruptured appendix, peritonitis, abdominal or pelvic operations, and (2) disturbances of the physiologic function of the tubes—failure of the ovum pick-up mechanism, delayed or too rapid ovum transport, endocrine disturbances and/or psychic stimuli; that is, if you are psychically disturbed, what goes on in your brain might inhibit certain necessary hormones from being released. Congenital anomalies also may be discovered.

If nothing yet has been found to be wrong, the doctor will then look into how sperm are placed on or near the cervix and how they pass through the cervical canal. The most well-known test is the Sims-Huhner, or post-coital test. Often it is the first test to find out how the sperm enters you. It is usually done six hours after you have had intercourse, though there's disagreement about that timing. When cervical mucus is taken and looked at under the microscope, the number of actively moving sperm is counted. There's also the semen-penetration (Miller-Kurzrock) test, in which a specimen of the man's semen is placed near a sample of cervical mucus. If the sperm can penetrate the mucus and live, then they are viable, they interact well. Sometimes the semen and cervical mucus are simply hostile.

Position of a couple during intercourse becomes important. For best results try making love lying under your partner with a pillow propping up your bottom, and *lie there for a while afterwards* to let gravity help the sperm.

Finally, there is psychogenic infertility. This means simply that because of your conscious or unconscious anxieties or fears, you will try in all kinds of ways not to have a baby. There is infertility due to no identifiable cause. And there is absolute sterility, which may occur, for instance, when both tubes have been seriously damaged.

The whole process of finding causes for infertility can be incredibly wearing and depressing. It takes a lot of strength for you to go through some or all of the above tests. But it's helpful to know some of the causes and some of the tests. It's essential to insist that the doctor tell you the exact nature of the procedures and tools s/he will be using, that s/he give you some idea of how the different processes will feel, and that s/he be responsive to your reactions.

And though it makes your struggle more difficult, if you are not satisfied with your doctor, try to find another doctor who is more sympathetic.

Often, when you least expect it, pregnancy will occur, almost by magic. This is most often seen when you "give up," change doctors, or "adjust" to being sterile. But there is no way to short-cut the studies. Most specialists will ask you to be patient and not be in too great a hurry; pregnancy can occur after almost any test, and further studies might not be necessary.

SECTION TWO: PREPARED CHILDBIRTH

INTRODUCTION: WHY PREPARATION?

Childbirth preparation means educating ourselves about what is likely to happen to our bodies, our minds, and our lives during the childbirth experience. It also means finding someone—husband, friend, or relative—to share this period with us. It is certainly not impossible to go through pregnancy, childbirth, and motherhood alone and unprepared, but it is difficult and unnecessary.

Above all, we must try not to be alone during labor. The companion we choose (early in our pregnancy) should be reading the same books, attending the same classes, and learning the same exercises and breathing techniques as we are. This person will serve as our coach during labor, and will stay with us throughout the entire birth process. Often the baby's father will be our coach. Sharing the labor experience and witnessing the birth with him is an important beginning to sharing the responsibilities and joys of parenthood. Some of us want to be with another woman during labor. We will find it most helpful to have as coach a woman who has already given birth. She will be able to support us with her firsthand knowledge, and her presence is a witness to the fact that it can be done.

If you have trouble finding someone to be with you during labor, contact one of the national prepared-childbirth associations listed in the appendix to this section. They will gladly send you information about classes and organizations in your area that can help you find a monitrice or trained labor companion.

However, there are hospitals that will allow only a registered nurse to be with you during labor, and many hospitals will not allow any outsider into the delivery room. We must work to change these rules, but until they are eliminated, search around until you find a doctor and a hospital that meet your requirements. Be particular, and make all the demands you feel are necessary to your best interests and your baby's security.

Prepared childbirth is often called natural childbirth. The only thing natural is that a woman's body is biologically equipped to bear and give birth to children. This doesn't mean that we have to have children or that we shouldn't be able to choose when we want to have children. It also doesn't mean that we should go through childbirth without preparation. Although much of our society considers it normal for us to have our babies while heavily drugged, in helpless ignorance and pain, and totally dependent on the medical profession, we believe it is much more natural for us to want to know what is happening to our bodies during labor. We want to give birth to our babies with confidence.

We are trying to find a way to have our babies safely and with dignity. The concept of dignity in labor was made popular in the West by two obstetricians. In 1932 Dr. Grantly Dick-Read, an Englishman, first introduced a method of concentrated relaxation during labor with the publication of his book *Childbirth Without Fear.* He understood that fear causes tension, and tension causes pain. Thus his approach was to try to eliminate the fear of labor through education and exercise. A French doctor, Fernand Lamaze, offered a different idea, called the psychoprophylactic method for childbirth. Lamaze asked that women respond actively to labor contractions with a set of prelearned, controlled breathing techniques. As the intensity of the contraction increased, so would the woman's rate of breathing. As a result, the laboring woman's posture and attitude changed. She was no longer flat on her back, to be pitied by all onlookers; now she was active, changing positions and breathing patterns as she knew she must. The onlookers cheered.

Marjorie Karmel introduced the Lamaze method of childbirth to the United States with her book *Thank You, Dr. Lamaze,* published in 1959. She had had her first child delivered in Paris by Dr. Lamaze, and when she returned to the States and tried to have her second child delivered by the same method, she ran into tremendous opposition and a great deal of ignorance on the part of doctors here. Mrs. Karmel finally joined with Elisabeth Bing, a physical therapist from Berlin, and founded the American Society for Psychoprophylaxis in Obstetrics (ASPO). The purpose of this society was to train doctors, nurses, and expectant parents in prepared childbirth techniques.

Now there are childbirth-preparation classes in every major city in the United States (see Appendix, p. 206). There are also many books, articles, and films on the subject. (You'll find a fairly complete bibliography at the end of this chapter.) Yet, as with everything else in our impersonal society, neither the classes nor the books will meet our very individual needs unless we demand

that they do. Many of the classes are too large, sometimes with ten to twenty couples attending at a time. So it's often difficult to learn more than just the fundamentals, such as basic anatomy and routine breathing techniques. These are essential to a prepared delivery, but they are sometimes not enough. If you look for them, you can usually find smaller, more personal classes, and the fee is generally the same as the fee for the larger, group classes. However, in either case the fee is higher than many women or couples can afford.

Furthermore, although physical preparation is necessary, psychological and emotional preparation can sometimes be more important. Often large classes are not conducive to discussions of personal problems. People should have the opportunity to talk to each other about all phases of childbearing, from the original decision to conceive a child to the all-too-neglected fears and feelings about child raising. Ideally there should be voluntary, free classes open to anyone who feels the need to talk to other people about any aspect of pregnancy and parenthood. Since these classes are nonexistent in most communities, we must organize ourselves to get them started if we want them.

It's up to us to seek the support we need. Until the time when we can persuade the medical profession to give us less mechanized care, we will have to find all the help we need from each other. But it's often hard to find each other! One way is to ask doctors and hospitals to provide us with the names of the pregnant women they are seeing. They cooperate with diaper services, so why shouldn't they cooperate with us? A way to find the names of women in your area who have just delivered babies is to check the town and state registries of births.

Once we have the people, we must have a place to meet. Hospitals and community centers can provide us with meeting rooms. As for books and teachers, one source is the department of public education. Information about pregnancy and childbirth is so vitally important to so many of us that we have the right to ask that it be supported by public funds. Surely if the state department of education can pay the salary of a person who teaches cake decorating in an adult education class, we might expect it to pay a teacher to prepare us for childbirth.

HOME OR HOSPITAL?

So far we haven't said anything about avoiding the hospital altogether by having our babies at home. Whereas in England over 50 percent of the women have their babies at home, in the United States almost all of us are hospitalized for delivery. In England there is an extensive system of midwives and traveling emergency units which makes home delivery routine, and it is often only the special case that is delivered in a hospital with an attending obstetrician. In the United States we have no such system, and thus home delivery can indeed be very risky. We feel that one of our demands must be to make home delivery feasible here in America. Many women have already experienced successful home deliveries, some with their doctor's help, and many without it. In northern California there is apparently a movement afoot to convince doctors to participate in deliveries at home. Some doctors themselves are behind this movement.* However, until our society is willing to break up the hospital's monopoly on safe deliveries by financing small traveling oxygen and emergency-equipment units for use at home, every woman must decide between hospital and home with their eyes wide open to the dangers as well as the joys.

Here are the personal accounts of two women, one who chose to have her baby in the hospital, and one who chose to have her baby at home.

* * *

Most of us [a group of women in New York] *are less certain than you* [Boston Women's Health Book Collective] *that deliveries should be done more frequently in the home. Obviously, this comes in part from the nature of our own experience in the hospital. Mine was pretty good. I got a lot of support from the nurses, especially over breast-feeding. This is, of course, exceptional. Still, I can't imagine a living situation, even a communal situation, where I would have had as much contact with women who were as experienced as the nurses. I was also glad to be in the hospital from the point of view of rest. I had a lot of lacerations, and I'm sure I wouldn't have been able to get as much rest at home—and this would be especially true of women with other kids.*

Obviously, much depends on the living situation and on the kind of preparation that the woman goes through during pregnancy. For a second birth the prospect of a home delivery is more attractive—I would not be frightened, would not be as much in need of support. Still, I must say the image of delivering eleven stories up over New York City does not thrill me. It does seem very isolated to me. I rather liked going out into society to have my baby, and bringing him home was sort of a rite de passage.

. . . As for safety, I can't quote statistics, but I know that in England they are getting away from the home births because of the higher rate of complications. I needed to have oxygen administered, and there was a

---

*At the 7th Biennial Convention of the International Child-birth Education Association held in Milwaukee in May 1972 it was reported by Lester Hazell that there were more than 100 home deliveries per month in northern California.

A HOME DELIVERY

while when they thought they were going to have to do a forceps delivery; the nurse-midwife was very nice, but very unsure of herself, and I was very glad to be in a situation where there were doctors and other midwives around.

* * *

It was a really beautiful thing to do—not only to be freed from the atmosphere and personnel of the hospital (and who knows what it means for a newborn to see wood walls and carpeted floor, to smell real human smells, to feel wool and cotton and flannel clothes instead of starchy, white, deodorized . . .) but also to know that my body and her body knew what to do, and probably did it better than any doctors could. She was crying before the push that sent her into the world had faded, and was wide awake from the start.

Now that it's over I can think of the risks we took—being an hour and a half from the hospital on a cold night if we needed help—and I can get angry again at the system and the attitudes that forced me to choose this risk. But still, the pride, the joy, the beauty, the wonder of it all overshadow the anger and fear. I hope lots more women do this—I feel strangely stronger (in terms of self, not physically) than ever before.

I didn't tell the doctor I was planning a home birth, since I felt I needed the information he had about my and my baby's health, and was afraid he wouldn't tell me even as much as he did if he knew what I'd planned. Have to go for a checkup next week—am more scared of facing him than I was of delivering my own baby—isn't that ridiculous?!!!

* * *

Whichever you choose, home or hospital, you owe it to yourself and to your baby to learn as much as you can

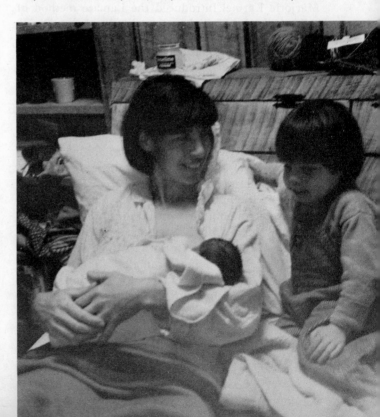

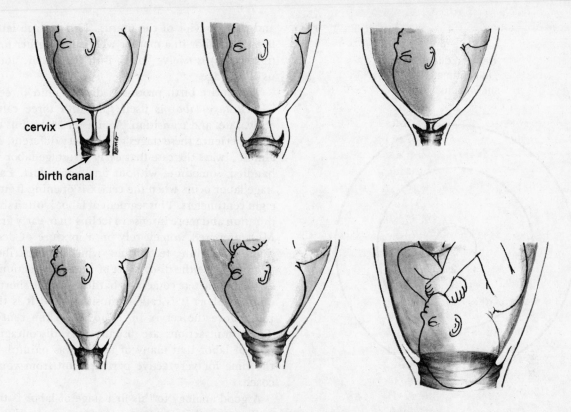

cervix

birth canal

THE CHANGING CERVIX: EFFACEMENT AND DILATION

about the process of labor and the means of preparing for it. If you would like more information about home delivery, contact the Association of Mothers for Educated Childbirth, whose address is listed in the Appendix to this chapter (p. 206). Also, be in touch with the childbirth-education associations in your own area. For the names and addresses of the associations see the Appendix.

WHAT IS LABOR?

Before we describe what labor feels like we should explain exactly what will be happening to our bodies during labor. Delivery comes only after the **effacement** (thinning) and **dilatation** (opening up) of the **cervix** (neck of the uterus). Effacement is measured in percentages. For example, at one of the last prenatal examinations your doctor might say that you are already 80 percent effaced. That means that the neck of your uterus is nearly totally thinned out or "taken up." Dilatation is the term used to refer to the size of the round opening of the cervix, which is exposing more and more of the baby's head. It is measured in centimeters, or sometimes in finger widths. When the cervix is ten centimeters, or five fingers, open, the first stage of labor is over, and the baby is ready to come down the birth canal to be born.

Many women begin to dilate even before labor begins. All through your pregnancy you'll probably feel occasional tightenings of your uterus. Sometimes these preliminary contractions are strong enough to make you catch your breath, but they are rarely painful. Although these so-called Braxton-Hicks contractions are painless, they aren't useless. Each contraction is exercising the uterus, getting it ready to function with utmost efficiency during actual labor. Also, these prelabor contractions are working to start the effacement and dilatation of the cervix. It is not unusual for a woman to begin labor already 90 percent effaced and one or two centimeters dilated.

Which brings us to the question, When does labor really begin? There is no general answer, and this helps to explain the enormous variability in the lengths of different labors. The only guide is that when labor finally does really get under way, one will feel contractions that are stronger and more regular than Braxton-Hicks contractions. They will begin with a gradual tightening of the uterine muscles and slowly rise in intensity. Then a peak will be reached, and the tightening will slowly relax. It reminds some women of the rising, breaking, and falling of waves on the shore. The first contractions are usually not too uncomfortable; they last anywhere from forty-five seconds to a minute. Then when the contraction is over, you feel nothing until the next contraction be-

Cervical dilation
in centimeters,
shown actual size

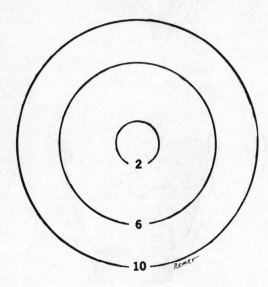

2

6

10 — Reimer

and the behavior of the uterus. The average length for first-stage labor in a mother who is having her first baby (primipara) is twelve hours. But, remember, not one of us is average.

The entire birth process is divided into three stages.

First-stage labor is itself split into three categories: **early, late, and transition.** Again, for each of us the way we experience these stages will be very different. But it is almost always the case that early first-stage labor is easily handled, sometimes without any discomfort. Late first-stage labor ocurs when the cervix is opening from five to eight centimeters. This segment of labor is often shorter in duration and more intense in feeling than early first-stage. Most prepared women rely on a mixture of deep- and shallow-breathing techniques—which are described later —to overcome the discomfort of these contractions. After eight centimeters comes the hardest and the shortest part of your labor. It is called transition, and it is the time just before the cervix opens to a full ten centimeters. These contractions are usually very discouraging, the part of labor that many of us felt was painful. This is the time for very active participation from your labor coach.

A good analogy to this first stage of labor is trying to pull on a turtleneck sweater. At first your head fits easily. Then, as you get closer to the neck opening, it becomes harder to push your head out. You tug at it and stretch it, and finally your head comes through. Similarly, the uterus is stretching and pulling open the cervix, until finally, when the cervix opens to its limit, the delivery of the baby begins. This is called second-stage labor.

gins. What is happening is that the lengthwise muscles of the uterus are involuntarily working to pull open the circular muscles around the cervix. This may take anywhere from two to twenty-four hours or more, depending on the size of the baby, the position in which the baby is lying, the size of the mother's pelvic area,

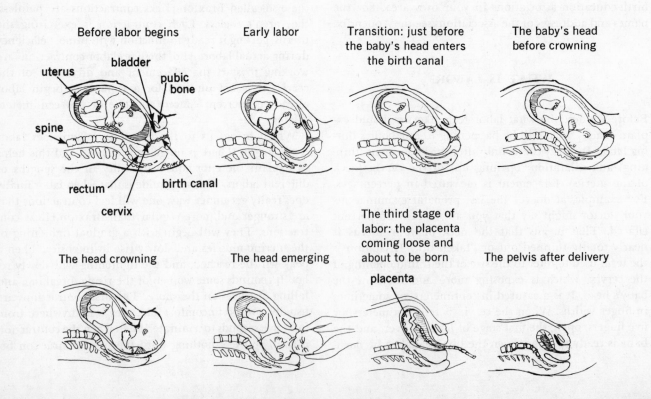

Before labor begins

uterus
bladder
spine
pubic
bone
rectum
cervix
birth canal

Early labor

Transition: just before
the baby's head enters
the birth canal

The baby's head
before crowning

The head crowning

The head emerging

The third stage of
labor: the placenta
coming loose and
about to be born

placenta

The pelvis after delivery

Second-stage labor begins when the cervix is completely dilated and the baby's head (or presenting part) moves into the birth canal, and it ends when the baby is born. It is during this stage that many women will experience a tremendous force inside their bodies. If a woman has learned to bear down correctly, she can help to push her baby down and out at this point. Doctors very frequently anesthetize women for the second stage of labor. Since second stage and delivery are usually not painful if a woman has prepared herself to know how to push and when to push, this unfortunate practice (anesthetizing) should be eliminated from routine obstetrical practice.

Second-stage labor may take anywhere from one half hour to two hours or more, but again this depends on the particular combination of circumstances in each labor. If the mother is unanesthetized, she can push her baby out, and this often speeds things up. In some cases —to be explained later—even mothers with certain types of regional anesthesia can push on direction from the attendant.

Just before the baby's head is born, the doctor will probably perform an **episiotomy** on the mother. This is an incision in the perineum, the area between the vagina and the anus, to enlarge the opening through which the baby will pass (see diagram). Although episiotomies are done routinely in the United States, there is often no need for them. If the mother is unanesthetized, she will feel when to stop pushing and when to start easing her baby gently out. Her doctor can direct her. The vaginal opening can stretch to very wide proportions without tearing.

We question the practice of administering episiotomies to all women before delivery. Some babies need more room to get out, and some lie in a position that calls for

AN EPISIOTOMY

mediolateral cut

median cut

anus

an episiotomy. Then it makes sense for a doctor to cut a straight incision, either to avoid a possible ragged-edged tear in the perineum or to ensure the birth of the baby as speedily as possible. Sometimes it is done, especially in this country, so that the woman's pelvic floor muscles and vagina will not stretch too much. This, doctors say, can create problems later on, such as uterine prolapse, and the like. This means a woman's reproductive organs begin to slip down through the pelvic floor, and sometimes into the vagina. However, prolapse can be avoided usually by perineal exercises, like the Kegel exercise, described in the section on exercises in this chapter.

Often male doctors are concerned that the woman's looser vagina will interfere with the man's sexual pleasure during intercourse.

* * *

I saw my doctor at the checkup six weeks after my baby was born. Full of male pride, he told me during my pelvic exam, "I did a beautiful job sewing you up. You're as tight as a virgin; your husband should thank me."

* * *

The episiotomy stitches are uncomfortable and they often itch. Many times the healing of an episiotomy is painful.

The birth of the baby under normal circumstances is gradual—head first, then shoulders, then body. With each of the last few contractions a new part is born. The baby may take a breath and cry before being completely born, especially if the mother has not been anesthetized, or s/he may take the first breath seconds after birth. The fewer drugs the mother takes during labor, the more active the baby will be at and immediately after delivery. At this point the baby will still be attached to the mother by the umbilical cord, which shouldn't be clipped until all the blood has emptied from it, except in very unusual cases.

Third-stage labor is the delivery of the placenta, the life-supplying organ that has kept the baby healthy and comfortable during the first nine months of life. There may be one or two more contractions before the placenta is released. The third stage may take no more than a few minutes, or it may take half an hour. After its birth the placenta should be examined by the doctor to make sure it is intact; if a piece is left in the uterus, the mother may subsequently experience hemorrhage.

Less Usual Presentations

In the above discussion we have assumed the baby's position in the uterus to be the most common—**left occipito anterior.** This means that the baby is head down in the uterus, lying on the left side, with the occiput, or back part of the skull, toward the mother's front. It is the most efficient way for a baby to slip past the pubic bone and into the birth canal. A baby in this position faces the floor at birth if the mother is lying flat on the delivery table.

Another position is head first but faced the opposite way, with the baby's face toward the mother's front. This is called **posterior presentation**. It often means a more tedious and more uncomfortable labor, since the baby will try to turn around during first-stage labor in order to be born in the more favorable way, facing the mother's back. This type of presentation usually means that the mother will experience labor pains in her back, and she should have this explained to her beforehand so she can prepare herself.

Some babies are born bottom down or feet first, in what is called **breech presentation**. This, too, can cause a longer labor, with contractions felt in your back. A danger in breech birth is that the baby will take its first breath as soon as its bottom is born, while the head is still inside the birth canal. To avoid this the baby's emerging body can be wrapped in a warm, clean blanket to keep the colder air from shocking her or him into a breathful of mucus. Also, the attendant may insert a finger into the birth canal to clear a passageway for air to reach the baby's face. An episiotomy is almost always done in the case of breech presentation so the baby's head can be delivered as quickly as possible.

There are other, very uncommon birth positions, such as **face presentation, brow presentation** and **transverse presentation**. In the first the baby's face enters the birth canal first; in the second the forehead is presenting; and in the third the baby is lying crosswise in the uterus so that a shoulder is usually presenting. A trained obstetrician should certainly be on hand to deliver these rare cases and to decide if a **Caesarean section** (explained later) is necessary. If the mother is fully awake, and if she has been prepared, she will be able to help the doctor by maneuvering as he directs. If it proves necessary for you to have a Caesarean section, try not to feel disappointed. As Sheila Kitzinger says in *The Experience of Childbirth* (pp. 148–49):

> In primitive societies a woman with this difficulty might find a fire lit on her abdomen to smoke the baby out, or be beaten with sticks to force the child to emerge, or have to confess adultery, which is usually considered a barrier to spontaneous delivery. We have a good deal to be grateful for in modern Western obstetrics!

Gravity is a woman's best friend during these unusual presentations, as indeed it is throughout any labor, and the laboring mother should sit as upright as possible to remain comfortable. If the labor bed cannot be adjusted to a sitting position, the woman should prop herself up with pillows, or the coach should support her back. The modern practice of having a laboring mother lie flat on her back throughout the entire birth process is unreason-

able and unnecessarily dangerous to the baby.* It is much less efficient to have to push our babies uphill to be born. If we could labor and deliver in a semiupright position, our voluntary muscles would work with gravity to push the baby downward and out (see diagram).

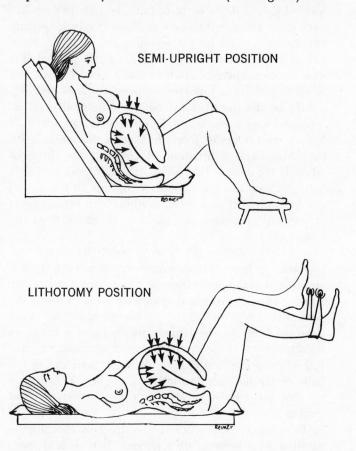

SEMI-UPRIGHT POSITION

LITHOTOMY POSITION

After the baby and the placenta are born, the doctor will sew up the episiotomy. If the woman is unanesthetized, the doctor will probably use a local anesthetic to eliminate the pain caused by the stitching. Many doctors give this local anesthesia even before they perform the episiotomy, and thus the drug reaches the baby. Since the pressure of the baby's head on the perineum creates a natural numbing of the area, the episiotomy can be performed without anesthetics. After the birth, when the numbing has worn off, a pain killer can be injected into the area to make the stitching-up easier on the mother.

*The dorsal position (lying flat on the back) causes the uterus to press on the *inferior vena cava,* involved with supplying blood to the uterus, which may cause shocklike symptoms in the mother and fetal distress in the baby. "Requiring the conscious, participating mother to give birth while in the dorsal or lithotomy position creates unnecessary stress on her respiratory and circulatory systems, which are already taxed by exertion and stress. These recumbent positions greatly hinder the mother's ability to give birth spontaneously" (Haire and Haire, *Implementing Family-Centered Maternity Care,* pp. III–6). Doris Haire is in the process of developing a labor bed that can also serve as a delivery bed.

Some Signs of Abnormal Labor and Delivery

However frightening or unrealistic such a discussion might seem to you, we feel it is important to know how to recognize some of the warnings your body gives you that there may be something wrong.

If complications should arise in your delivery, it is of course of vital importance that you be aware of them and make your doctor aware of them. Here are a few signals that should warn you to contact your doctor immediately.

1. A continuous and severe lower abdominal pain, often accompanied with uterine tenderness (different from the pain of normal labor contractions, which comes on with increasing intensity and then gradually disappears until the next contraction).

2. Discontinuance of good, strong contractions (labor contractions usually get more and more intense as you approach delivery).

3. Excessive vaginal bleeding (although it is not uncommon to have a heavy, bloody mucous discharge during transition).

4. An abnormality in fetal heartbeat (the nurse should be checking fetal heartbeat throughout labor).

5. Abnormally slow dilatation of the cervix.

6. An abnormal presentation or prolapse of cord, placenta, or extremity.

7. Any adverse change in condition of mother or baby (heartbeat, blood pressure, onset of fever).

Any one of these signs does not indicate the need for immediate Caesarean section. In many cases the doctor will simply try to speed up labor by rupturing the membranes (the bag of amniotic fluid in which the baby is floating) or administering a solution of oxytocin* and dextrose.

Occasionally, in the case of a very long, hard labor that seems to be accomplishing little in terms of cervical dilatation, a Caesarean section will be advised. The operation is also necessary if the mother's pelvic structure is too small to allow the baby to move into the birth canal. Other possible situations calling for a Caesarean are those in which the placenta comes loose and begins to prolapse; the cord prolapses; the mother or baby suddenly has an adverse change of condition; or there is excessive bleeding. In all these cases a trained obstetrician should be present to judge the situation and make the decision.

If the doctor recommends a Caesarean section, you must trust that judgment if you haven't enough medical knowledge to argue. Almost always the operation is done

*Oxytocin is a hormone that causes the uterus to contract, sometimes violently. It is used to induce labor, and it is sometimes used postpartum to aid the involution of the uterus. (See "Induction of Labor," p. 191.)

to save your life or your baby's. The procedure is to give the mother anesthesia so she will not experience pain during the operation. She may request regional anesthesia, a spinal type, and thus she can be awake when her baby is delivered. The actual operation may be hidden from her behind sterile drapes. An incision is made through the abdominal wall and into the uterus. The baby is then removed from the uterus by the doctor's hands. After baby and placenta are out, both incisions, uterine and abdominal, are repaired by stitches.

The following is a discussion of Caesarean section by a woman whose first baby was delivered that way.

* * *

My doctor knew when he first examined me that there was a chance that I'd have to have a Caesarean, but he didn't tell me. He didn't want to scare me. So I wasn't at all prepared for it. He did tell me that I'd have a long labor, and toward the end of my pregnancy he said he was worried because the baby's head was so big, but he didn't tell me why he was worried. Then after eighteen hours of labor he told me I'd have to have a Caesarean because I wasn't big enough. I didn't believe what he said; I thought there was something wrong with the baby. Part of me believed it was because I hadn't labored hard enough. Part of me believed I had failed because I hadn't been able to deliver normally (that's one thing Lamaze training doesn't prepare you for, how to deal with a childbirth that doesn't work out normally). I was given an epidural, and I was terrified that something was wrong with the baby. (In the middle of the operation they put an oxygen mask on my face. I didn't know what it was. I thought it was ether, so I didn't breathe for a while. Apparently, giving oxygen is common.)

"Caesarean" shouldn't be such a scary word. Caesareans always take place in operating rooms, not in delivery rooms. You have to be prepped (pubic hair shaved), and you don't have to be completely knocked out. It's good to have an epidural; you can feel your waist and your knees (although not always), and you can remain completely awake if you want to.

A cut is made in the uterus, and the baby is lifted out. I saw my baby being lifted from my stomach in the reflection of a lamp over me. That was very nice. I think my operation took longer, too, because I had a punctured bladder. (I found out later that that was a fairly common thing to happen, and I didn't find out until after the operation that it had happened to me.) My baby was very bloody, a lot bloodier than I had seen in pictures, I think because it was a Caesarean. As soon as they lifted him out he started yelling. That made me very, very, very happy. They flashed him past me, and because Caesarean babies are more susceptible, they put him in intensive care for twenty-four hours in an incubator. I didn't understand why they took him away so quickly, because they kept telling me he was very healthy. They didn't tell me before the surgery that he would automatically be put in intensive care, so I didn't understand why I couldn't see him the next day. I thought something was wrong. Finally I got to see him that night, and he was put into the regular nursery.

Afterward I had a lot of happy, normal birth feelings. I was very proud. I got over being ashamed. The day after he was born I had to walk, and my stomach hurt. One thing that helped me was that I was in a bed next to another woman who had had a Caesarean six days before. Breast-feeding was a little hard, because I had to have this thing to prop him up, and for the first few days I couldn't turn on my side. After that I could put him next to me while I nursed.

Part of my easy postpartum adjustment was that I stayed in the hospital for eight days and was well taken care of because I'd had surgery. (I was a "sick" person and had a reason to get good nursing care.) Also, I had no episiotomy, and I was well rested. And when I got home, people took good care of me.

* * *

We have a right to know beforehand if the doctor suspects there might be complications in our delivery, but too often the doctor will keep that information from us for fear of scaring us.

It is very unlikely that your coach will be allowed into the room during your operation even if you are awake. Talk this possibility over with your doctor during a prenatal visit. Usually it is a last-minute decision to perform a Caesarean section. If, however, a woman has delivered once that way, all future births may have to be conducted by operation, although each successive pregnancy can be judged individually.

Be sure to discuss this operation with your doctor beforehand, and understand all aspects of it. A Caesarean hysterectomy should only be performed in the most severe emergency, when the uterus has become seriously infected or ruptured. Routine hysterectomies during a Caesarean operation are deplorable (and even criminal), and your best weapon against them is knowledge and forewarning.

A Caesarean delivery is not as safe for the mother or baby as a normal delivery.* It is a major abdominal operation, and as such carries with it the risk that any major operation involves. If, however, complications during labor call for a Caesarean, the operation is usually safer for the mother and baby than a vaginal delivery would be under those circumstances.

Another deviation from the normal spontaneous vaginal delivery is delivery by **forceps**. This means that the doctor pulls the baby gently out of the mother's body by

*Nicholson Eastman, *Expectant Motherhood*, p. 153.

the use of a double-bladed instrument. There are many varieties of obstetric forceps, but in general they resemble salad tongs, except that the blades are longer and curved to fit the shape of a baby's head. Each blade is introduced into the vagina separately and placed carefully on the side of the baby's head, usually over the ear, but sometimes at the temples. Then the two blades are clamped together outside the vagina. Depending on where the baby's head lies at the time of delivery, the doctor will use high or low forceps. The higher the forceps, the more dangerous the delivery, since that indicates that the baby will have to be pulled out a longer distance. Here is what an obstetrical text says about the use of forceps:

> The function of the forceps in general is to terminate labor when the second stage is unduly prolonged (dystocia) and when the mother or the baby is endangered. The instrument is used too often without proper indications as a matter of convenience and because of the importunities of the patient or family for relief. However, in recent years the widespread use of regional block anesthesia (spinal or caudal) has greatly increased the need for low forceps delivery, because a very high percentage of women thus anesthetized are unable to exert the voluntary muscular action needed to complete the second stage of labor.*

We know that delivery by forceps has saved the lives of many infants and mothers, but we also know that many forceps deliveries are performed simply for the sake of teaching young obstetricians the technique. Discuss forceps with your doctor before delivery and find out his or her views on the subject.

The usual reasons for a forceps delivery are:

1. To speed up second-stage labor if there is severe fetal distress.

2. If the umbilical cord is wrapped tightly around the baby's neck or if the cord prolapses.†

3. In case of unusual presentations.

4. If regional anesthesia doesn't allow the mother to push out her baby.

5. To shorten a very long second-stage labor.

It is uncommon for a prepared, unanesthetized mother to have to have her baby delivered by forceps, but should the occasion arise, the breathing techniques may be enough to carry you through without anesthesia.

*Charles E. McLennan with collaboration of Eugene C. Sandberg, *Synopsis of Obstetrics*, ed. 8, 1970, St. Louis, The C. V. Mosby Co., p. 432.

†"The problem of the cord around the neck is common and occurs in 25 or 30 percent of deliveries" (*ibid.*, p. 166). Usually the doctor can loosen the loop and gently slip it over the baby's head. If the cord is prolapsed and actually falls into the vagina, there is danger that the cord might be compressed between the presenting part of the baby and the bony structure of the mother and thus cut off the baby's circulation.

Premature Labor

A newborn is considered premature if his or her birth weight is less than five and a half pounds. More than half the deaths of newborns in the United States are due to prematurity. The tragedy is enhanced by the fact that much prematurity can be prevented through good nutrition, proper prenatal medical care, and adequate birth control, which is especially important for young teenagers, whose bodies may not be developed enough to carry a fetus to term. As one maternal nursing text stated, "If an equal amount of the money expended on premature care were applied to preventive care, it would be interesting to prognosticate the results."*

Some specific causes of premature labor are infectious diseases (such as syphilis), toxemia, diabetic diseases, thyroid disturbances, fetal abnormalities, placental abnormalities (placenta previa, abruptio placenta, etc.), and multiple pregnancies. It has been shown that good nutrition and excellent prenatal medical care can eliminate many of these problems before they lead to premature labor and possible neonatal death. (See section on "Pregnancy.") There is little knowledge about what causes prematurity in nearly half the cases; however, it is known that race, ethnic group, economic status, social class, and nutritional status all influence the statistics. Seven percent of white women in America deliver prematurely, compared to 12 percent of nonwhite women. We can infer that poorer women receive poorer prenatal care.

Premature labor proceeds as does normal, full-term labor, although it may be a little slower due to weaker contractions. There is often much more anxiety involved in a premature labor if the mother is wondering if her baby will survive. Most premature babies who do not survive succumb to hyaline membrane disease,† although the premature infant in general is much more susceptible to all infections.

The smaller and more feeble the baby, the more need there is for immediate care. Premature infants are placed in oxygen-, temperature-, and humidity-controlled incubators, and they must be constantly watched and carefully protected from every possible source of infection. Feeding the premature infant is a problem because of the baby's underdeveloped intestinal tract. A study by V. Crosse and others showed that "premature infants fed human milk not only had the lowest incidence of major infection and mortality during the hospital stay but also proved free from infection after leaving the hospital

*Elise Fitzpatrick *et al., Maternity Nursing*, p. 407.
†"Hyaline membrane disease is a syndrome of neonatal respiratory distress in which the alveoli and the alveolar ducts are filled with a sticky exudate, a hyaline material, which prevents aeration" (*ibid.*, p. 532). It is seen mostly in premature babies and those delivered by Caesarean section. There is recent evidence to suggest that hyaline membrane disease may be determinable before birth.

when breast-fed at home."* A mother can pump her own colostrum and milk using a hand or an electric breast pump, and this milk can be supplied to her infant in the nursery incubator. Human colostrum is so full of antibodies to fight the very infections to which the premature infant might succumb that it seems foolish not to insist that colostrum be an integral part of the premature baby's diet.

Another reason to feed the premature infant breast milk is just as important. That is the mother's need for contact with her newborn. The birth of a premature baby comes usually before the mother has prepared herself psychologically for delivery and motherhood. Guilt feelings and emotional uncertainty are almost an inevitable aspect of prematurity. The hospital staff, nurses and doctors alike, should be aware of this and should encourage the mother whenever possible to visit her baby, hold her baby, and even feed her baby. If the mother feels that it is her milk that is sustaining the infant and her efforts that are helping the baby to grow stronger, then she will begin the postpartum period with a much stronger and more confident attitude.

Induction of Labor

Induction is the term used to refer to a preplanned delivery, whereby labor is artificially induced, usually with chemical substitutes for the hormones present in natural labor, oxytocics (from oxytocin, the hormone) or "pit," short for pitocin, the chemical substitute. Induction may also refer to any deliberate attempt to get labor started—for example, rupturing the membranes with instruments.

There is still considerable controversy over induction, and in some hospitals induction for convenience (either the mother's or the physician's) is not permitted. Unfortunately, induction for convenience is growing more and more common. Some obstetricians have their delivery schedules arranged in advance. One of the reasons for the controversy over induction is that it is in many cases difficult to tell the true maturity of the fetus, since conception itself can rarely be pinpointed with accuracy. Without knowing the true age of the baby, it's difficult to know if s/he is ready to endure extrauterine life or the stresses of labor and delivery. In most cases there must also be evidence that the mother's body is ready for labor, such as considerable effacement and a certain amount of dilatation. Often if a mother has a previous history of extremely short labors and lives some distance from the hospital, induction will be chosen. Or if there is some question about the baby, such as toxemia of

*V. Crosse *et al.*, "The Value of Human Milk Compared with Other Feeds for Premature Infants," in Haire and Haire, *Implementing Family-Centered Maternity Care*, pp. V–42–43.

pregnancy, hemolytic disease, or maternal diabetes, which might require emergency mobilization of the hospital team, it might be wiser to induce labor.

However, induced labor poses a special problem for the laboring mother because of the peculiar character of induced contractions. They frequently do not follow the normal wavelike course, but reach intensity instantaneously, remain intense for a long period, and are often described by women who can make comparisons as much more painful than ordinary, normal contractions. If the mother is not prepared for this, it can prove very discouraging indeed. If she is prepared—which means being told beforehand by her doctor what to expect—she can usually carry on, using her breathing techniques without medication. Even women whose membranes are artificially ruptured may have very hard, although shorter, labors.

A mother whose labor is induced will probably require extra support and definitely needs good information on the progress of her labor. Naturally, she must be closely monitored to make sure that the uterus is not overstimulated or the baby is not distressed by the use of the drug.

There are some risks involved with induction, such as uterine rupture, hypertension, possible water intoxication, prolapse of the umbilical cord, and fetal distress. Careful and judicious administration of the oxytocin drip greatly reduces the chance of these potentially fatal complications.

The following is the story of one woman whose first labor was induced.

* * *

At the hospital I got some injections of what I thought was pitocin. My labor was very intense and unexpectedly short—four hours. I felt pretty much in control. My daughter had to be delivered by forceps because her heartbeat was slowing down and I couldn't push her out quickly enough. I was told her life had been endangered because my contractions were too strong and the placenta had separated from the uterine wall too early. My doctors were heroes! They had saved her life.

Three years later, seven months pregnant, I asked my doctor a casual question about my first labor and delivery. He began reading my record to me. He read about injections of Demerol. I was amazed and said, "That doesn't sound like my labor." It turned out that I had gotten pitocin to induce my labor for a time, then Demerol to slow my contractions down, because they were going too fast.

Now that I look back, I think that perhaps the pitocin stimulated my labor too strongly so that indeed it wasn't natural, and was even dangerous. And I think that my strong contractions made the placenta separate early. I'm sure that the Demerol slowed my daughter's heart-

beat and oxygen intake. It also explains why she was so sleepy the first three days and didn't immediately nurse. Now I know that unmedicated babies are not sleepy at birth.

In other words, now I don't feel the dangers would have happened if I hadn't been induced and then slowed down. My doctors gave me the feeling that they were responsible for saving my daughter's life, and if they hadn't been there . . . ! Now I feel they were responsible for the dangers to my daughter's life—if not completely, at least in great part. Induction complicated my labor and delivery.

* * *

DRUGS

One goal of a prepared mother is to allow drugs and/or instruments to be used in her labor only when a real medical emergency arises. The exercises described in the following section will give you appropriate, safe, and manageable tools to help you keep in control of yourself during labor. They are not guaranteed to bring us "painless" childbirth; they are designed to help us overcome the pain that may be involved in our labors.

Drugs can also help us overcome the discomfort of labor, and there are times when the use of obstetric drugs is appropriate. However, a completely drugged woman is sensationless. She feels nothing during labor, or in some cases when amnesiacs are used, she just remembers nothing about what she felt during labor. Although she may have eliminated painful contractions, she has also eliminated the excitement of participating fully in this most joyful of human experiences. Furthermore, as Dr. Nicholson Eastman says in his book *Expectant Motherhood* (p. 64) of the drugs employed in childbirth, "None are without their drawbacks; none are applicable in all cases; and none are without some slight risk to the mother or child under certain circumstances. Moreover, with a few exceptions, none can be employed except in hospitals with a special nurse in constant attendance."

According to one obstetrics text, "About 10 percent of maternal deaths now are attributable in some way to the anesthetic used. Aspiration of vomitus and excessively high levels of spinal anesthesia are the chief problems."[*] Furthermore, there is evidence to indicate that almost all if not all drugs taken by the mother cross the placenta and reach the baby.[†] This can be especially harmful if the baby is premature or just very small. Narcotics and barbiturates can cause depression of fetal respiration as

[*]*Synopsis of Obstetrics*, p. 174.
[†]Haire and Haire, pp. III–8–14.

well as decreased responsiveness in the newborn infant. A study by Brackbill and Conway and others shows that infants whose mothers received various medications during labor and delivery can give significantly retarded muscular, visual, and neural development in the first four weeks of life.* Of course, not every baby will be so affected, nor will the babies affected be permanently retarded in development, but four weeks is a very long time in an infant's life, and many imprinting patterns† can be set during that time. It seems to make sense to try to give your baby the very best head start you can.

Labor to a woman who has not prepared herself for it can of course be a very frightening experience. Even if you have learned generally what to expect, the actual process of labor may not approximate your vision of it. We must not set ourselves up for an endurance test. Instead we must educate ourselves realistically and thoroughly as to how we can best manage our labors. Exercises and breathing techniques, and constant companionship, will be all many of us need to master the occasion. Some of us will use drugs to help us during labor. We must not feel that one way is "better" than the other. We should, however, understand what drugs might do to our babies as well as what they can do to ease our pain during labor, and we should know that different drugs and different amounts of the same drug can have significantly different effects on us and our babies.

We'll list here some types of drugs most commonly used during labor and discuss some of the possible complications these drugs might produce. Never accept a drug without first asking what it is and knowing in advance what effect it might have on you and your baby. The hospital staff is obliged by law to tell you, if you ask, what drugs they are administering. They probably won't tell you anything if you don't ask.

As soon as labor begins to become serious business, and you find you have to work hard to keep yourself in control, the doctor or nurse will probably offer you a tranquilizer or a narcotic. According to a survey by Doris and John Haire, tranquilizers such as Equanil, Miltown,

Librium, and others, may have little untoward effect on a human fetus. Tranquilizers, however, if given in too large a dose, can hinder the mother's efforts to remain in control of her contractions. She may find herself falling asleep until the contraction reaches its peak, and then she may panic, forget to breathe appropriately, and actually experience more pain than she would have without the drug. With a good coach by her side reminding her of the breathing techniques and keeping her awake from the start of the contraction to the finish, that shouldn't happen too often. Narcotics have a similar effect on the mother, but all such narcotics as Demerol, Dolophine, or Nisentil, for example, have a depressant effect on fetal respiration, and the newborn's responsiveness may be seriously decreased by these drugs.

Barbiturates, derivatives of barbituric acid, have been used to produce sleep in the laboring mother. Nembutal and Seconal fall into this category, as do Luminal, sodium Amytal, and barbital, to name a few. These drugs are dangerous to the fetus; they cross the placental barrier readily, and they can depress fetal respiration and responsiveness. Furthermore, a study by Ploman and Persson found that

. . . the selective tissue storage of depressant drugs such as barbiturates was many times higher in the midbrain than in the circulating blood [of the newborn]. This selective storage lasted for as much as a week in the immature brain, affecting the midbrain-mediated behavior of the newborn for the entire time. Since the newborn's behavior is primarily midbrain in origin, this means that his behavioral repertoire is influenced for the entire important first week of his life by medication given innocently to the mother in the few hours just prior to delivery.*

It is often the case that barbiturates are given to the laboring mother early in labor in combination with a small amount of scopolamine. Scopolamine, sometimes called Twilight Sleep, is an amnesiac and a hallucinogen that has the effect of making the woman forget what she experienced during labor, but does not stop her sensations at the time. In other words, she goes through labor in a kind of nightmarish sleep, and then when she wakes up, her conscious mind forgets what she has felt. Like other hallucinogens, scopolamine can cause some women to become physically violent and others to become stuporous. A woman under the influence of scopolamine can cause herself physical damage by thrashing about wildly during contractions, and as a result, she must be constantly watched. Hospitals once used this drug routinely as the answer to pain in labor; too many hospitals in New England and in the South still use it. The use

---

*In *Ibid.*, pp. III–10; from W. Bowes, Y. Brackbill, E. Conway and A. Steinschneider: *The Effects of Obstetrical Medication on Fetus and Infant*, Monograph of the Society for Research in Child Development, Vol. 35, No. 4, 1970, University of Chicago Press. Control groups showed that this effect was directly related to the obstetrical medication used. Furthermore, R. Kron, M. Stein, and K. Goddard show in "Newborn Sucking Behavior Affected by Obstetrical Sedation," *Pediatrics*, 37:1012–16, 1966, that newborn sucking behavior may be depressed for as long as four days after delivery by medication used routinely on the laboring mother.

†Imprinting refers to certain bonds of a psychological nature that create patterns for future action and that either take place at a specific time or do not take place at all. For a discussion of the subtle effects of depressant drugs used during labor see T. Berry Brazelton, "Infant Outcome in Obstetric Anesthesia," in the *ICEA News* (November-December 1970).

*L. Ploman and B. Persson, "On the Transfer of Barbiturates to the Human Fetus and Their Accumulation in Some of Its Vital Organs," J. Obstet. and Gynaecol. Brit. Emp., 64:706–11, 1927, as discussed in Brazelton, *ibid.*

of scopolamine is described in an obstetrical textbook:

> This method can be properly used only in a hospital in a quiet, darkened room; the mother must be watched carefully to guard against injury or falling from the bed if she becomes excited. Some physicians believe that a woman who is spared the recollection of her labor may be harmed psychologically and may even reject her off-spring. This method has very largely fallen into disfavor because of the associated pulmonary edema, swallowing of the tongue, and maternal excitement.*

Needless to say, scopolamine, or "scope," as it is sometimes called, is a drug to avoid.

In another category of anesthesia are gas and volatile anesthetics. These are inhaled by the mother and produce intermittent analgesia during contractions. Included in this category are ether and nitrous oxide, or laughing gas. They can be used during second-stage contractions but not before. Ether can retard labor, and it may "provoke vomiting, excessive uterine relaxation, and bleeding."† Nitrous oxide is a safer substance, for mother and baby, as long as it is administered in combination with 20 percent oxygen.‡ Trilene, or trichloroethylene, is a similar type of anesthesia, because it is inhaled and has a temporary analgesic effect.

Lester Hazell describes Trilene in her book *Common-sense Childbirth*:

> [Trilene] is a volatile liquid that is placed in a special inhaler. The mother holds the inhaler herself, breathes in the vapors as she needs to. If she gets enough of the vapor to make her drowsy, her hand falls away and she will soon have her head clear from breathing fresh air.§

The problem is in learning how to breathe in these inhalation anesthetics just in time to have them working when they are most needed, during the peak of a contraction. It usually takes about fifteen to thirty seconds for Trilene to start working, and Trilene apparently has no depressing effect on the fetus.¶ Furthermore, since it is self-administering, you have control over how much to take, when to take it, and if to take it. This would be a particularly good drug for a woman with painful second-stage contractions, but for some reason doctors rarely offer it.

More and more women and doctors these days are rejecting such general anesthesias as those previously mentioned in favor of regional anesthesia, which, for the purposes of labor, is injected into the spinal area and serves to anesthetize the lower body. The drugs used in spinal anesthesia vary as do the dosages.

*Synopsis of Obstetrics, p. 175.
†*Ibid.*, p. 176.
‡Haire and Haire, pp. III–34.
§P. 179, paperback edition, New York, Tower Publications, Inc., 1970, originally published by G. P. Putnam's Sons, 1969.
¶Haire and Haire, pp. III–34.

In spinal anesthesia, [saddle blocks] the drug is introduced directly into the spinal canal in the region of the small of the back. It is employed chiefly for actual delivery but is sometimes used to cover the last few hours of labor. In caudal anesthesia the drug is introduced somewhat lower and into a bony space at the very lower end of the vertebral column. By renewing this anesthetic solution from time to time, as its effects wear off, it is possible to make caudal anesthesia "continuous" for as long as six or eight hours, sometimes longer.*

Both saddle blocks and caudals cannot be administered to every woman in labor for various reasons. Both rely heavily on obstetrical intervention, especially in the use of forceps during delivery, since the mother's bearing-down urge is obliterated. Furthermore, there are some women who suffer from serious aftereffects, such as postpartum headache. Only an experienced anesthesiologist is able to administer spinal anesthesias, and the laboring mother must be kept under constant supervision because of the possibility of complications.

A type of caudal anesthesia, known as an epidural, seems to be safer and more reliable than the others. It is administered through a catheter placed in your lower back, into the epidural space outside the spinal column. Its effects wear off in about forty-five minutes, but it can be renewed throughout labor. Unlike some other forms, the epidural can be given to a laboring woman from about four centimeters' dilatation until delivery. Under the influence of an epidural you are awake, but you just can't feel anything from your breasts to your knees or ankles.

Why shouldn't everyone have an epidural during labor then? Well, first of all it isn't available everywhere, and only a very experienced and highly skilled anesthesiologist can administer it properly. Secondly, it is very expensive, and thus not everyone can afford it. Third, because a woman under regional anesthesia has to be monitored continuously—due to the risk of hypotension or fetal distress—trained personnel have to be on hand at all times during the labor. Since hospitals are usually short of staff, a number of women under this anesthesia are often placed together in a room to be monitored jointly. That means that except under very specific conditions (for example, if you're the only woman laboring at a given time) your coach cannot be with you during labor. In some hospitals the coach may be allowed into the delivery room to witness the actual birth, though he or she couldn't be with you during first-stage labor. During delivery you won't be able to feel when to bear down and push the baby out, but you may be able to push on direction from the doctor. A new study by Dr. Wayne L. Johnson seems to have confirmed the theory that all regional anesthesia can prolong

**Eastman, *Expectant Motherhood* (Little, Brown and Company), p. 163.

second-stage labor and result "in an increased use of oxytocin and an increased incidence of forceps deliveries."* In many teaching hospitals the use of forceps on women with regional anesthesia is still routine. Studies have yet to be completed to show the full effects of this type of anesthesia on the newborn, but thus far a brief slowing of the baby's heart rate is one demonstrated effect. Also, the longer the drug is continued, the greater is the risk to the baby.

If you are given a regional anesthesia you will feel nothing during labor, and you will have none of those thrilling and unforgettable sensations related to the birth of your baby. Also, as we have seen, the use of any drugs immediately increases the risks involved in childbirth.

Many doctors like to give us anesthesia during the second stage of labor so that they can complete any obstetrical maneuvers they deem necessary to deliver the baby quickly, including episiotomy and repair. We know that second-stage labor is rarely painful if we have learned how to push effectively. We know that we can control the force with which we push our baby into the world if we are unanesthetized. Furthermore, we know that in most cases babies can be delivered spontaneously, and forceps should be used only if there are complications. During childbirth any unnecessary procedure should be omitted, the birth of a healthy baby being the uppermost goal.

If we are skeptical about the use of drugs and instruments during normal childbirth, we must have some other tools to cope with labor and delivery. The tools that have worked for so many of us are preparation, exercise, breathing techniques, and companionship. In the next sections we will discuss these tools in detail.

EXERCISES

The work of labor centers on the pelvis and uterus. The function of our preparation, then, is to help these parts work most effectively during labor.

In terms of the physical aspect of labor we have to learn two basic things: first, how to breathe in a way that will give our body the necessary oxygen it needs to function most efficiently; and second, how to allow one part of our body to work while keeping the rest of our body relaxed.

One idea behind these two techniques is efficiency. If we can teach ourselves to pace our breathing according to how vigorously our body is working, we can help it do its work well. Controlled breathing, sending the right amount of oxygen to our laboring muscles, will give those muscles the fuel they need to keep functioning.

*"Regionals Can Prolong Labor," p. 41.

The same principle of efficiency can be applied to the disassociation technique. By voluntarily relaxing all our muscles except those of the uterus, we will not be taking needed energy away from our laboring parts.

Another idea behind the techniques is selective attention. We all have experienced selective attention. If we receive too many outside stimuli at once, we can't incorporate them all into our consciousness, and so some go unnoticed. It's like trying to listen to two conversations at once; we either confuse them or let one surface to the disadvantage of the other. Well, by concentrating as hard as we can on what our response to the contractions will be, we don't give our minds time or room to register that we might be feeling pain. It's not that prepared childbirth is painless, it's just that we are taught how to interpret the sensations associated with contractions. As a result, some women say they never really felt any pain during labor; other women say that feelings of pain kept surfacing, but they were almost always able to control those feelings with increased concentration on the breathing techniques. One woman wrote that there was a kind of beauty in her acceptance of the pain she felt:

* * *

I don't think pain is necessarily bad. I had a short, hard labor and it was clear to me that the incredible euphoria that I experienced afterwards was in part a function of the fact that it was very painful. It really was almost positive pain, really worth it in retrospect. I just think that pain is pain, and childbirth is painful.*

* * *

The way in which each of us will experience her own labor is impossible to predict, but it is certainly true that we needn't be afraid of labor.

It can only be to our advantage to learn how to use the tools that can help us during labor. There are many exercises that we can do even before our pregnancies begin, to get our bodies into condition, and there are many others that we can practice during pregnancy. You can find exercises in some of the books in the bibliography. Four books are particularly helpful: *Commonsense Childbirth,* by Lester Hazell (a woman); *The Experience of Childbirth,* by Sheila Kitzinger; *The New Childbirth,* by Erna Wright; and *Six Practical Lessons for an Easier Childbirth,* by Elisabeth Bing.

Here we will be concerned mainly with the **disassociation techniques** and with **controlled breathing.** First, however, there is one very simple exercise, called the Kegel exercise or the "elevator," that can be done at any time and in any place. It involves gradually tightening the muscles around your vagina, the perineal area, and then loosening them just as gradually. You can really

*Excerpt from a letter to Boston Women's Health Book Collective.

feel this working during urination. If you can stop the flow of your urine by tightening your vaginal muscles then you will know how this exercise is supposed to feel. Do it first to a count of six, and work up to a count of ten. Once you become proficient at this, try to imagine the muscles up farther inside of you, those on the pelvic floor. See if you can repeat this exercise using those muscles.

Try to do it whenever you think of it. It's an important exercise, for it teaches you how to relax the muscles of the pelvic floor and perineum—which have to be relaxed to allow the baby to pass through at birth—and it also teaches you how to tighten those muscles so that after the birth you can return to your naturally firm condition.

We shall now describe some disassociation techniques. Since we have learned to use muscles, not singularly, but in combination with one another, we have to learn to dissociate the muscles from one another if we are going to be able to allow the activity of the uterus to be as unhampered as possible. We do not want any muscles other than those that work automatically to be using up energy during labor. Our goal in these exercises is to learn what a tight muscle feels like and how to relax it. Try doing these exercises with someone around to check your relaxation.

Lie flat on the floor with pillows comfortably under your head and knees. First relax all your muscles as much as you can, and then, starting with your toes, begin to tighten them, one at a time: first your toes, then your feet, then your calves, then your knees, thighs, vagina, rectum, abdomen, chest, shoulders, neck, and face. By the time you reach your scalp you should be one mass of tensed muscle. At this point we want to reverse the process: starting at the top of your head, begin to relax, one muscle at a time, until, when you relax your toes, you feel totally limp. This exercise should be done at least once a day—before bed is a perfect time—and perhaps two or three times a day if you can comfortably manage it.

A variation on that exercise is to lie comfortably relaxed; then think of one part of your body and tense it. Make sure that all your other muscles stay loose. Then relax again, and tense another part.

Another variation is trying to tighten two muscles on opposite sides of your body while keeping all your other muscles relaxed. Lie on the floor again, with pillows arranged for your comfort. Make sure all your muscles are relaxed by checking them from head to toe in a mental rundown. Then tense your left leg and your right arm at the same time while everything else is relaxed. After a slow count of five, loosen up and switch to your right leg and left arm.

Try doing these exercises in different positions. During labor you may be on your back very little, and you should be able to keep your muscles relaxed no matter what your position. Also, check yourself from time to time when you're not doing these exercises to see which parts of you tend to tense up without your knowing it. If you locate specific areas, like your mouth or your hands, you can concentrate especially on keeping them relaxed during labor.

Before we describe the four main types of breathing we should state that these have evolved over the years and are still subject to change. For that reason it is worthwhile to check with a childbirth-education class to find out the newest techniques. To find a class near you, contact the national childbirth association offices listed in the Appendix.

The first type of breathing is a deep, full abdominal breathing. You breathe in with your nose and out with your mouth, trying to make your abdomen rise as you inhale and fall as you exhale. Do this breathing slowly and rhythmically, counting forward (to five or eight or even ten) as you breathe in, and backward as you breathe out. This type of breathing will be very helpful during early first-stage labor. It will help to relieve some of the pressure around your abdomen.

The second type is a chest breathing. This is also a very deep breathing, but it sends all the air into your chest. Place your hands under your breasts on your rib cage as you breathe this way, and feel your ribs rise and fall. Again breathe in with your nose and out with your mouth, just as with the abdominal breathing. Make sure your abdominal muscles are as relaxed as you can make them. During early and late first-stage labor you will use this second technique to meet the first contractions, which involuntarily make your abdominal wall rigid. You needn't keep your hands on your ribs during this exercise once you are sure you are doing it properly. Breathe regularly and rhythmically.

The third type of breathing is a shallow chest breathing. It is sometimes called the "out" technique. Take a short breath in with your mouth and then push it out by making the sound "out" in a whisper (in some classes the word is "hut"). Try doing this exercise for thirty seconds at a time. Pace yourself comfortably, and try not to breathe too quickly. During labor this exercise will be very helpful. Some women use it from the moment labor begins to get serious until the baby is ready to be pushed out. You will probably not be using "out" throughout an entire contraction. It is more likely that you will begin with a few deep chest breaths, and then, as the contraction becomes more intense, you will switch to this more rapid breathing. Then, as the contraction eases, so will your breathing. At the end of each contraction you should remember to take a long, deep breath and exhale it fully. This will help you to relax while awaiting the next contraction.*

It's very useful to practice this shallow chest breathing with someone there to time you with a clock or stop watch. Your companion can give you the signal: "Contraction begins." You take a deep breath, and exhale it completely. Then you breathe deeply, as described in the second technique. When your companion calls "Fifteen seconds," switch to the "out" breathing, and keep that up until she calls "Forty-five seconds." At this point your breathing should return to a deeper chest-centered breathing. Finish your practice after one minute is reached with a deep breath, and exhale it completely. When they occur, use Braxton-Hicks contractions for practice purposes.

The fourth type of breathing is a very shallow, mouth-centered panting. It takes a lot of practice to learn this technique well, and some of us never master it in practice, but find that it often comes naturally during labor. Actually, it doesn't matter; do what you can and what keeps you comfortable for as long as possible. Panting will be most useful during transition, when you might vary it by a combination of panting and blowing. To learn the pant, relax your body, drop open your jaw, and breathe in and out through your mouth so that you feel the air going only to the back of your throat and then out again. You will probably hear a very quiet panting noise during this, but it should not become too loud. Try to keep the breaths regularly spaced, perhaps three or four a second, and don't pant too rapidly, or you might become hyperventilated. The best way to avoid **hyperventilation**† is to make sure that for every breath you inhale, you exhale completely. To pant correctly requires a certain amount of concentration, and that is helpful to take your mind off your uterus. Sometimes, however, even panting might not be sufficient—for example, when you are trying to control the urge to push at the end of transition. Here are two techniques to help you through those times.

Pant-pant-blow: Many women who have trouble panting have no difficulty at all with this technique. All you do is take two, three, or four panting breaths and on the last one blow out. In-out, in-out, in-out, in-*blow*. Make sure to blow out with force.

Whoo-ha: This is a rapid, shallow pant done saying the word "whoo-ha" and moving your head slightly from side to side (another thing to keep your mind busy) at the same time.

There are some other tools that you or your labor coach can use to make labor manageable. One of these is **effleurage**. Elisabeth Bing describes it in *Six Practical Lessons:* "Cup your hands lightly, place them under your abdomen. Then massage gently with your fingertips, leading your arms out and up while you inhale, completing the circle down again as you exhale."* This light massage helps you to relax, it relieves some of the tension you might feel in your abdomen, it gives you something to do, and it feels good.

It is often very helpful to you if your coach gives you a gentle massage on your legs, usually around your thighs, or on your back. Some women with backache labor rely on this massage to keep them comfortable. Unfortunately, during transition, you will probably be so irritable—a common symptom of transition—that you won't allow anyone to touch you. This, of course, may not be at all what happens to you, so remember massage as an effective technique. Sheila Kitzinger gives a detailed account of massage in *The Experience of Childbirth* (pp. 94-95).

Finally, there are many ways you can be made to feel more comfortable during the intervals between contractions. Sucking ice chips or a wet washcloth, sipping water, licking a candy stick, or feeling a cool washcloth on your forehead can all help to relax you and give you the confidence you need to keep on working.

The preceding discussion applies to the first stage of labor. It suggests ways to keep yourself comfortable during the tedious process of dilatation. Now we can talk about the much more exciting work of labor, the expulsion of the baby. Once second stage begins you'll probably feel terrific, because finally you'll be able to actively help in your baby's birth.

To push effectively you should be in a semisitting position, or if you are in the delivery room, with your feet in stirrups, your back should be raised off the table at about a 45-degree angle. Either your coach can support your back or you can prop yourself up on two pillows, brought from the labor room for this purpose. As soon as you feel the contraction coming on, get into the pushing position by curving your back, holding your legs up under the knees, pointing your elbows out, and bending your head down with your chin on your chest. Then take two deep, cleansing breaths and exhale them each completely. Take a third deep breath in, and hold it. At the same time, bear down with all your might, thinking about how you are helping to push the baby through the birth canal. Continue bearing down with this first breath for as long as you can comfortably; then lift your head, blow the air out, take another deep breath, and bear down again. Keep your legs up while you change breaths. You will probably have to take at

*Contractions are different for everyone, and even within the course of your own labor your contractions may follow different patterns.

†Hyperventilation is caused by an improper oxygen-carbon dioxide balance. If you become hyperventilated you will feel dizzy, and your fingers and toes will tingle. You may even faint.

*Bring along some talcum powder to rub on your stomach. It makes effleurage easier.

least three breaths during each second-stage contraction. Try to keep your vagina and perineum relaxed. (*Note:* While you are learning the pushing technique during pregnancy, practice the position and the breathing sequence, but *do not push or bear down very hard.*)

There are some women who have reported that they never felt the urge to push. This means that you will have to push when directed to push by your doctor or coach, who will have a hand on your abdomen to feel when the contraction begins its tightening. Keep pushing until they tell you the contraction is over.

As the baby's head crowns, you will have to stop pushing, and you can use the pant-pant-blow technique to control your urge. You want to ease the baby out without tearing your perineum.

It is of course best to be as awake and aware as possible during labor. If you can feel your contractions, you will know how to work with them. During first stage you will know when to switch from one breathing level to another, and you will be able to feel your contractions increasing in intensity as second stage approaches. When, finally, the urge to push becomes utterly uncontrollable, you will be in second stage, and you will be able to start pushing your baby out.

BEING IN LABOR

You've gone through a lot from the time you decided to have a baby until now. You feel you are well prepared both physically and emotionally, and you're really excited that any day you'll be meeting that unknown bump in your stomach. But then it hits you. You're scared, and the most frightening thing of all is that at this point there's no turning back.

You'll have a few signs at the end of your pregnancy that labor is about to begin. Sometimes you'll find some blood-tinged mucus on your underclothes. This is the mucus plug that has been in the end of the cervix (like a cork in a bottle), whose purpose it was to keep the uterus free from germs that might have entered through the vagina. Many women never notice or never have a bloody show, as it's called, before labor. Others have an increasing amount of show all the way through the first stage of labor. This is another indication that each labor is unique.

Some women begin labor when their membranes rupture. This means that the bag of waters, amniotic fluid, in which the fetus has been floating, breaks, and water begins to trickle out of your vagina, quite uncontrollably. That's the way you can tell it isn't urine; you can't stop it. In most cases the bag doesn't break until the second stage of labor is ready to begin, but occasionally a strong contraction will force the bag to burst

before then. Sometimes the doctor will artificially break the bag of waters. This is a device used to induce labor or to speed up a long or inefficient labor.

Once the bag of waters has burst, there is a good chance that the baby will be born soon. For that reason it is very important to contact your doctor or hospital if you think your membranes have ruptured. Even if you aren't in labor, the doctor will most certainly have specific instructions for you. Demand them, if you are in doubt. Remember, if the bag has burst, it doesn't mean that all the water will empty from it permanently; the amniotic fluid is continually manufactured by your body. But it does mean the chance of infection is increased.

Diarrhea is another sign that labor is approaching. Many women have a diarrhealike urge for about three days before labor begins. This is nature's way of emptying the rectum before the birth process, so that there will be no unnecessary pressure on the birth canal. Frequently, women feel an increased number of Braxton-Hicks contractions for some time before labor actually begins, and often these contractions are confused with real labor contractions. Most books say that the difference between false and real contractions is that the former are erratic and the latter are regular, lasting for a specific amount of time, with a regular interval between them. This isn't the case for many of us.

* * *

I didn't begin to feel regularly spaced contractions until I was four centimeters dilated. My doctor had told me to call him as soon as my contractions were lasting about forty-five seconds and spaced about five to ten minutes apart. That just never happened. My contractions from the beginning were anywhere from two to five minutes apart, and the spacing stayed that way throughout much of my first stage. Only the intensity of the contractions changed.

* * *

Probably the best sign that you are in labor is that you have to do your breathing techniques to stay comfortable during a contraction. If you suspect you are beginning labor, eat very lightly, perhaps some clear bouillon and some gelatine. This will give you a little extra energy, but it won't fill your stomach enough to make you nauseated as labor progresses. Bring some barley-sugar lollipops with you to the hospital to suck on for added quick energy between contractions. If you live far from the hospital, check with your doctor about the clues you'll need to get you there on time. By the way, it's a good idea to register at the hospital early, so that you won't have to go through all the impossible red tape while you're in heavy labor. Most hospitals have forms that you can fill out ahead of time and bring with you when you enter.

When you arrive at the labor room the nurse will

prep you and give you an enema. Both of these procedures are of questionable importance. As we've said, a natural diarrhea may have already cleaned out your bowels, so there may not be very much anyway for the enema to do. Also, if you're in hard labor, it can be quite uncomfortable. The prepping in itself is not painful. The nurse shaves off your pubic hair, and when she finishes, you feel very naked indeed. However, when the hair begins to grow back, it can be awfully itchy and most annoying.* If you arrive at the hospital before late first-stage labor gets under way, you'll have a much easier time handling these and other routine procedures. Every outside demand becomes more of a hassle as labor progresses toward transition. While in heavy labor, do not hesitate to insist that people wait until your contraction is over before they do anything to you or ask anything from you. A good, sensitive coach can serve as a go-between here.

You will probably be given a vaginal or rectal exam to see how far your cervix has dilated. The person doing this may be the resident doctor and not your own doctor at all. Your doctor may not show up until forty-five minutes before your baby is born, as mine did! But don't let this stop you from asking questions. You have to let them know from the beginning that you are very much interested in what your body is doing, and that you are going to be actively involved in your labor from start to finish. Be sure the doctor or nurse checks the vital signs, like fetal heart rate, your temperature, blood pressure, and pulse. Remember, you have learned what should be happening during labor, and you are aware of what is happening to you. Putting these two together should give you enough indication that your labor is going normally, or that something is seriously wrong. If you suspect the latter, keep complaining until someone listens to you!

Although your contractions up until now have probably been fairly easy to handle, they may get stronger after your enema. This doesn't always happen, but you should be prepared to use more rapid breathing if it proves necessary. Often your contractions will fall into a pattern and you will be able to anticipate the intensity of the next one from that of the previous one. However, you must constantly be on guard to switch to another kind of breathing without forewarning. If you practice breathing for weeks beforehand it makes this easier. Relax between contractions, but keep very alert during them.

By this time you are probably four or five centimeters dilated. That means soon you'll be meeting heavier contractions of longer duration with shorter spaces between. Deep abdominal breathing may not work for you

*Try some soothing cream on the area when your hair begins to grow back. Ask your doctor to give you some.

now, and you should switch to another level, rib-cage or "out," to keep yourself comfortable. Again, remember the point of the exercises is to keep you feeling okay, so do whatever breathing you feel meets your needs. You may still be able to read, sing, play cards, and talk to people around you if that helps you to relax between contractions. You may just want to sleep. Sleeping can be a hindrance, however, unless you are alert enough to jump into your breathing as soon as the next contraction starts. Usually if you don't ride the contraction from the start, it is difficult to remain in control when it reaches its peak. If the people in your room are bothering you or keeping you from relaxing between contractions, ask them to leave. If, because of sleep or someone annoying you, you lose control in the middle of a contraction, do the following: relax, pant rapidly, and use the time after the contraction is over to relax completely. At this point a back rub or leg massage can help immensely to give you confidence.

By the time you are six centimeters dilated, your contractions will in most cases be very strong, and you will probably feel a definitely uncomfortable rise of pressure and tension at the peak of the contractions, and then a gradual lessening of the tension until the contraction is completely over. It usually feels like this: ⌒ . You will need to be alert at all times, although you should take full advantage of your vacation time between contractions to rest. Many women ask for medication at this point. A tranquilizer is often enough to keep you very comfortable, but sometimes you will have to specify a tranquilizer by name or you might be given something stronger than necessary. Specifying makes all medical people angry, so be prepared. Discuss drugs beforehand with your doctor at a prenatal checkup (he or she may not be with you at this point), and as we said before, always ask the name of every substance you are offered.

* * *

As soon as the going got a little rough, I asked the nurse for "something." She quickly brought me Nisentil, a narcotic. It began to take effect very soon after she administered the shot, and it helped me to relax between contractions so well that I often found myself on the verge of sleep. I think that total relaxation in between gave my body the energy it needed to work doubly hard during contractions. I had a very fast, hard labor. But if I had known then the dangerous effect a narcotic can have on a baby, I would not have accepted it. A tranquilizer would probably have worked just as well.

* * *

The closer you get to transition, the more intense your contractions will become, and the more help you'll need to cope with them. But that help doesn't necessarily mean medication. A good coach will be sensitive to your

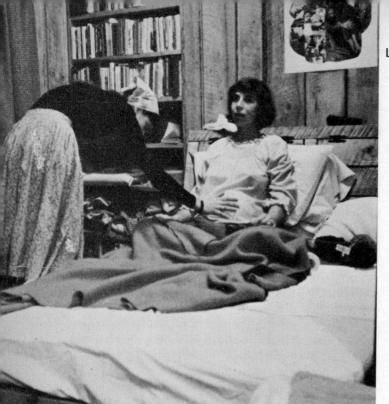

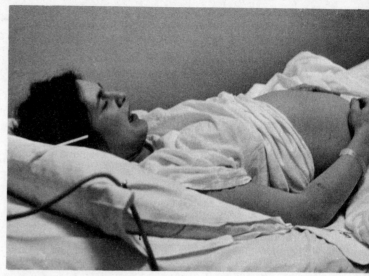

LABOR BEGINS (HOME DELIVERY)

LATE FIRST STAGE

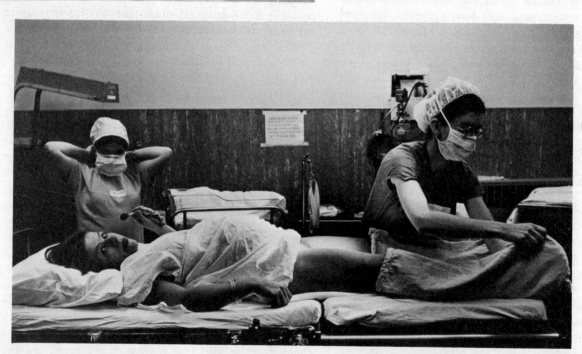

IN THE
DELIVERY ROOM

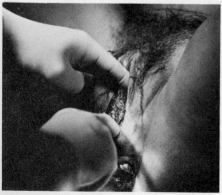

THE BABY'S HEAD
BEGINNING TO SHOW

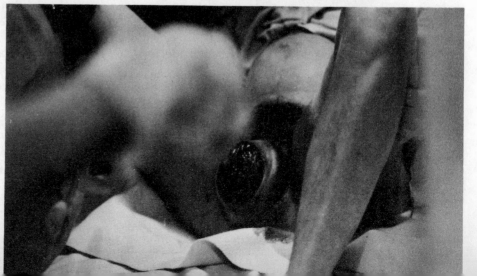

THE BABY'S HEAD CROWNING

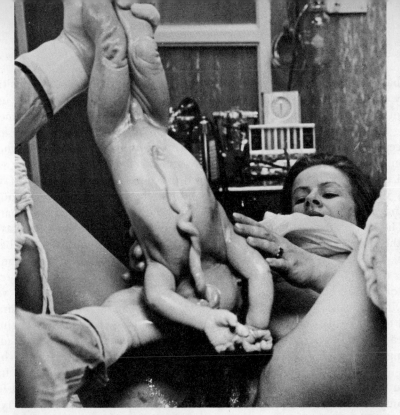

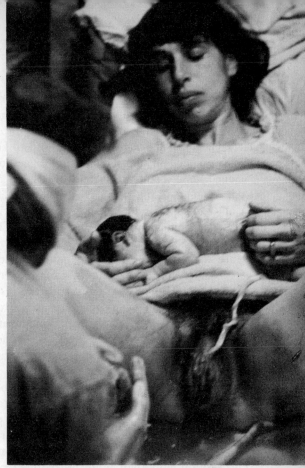

THE BABY IS BORN.

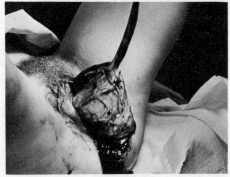

THE BIRTH OF THE PLACENTA

THE CORD STILL CONNECTING BABY
TO PLACENTA (HOME DELIVERY)

THE TINY NEWBORN NURSING (HOME DELIVERY)

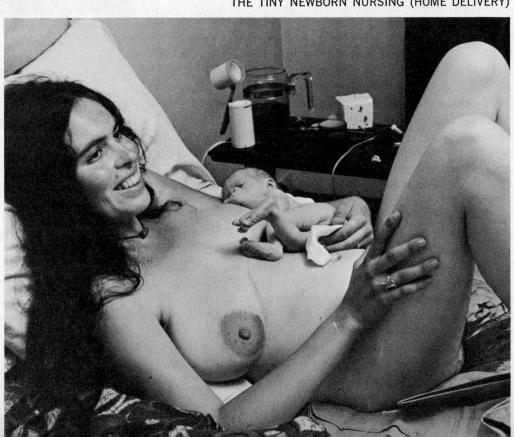

needs and will remind you gently that a change of position might help, or perhaps a temporary switch to a deeper breathing, or even more important s/he could begin to breathe with you throughout the contraction. That helps you to pace yourself and to keep alert. Unfortunately, you may resent any suggestion from someone else and stubbornly remain fixed to a certain position or breathing style. This irritability is very normal and probably indicates that you're entering transition, the very end of the first stage of labor. The more you begin to worry that you'll never make it, the closer you are to making it. The long middle phase of labor is over. Now you are about eight centimeters dilated, and you will feel the most intense contractions of all. But be encouraged! If you've come all this way without drugs, you can overcome transition on your own too. It is the shortest part of a normal labor, and it means that very soon you'll be in second-stage labor, during which you will want to be wide awake.

Transition is different for everyone, but some common signs are: nausea and vomiting, leg cramps, shaking, severe low backache, pressure deep in the pelvis, increasing apprehension, irritability, frustration, and an inability to cope with contractions if left alone. It is during transition more than at any other time that your coach's presence is essential. Your coach should actively participate in your labor by breathing with you, comforting you, and continually reminding you that this is the most difficult and the shortest part of your labor. Try to change your position if you remember. Try sitting almost upright, with the soles of your feet together and your legs relaxed. Prop pillows behind you to support your back. Use your most comfortable rapid breathing techniques—pant-pant-blow, or four pants and a blow, or anything else you've practiced and can do automatically. A sip of water or some ice chips to suck between contractions may be the thing to lift your spirits.

You will feel very vulnerable during transition, and you'll be very tempted to accept medication at this point. Be careful—because by the time you ask for it, and by the time it is administered and takes effect (depending on which type of anesthesia you are given), you'll be very near to second stage. And you don't want to be asleep when it's time to push. Also, the closer to delivery a drug is given, the more effect it has on the baby's responsiveness.

* * *

My legs shook all the way through transition, not just during a contraction. My husband gently held them, and that really helped. He also offered me ice chips after each contraction, and wiped my forehead with a cool washcloth. I couldn't have made it without his being there every minute.

* * *

Someone should be with you throughout transition. If you are alone, call the nurse and make her stay until transition is over. Sometimes your doctor will come in time to help you through. You'll have a hard time concentrating on your breathing now unless someone is being very directive and doing the rapid breathing with you. Be careful not to become hyperventilated. If it happens, slow down and breathe into a paper bag (brought from home for this occasion) or into your cupped hands. If your oxygen-carbon dioxide balance is off, so may be your baby's, so try to avoid hyperventilation by being sure to breathe out fully for every time you breathe in.

Just when it seems that transition will go on forever and all you want to do is leave the hospital and your coach and forget completely about this baby business, something remarkable will happen. You will begin to feel, slightly at first, and then with more and more urgency, the need to push, or bear down. It's a hard feeling to explain, but it is amazingly different from anything in the preceding contractions. Actually, it feels like what it is, a tremendous pressure inside you, trying to push its way out.

It would be terrific if at this point we could simply follow our body's demand and *push*. However, unless the doctor or midwife tells you your cervix is completely dilated (a full ten centimeters open) you must not push or you might tear yourself and perhaps hurt the baby's head.

* * *

All of a sudden my body told me to push. I kept shouting to everyone around me, "I have to push, I have to push." They all said, "That's impossible. You were just five centimeters dilated an hour ago." Nonetheless, I had to push! Controlling that urge was the most difficult part of my labor. For about five contractions I panted and blew and sweated for all I was worth. Why weren't they letting me trust my body? It was ghastly. Until, just when I was sure I couldn't control the urge to push one more minute, my doctor appeared in the doorway. He took one look at me. "Push," he said, "go ahead and push." I was too happy at that moment to ask him where he'd been until then.

* * *

With the onset of pushing, second stage has begun, and in about forty-five minutes you'll be holding your baby. The delivery of the baby will probably be done in the delivery room of the hospital, and to get there you'll be wheeled on a kind of movable bed table. Ask the nurse not to transfer you from one bed to another in the middle of a contraction. In the delivery room your bed will have stirrups and arm straps and many other medieval-looking contraptions that may scare the wits out of you. Don't panic. The arm straps are completely unnecessary, since you are awake and not thrashing wildly about as a totally drugged woman might be. Also, the stirrups are not too uncomfortable if you insist they be adjusted to your satisfaction, and they can in fact make pushing a little easier, since you won't be supporting the full weight of your legs any more. Be sure you or your coach brings some pillows along to keep your back propped up. Pushing while lying flat on your back is nearly impossible. Your coach, too, can help support your back during contractions.

For almost everyone the second stage of labor is thrilling and not painful. Once you are allowed to push along with your body, you will finally be able to help actively in your baby's birth. It feels great, and you feel exhilarated. You push only during contractions—your body will give you no choice then—and between contractions you relax. Make sure you blow out all your air at the end of the contraction, and try to remain as limp as possible.

The delivery room can be a very pleasant place between contractions. If everything is going normally, there'll probably be a lot of laughing and exciting chatter during the rest intervals. There is about five minutes between these second-stage contractions, and soon the next one will come. Breathe in, breathe out, breathe in, breathe out, breathe in and hold. Sometimes your obstetrician or your coach may keep up a running commentary as you're pushing: "Good, good, keep it up. Push, push, push, come on, come on, push, push. Good." Although some women appreciate this encouragement, others resent it and find it interferes with their concentration. Tell everyone to keep quiet if you have to. Or perhaps, since you'll be working so hard, your coach can tell them all for you.

By now you're probably very tired, and perhaps you're beginning to feel a burning sensation around your perineum. This means the baby's head is about to crown and the birth is imminent. It's your body's way of saying, "Don't push so hard; ease the baby out." Try to keep your perineum relaxed by releasing those muscles. Also, keep your mouth loose between contractions; you may find this influences the relaxation of your vagina.

Just before the baby is born your doctor will probably give you local anesthesia in the perineal area. This is so you won't feel the episiotomy and subsequent stitches when s/he closes you up again. Actually, the baby's head pushing against your perineum will have numbed it enough so you wouldn't have felt the episiotomy anyway, but the anesthesia is given just to make sure the natural numbing doesn't wear off before all the stitches are in. The particular brand of anesthesia may vary from doctor to doctor, but all these drugs cross the placenta readily and may have a direct drug effect on the fetus. As we stated above, we don't see why episiotomies

are done so routinely when there is always the chance, no matter how minor, that the anesthetic used will harm the newborn. Perhaps, if we can't persuade doctors to give up episiotomies, we can at least ask them to give us our anesthesia after the baby is born.

When the last contraction comes, the doctor will tell you to stop pushing and to use some rapid breathing to control your urge to push. Then, in the middle of the contraction, out will come your baby's head, usually facing the floor and then rotating to the side. Before you know it, the body will come sliding out.

* * *

Although there was no mirror, so I couldn't see my baby emerge, I could feel everything. It was the most thrilling experience I'd ever had—a perfectly formed baby slithering out of my body.

* * *

Probably the baby will take a breath as soon as the head hits the cooler air of the delivery room. Or s/he may not cry until her/his whole body is born.

* * *

There he was, our new son, facing us for the first time. He breathed in some of our worldly air and began to cry, loudly and unremittingly. We cheered to hear him and to know that he was really, finally, alive.

* * *

If your baby cries before s/he is completely out, s/he may be born with a normal flush. Otherwise s/he will probably look bluish-yellow. Soon his or her breathing will become regular and sustained. No one knows for certain the cause of the onset of respiration in the newborn, but whatever the reason, the first real breath is a time for rejoicing!*

Ninety percent of all babies born in American hospitals are considered to be in excellent condition at birth, and this is especially true of babies born to unanesthetized mothers. Some infants, however, will require help. The doctor in a hospital has various instruments and equipment at hand to encourage the baby's respiratory functions to begin. This is vital, since lack of oxygen can cause brain damage to the infant. Also, the attendant will look for normal color, body tone, and immediate urination.†

Your baby will be wet-looking, possibly covered with a milky substance called vernix, and usually not very bloody. Her/his head may look very strange at first, due to its molding during the birth. This odd shape is tempo-

*L. S. James, M.D., "The Importance of Observations of the Newborn at Birth," in Nancy Lytle, ed., *Maternal Health Nursing*, p. 97.

†*Ibid.*, p. 101, Irving and associates showed that while less than 2 percent of infants delivered of mothers having no sedation had a delayed onset of respiration, 35–67 percent had delayed respiration if sedation was used.

rary, and the baby's head will look normal soon. You may want to reach down and touch her/him immediately, but the hospital attendants probably won't let you. A baby born to an unanesthetized mother will be very active from birth if the delivery has been normal, and s/he may be grabbing onto everything in sight. You wish s/he could be clutching you.

The umbilical cord is still connecting you to your baby via the placenta, which is still inside you (except in the case of placenta previa). As soon as the blood is emptied from the cord, the doctor will clamp it, and then he will cut it a few inches from the baby's navel. In a week or so the cord will dry out completely and fall off, leaving the baby with a normal navel.

* * *

The cord struck me as exceedingly strong and beautiful—translucent, blue, and in the shape of a telephone cord, but thicker. The doctor gave my baby to the nurse to suck out more mucus, wipe and wrap her, and only then did I get her. I was shaky, chilly, exhausted, and happy. I wanted to hold and nurse my baby, but had no energy left. So my husband held her close to me. I felt so close to him at that moment, and also to the woman who had been my monitrice.

* * *

After a short interval you will begin to feel a contraction coming. This is the third stage of labor, the birth of the placenta. After a few minutes the placenta will separate from you completely, and you will push it into your vagina and out. The whole process might take from five minutes to thirty-five minutes. Sometimes the placenta will actually follow the baby almost immediately, and sometimes the placenta will have to be extracted manually by the doctor. With the birth of the placenta, labor is ended.

The doctor will examine the placenta carefully to make certain it is whole. If there is any doubt, he may explore inside your uterus to see that no fragments are remaining. If the doctor will let you walk from the delivery room to your bed, gravity will probably eliminate any foreign particles.

Next, your episiotomy will be sewn up.

* * *

I didn't have any medication whatsoever, and that was the only thing that hurt me. It could have been less painful if he [the doctor] had put in the stitches loosely before the numbness of the area wore off, and therefore before the placenta was even removed. It was a sensation of pin pricks. It was especially bothersome, because by that time I didn't want anyone to touch my body.

* * *

You will probably then feel afterpains, which are caused by the uterus beginning to return to its normal shape and size. The whole involution process takes, on the average, six weeks. In addition to these cramps you'll have a bloody discharge lasting for several weeks. This is called lochia. Have a good supply of sanitary napkins at home waiting for your arrival.*

If you are planning to breast-feed your baby, now is a good time to start if you feel up to it. The sucking reflex of a baby born to an unanesthetized mother is very strong indeed, and the colostrum in your breasts is full of protein, minerals, vitamin A, and nitrogen, as well as antibodies that help to keep the newborn immune from harmful germs such as several staphylococci and *E. coli*. So if your doctor has agreed to it, let your baby suckle right on the delivery table. Your real milk won't come in for a few days, but the newborn can certainly benefit from the colostrum so soon after birth.

In most hospitals the baby will be taken from you very soon after birth and placed in a separate nursery room for anywhere from six to twenty-four hours.

* * *

I remember feeling very strange, to have experienced the most remarkable of all things, the birth of my first child, and then to be left all alone. First they took the baby into the nursery. Then I was wheeled into my room, where my husband was able to stay and chat for a while. But he had to work the next day, so he needed some sleep. I was tired, but too excited to sleep. So there I was, alone, remembering the experience full of wonder and amazement that we had all shared. But for the next few hours we were not sharing. The hospital had separated us.

* * *

It is now possible to find hospitals that believe in family-centered childbirth and permit modified rooming-in. This is an attempt to keep the new family as together as possible during the hospital stay. Of course, this is expensive, and now usually only the luxury of private patients. We shouldn't feel satisfied until family-centered childbirth is possible for all women who desire it.

Modified rooming-in. When you are looking for a hospital, be sure to find out about its rooming-in policy, if that interests you. In some hospitals the mother is allowed to keep her baby in her room whenever she desires and for as long as she desires. When she is too tired to be entirely responsible for the baby, the baby can be brought back to the nursery. This is called modified rooming-in. Some hospitals, however, work under an all-or-nothing plan, meaning that if the mother chooses rooming-in, she must keep the baby with her in her room at all times. This can prove to be a tremendous burden, especially for a new mother. Also, some hospitals do not

---

*For the first few weeks at least, don't use tampons.

allow the father or other family members to visit except during the regular, restricted visiting hours, even if the mother and baby are in the same room.

Rooming-in provides the right atmosphere for breast-feeding and feeding on demand rather than according to a rigid schedule. The baby usually cries less and gains weight faster if s/he is fed when s/he feels hungry and not when the hospital staff thinks s/he should be hungry.

THE IMMEDIATE POSTPARTUM PERIOD

During the first few hours after the birth of your baby your body will already be beginning to get itself back into its normal condition. Your uterus will be firm and contracting, reducing its size, so that by the tenth day after delivery it will have descended from your abdomen into your pelvis again. Breast-feeding your baby will naturally speed up this involution process by releasing the hormones you need to trigger the uterine contractions and keep them working. These postdelivery contractions of the uterus are often strong and may startle you. Your doctor can prescribe drugs, such as Darvon, to reduce the pain, but remember, if you are breast-feeding, all drugs you take will reach the baby through your milk.

While you are in the hospital they will be checking your temperature often to make sure you are not developing a puerperal (*puer*, "child," + *parere*, "to bear" = puerperal: "pertaining to childbirth") infection. Also, your pulse will be checked, and you will be given a blood test after a day or so.

As we have already mentioned, you will have a postpartum uterine discharge called **lochia** which will change in color over the first couple of weeks from red to pinkish-brown to yellowish-white. This lochia should not smell bad. If it does, that is a sign that an infection is developing, so warn your doctor. Sometimes bits of the placental tissue are left inside the uterine area. So if you experience persistent bloody lochia, inform your doctor, because it generally indicates that something is in the uterus that shouldn't be there.

One thing many of us worry about during the immediate postpartum period is how we will ever be able to move our bowels. As long as you don't strain, you won't tear your stitches or dislodge your recovering organs (a common fear). Drink a lot of liquids to keep your bowel movements soft. Hospitals worry a lot more than they ought to about your particular bowel functions. Don't you worry. Relax and let your body take over. If necessary, you can always have an enema or a suppository to stimulate your bowels.

Urinating should not prove difficult, but if you experience pain, tell your doctor about it. For that matter, if you experience pain anywhere, let your doctor know, and make sure s/he checks it. The immediate postpartum period is a time when infection can occur easily, and you must be on the lookout for signs that something might be wrong. Depend on the hospital and the doctor only so far; they are busy supervising the recovery of many women and may overlook the very thing that might bother you later on. Women who experience the most bowel and bladder trouble after delivery are the ones who were totally anesthetized. It takes their bodies a lot longer to get back to normal functioning.

Your breasts may become markedly engorged when your milk first comes in, during the second or third day after delivery. Breast-feeding on demand should relieve this situation quickly.* If you do not plan to breast-feed your baby, the hospital staff will be around to suppress your milk supply with shots of estrogen or androgen (male hormone). Tell your doctor and the hospital if you would like to breast-feed so they'll know not to give you the shots, which are often given routinely.†

When you are released from the hospital, you will probably be given instructions about what you should and shouldn't do in the next few weeks. Remember, don't overexert yourself, and don't try to return to your normal routine until you feel absolutely ready for it. Many women continue to feel tired and lethargic for six months or more. Trust yourself, and try to accept postpartum as the total readjustment period it is.

Some important things to remember are:

1. Get plenty of rest.

2. If you are breast-feeding, drink a lot. Usually a quart of milk (or two cups of milk and two cups of another liquid) per day is recommended.

3. Take very shallow, warm-to-hot baths often to help your stitches dissolve (only a few inches of water in the tub).

4. Overexerting yourself can be dangerous. Take advantage of this short time to pamper yourself for a while and concentrate on your new baby.

5. If you have any sign that something is wrong, call your doctor immediately, especially if there is a marked increase in vaginal bleeding.

6. Try to share your fears (they're just about inevitable). Talk to your husband, your friends, your doctor, your mother, or whoever is available and willing to listen, about what may be bothering you. If you don't feel any better, call your prepared-childbirth instructor for help. There may be postpartum groups organized in your area.

---

*If you nurse your baby from birth onward without the usual twelve-to-twenty-four-hour wait, and if you nurse according to the baby's demand for food, engorgement will probably not occur.

†Even if you are given the shots to suppress your milk, you can nurse. Just put your baby to your breasts regularly and persistently and the suckling will cause your milk to come in.

7. Most doctors say sexual intercourse can be resumed after six weeks, but this is an individual thing. You may be ready before then, or you may not feel like making love for a while after that time. Follow your own emotions and see how you feel physically. Anyway, good sex need not necessarily mean intercourse only. (See "Sexuality" chapter and "Postpartum" section of this chapter.)

Whatever you feel immediately after the birth, you will know that because you were prepared you did the best you could to help your baby into the world. You may not experience that "gush" of motherhood you've heard so much about. Don't feel guilty. It takes time for you and that beautiful little being who just emerged from your body to get to know each other. And besides, you may feel overwhelmed by all sorts of emotions. You're excited and proud of yourself, and rightly so, for having succeeded so well. You may feel very scared and depressed when you think of the enormous responsibility you now have with a new baby. You may have an urgent desire to talk about how you are feeling, or you may just want to be alone. Remember, all your needs are legitimate and you have the right to expect those needs to be met. If the hospital situation is miserable for you, ask to be released as soon as possible. The usual stay is three to five days for a normal delivery. Make sure that you will have family or friends to help you when you return home. You'll want to share your excitement with them, but it will also help to share the burden of brand-new motherhood.

Your baby is born, and you have done all that was in your power to give that baby the safest and healthiest birth possible. As women we know that the experience of childbirth is an extremely important experience in our lives. If we are prepared and unanesthetized during childbirth we are in touch with our entire self, mind and body, and we are working intelligently along with this inevitable biological process. We are in control. Childbirth is an experience that can have a positive effect on all the other aspects of our being. We can feel freer sexually, having experienced such a massive physical and sexual event. We can feel more independent, having survived on our own merits this incredibly powerful experience. We can feel more in control of ourselves as whole people, having used both our mind and our body together to see us through labor and delivery. We can be more confident mothers, having done our best from the start to give our children a safe and satisfying birth. And finally, we can be sure that as women we are strong, competent, and beautiful!

Yet motherhood need not be our biological destiny. As women we must come together to support each other. Those of us who have decided not to have children and those of us who have decided to have children must no longer stand by while others control our lives. To give birth only to a child we have wanted and will cherish is not our privilege, it is our right.

APPENDIX

Associations Concerned with Childbirth Education

American Society for Psychoprophylaxis in Obstetrics (Lamaze)
  36 W. 96th Street, New York, New York 10025
Association of Mothers for Educated Childbirth (concerned with home delivery)
  Box 9030, Far Rockaway, New York 11691
International Childbirth Education Association (modified Lamaze)
  Box 5852, Milwaukee, Wisconsin 53220
International Childbirth Education Association/Education Committee
  Box 22, Hillside, New Jersey 07205
La Leche League International (concerned with breast-feeding)
  9616 Minneapolis Ave., Franklin Park, Illinois 60131
The above organizations will provide you with information about childbirth classes and labor coaches and will give you the names of the local childbirth organizations in your area.

How to Choose a Childbirth Class

A good course in childbirth preparation, along with good prenatal medical care, is one of the most valuable investments a pregnant woman can make.

1. Make sure the class is small—although it's hard to find a class with fewer than ten couples.

2. Compare the prices of the classes with the quality of teaching and attention to your needs as an individual.

3. Make sure the class will include adequate discussion, detailed information, plenty of rehearsal to learn physical techniques. Six weeks is minimal; eight to ten weeks better. Usually classes are two hours long.

4. Be sure the class encourages fathers and/or friends to participate. The class should be built around the expectation that someone who is as trained as you are will always be with you throughout labor and delivery.

5. The class should discuss feelings and attitudes as well as techniques. It should not only prepare you for labor but also for parenthood, breast-feeding, etc.

6. Find out as much as you can about the organization that sponsors the classes. If it is a hospital class, make sure they aren't simply trying to get you to accept all hospital procedures as normal and inevitable. If the organization is profit-making, find out why. Most classes are too expensive as it is.

7. If your class is to be part of any research study, find out as much as you can about it. Don't consent to anything you don't feel comfortable with.

8. Look at the qualifications of the instructor. A reputable teacher needn't be an R.N. (registered nurse), but she should have a detailed sheet of her qualifications and experience ready to give you. She should be able to provide references (students who have taken her classes previously), and she should either have had personal or professional experience with prepared childbirth during delivery. Find out how the instructor is supervised. Be cautious of independent instructors.

9. Find out whether any professional board is affiliated with the class program and who is on it. Both doctors and nonmedical professionals should be represented, especially mental-health workers. Psychological and emotional problems are too often overlooked.

Readings in Childbirth Preparation

See the Bibliography at the end of this chapter.

SECTION THREE: POSTPARTUM—
AFTER THE BABY IS BORN

The initial phase of motherhood, the weeks and months following childbirth, commonly known as the postpartum period, is for most of us a time of significant emotional upheaval. Some of us are high, some are mellow, some of us are lethargic and depressed, or we are irritable and cry easily. Mood swings are common. We are confused and a little scared, because our moods do not resemble the way we are accustomed to feel, let alone the way we are expected to feel. If this is a first baby we may feel lonely and isolated from adult society. The special attention and consideration many of us receive as expectant mothers shift to the baby and we too are expected to put the baby's needs before our own. We may find ourselves, at first, with little time for even our simplest personal needs. Some of us have difficulty staying awake in social situations during the first weeks and months and find it hard to maintain involvement in outside interests. With subsequent children we often feel an inability to cope with daily household routines, finding ourselves suddenly with a family too large to manage. Often we feel that we have lost control over our lives, and dread that life will always be this way.

We often feel guilty, because we think our own inadequacies are the cause of our unhappiness. We rarely question whether the roles we have are realizable. Because of the societal pressures surrounding motherhood, and the mystique of the maternal instinct (joys of child care, fulfillment through others), many women are unable to pinpoint their feelings of confusion and inadequacy or are unable to feel that it is legitimate to verbalize their hesitations and problems.

What little research has been done suggests that over half of all women who bear children experience a marked degree of emotional upset in the weeks and months following childbirth.*

KINDS OF POSTPARTUM EMOTIONAL PROBLEMS

For the many of us who experience some form of postpartum emotional disturbance it can vary in the form it takes as well as in length and intensity.

There is commonly a mild depression between the sec-

*A British survey of 137 obstetrical patients postpartum found that 64 percent displayed such symptoms as anxiety, depression, mood swings, distractibility, and shortened attention span. (Kane, Harmon, *et al.*, "Emotional and Cognitive Disturbance in Early Puerperium," pp. 99–102.)

ond and fourth days after delivery. Many people believe that the initial twelve-to-twenty-four-hour separation of the mother and the child (which is the policy at most hospitals even when the mothers nurse and/or have rooming-in) may contribute to the depression.*

Both in the hospital and afterward we can be frightened by dreams and fantasies—suicidal fantasies (anger turned inward), or fantasies of leaving the baby or its father (anger turned outward), or thoughts and dreams about hurting or neglecting the baby. We resent and/or worry about the baby's helplessness and vulnerability, and question our own ability to take care of an infant.

* * *

Immediately after the birth of my first baby I felt high and exhilarated. But that night I got sad. I cried all night long. During the next few days I lay on my bed thinking of how I would kill myself. I looked at how the windows opened and I concentrated on figuring out times when no nurses were on duty. I couldn't sleep at all. I tried to tell them I was depressed, and all they gave me were sleeping pills. I felt like I'd never feel anything again but this incredible despair, that it would never end. I had nightmares. The one I remember best is where I would be feeding the baby. I would fall asleep and the baby would fall off the bed and be killed. I don't know why I had these dreams and impulses. I have a happy marriage and it was a wanted pregnancy.

* * *

This same woman talked about meeting another woman who had gone through a similar experience, including a dream that she had slit her new baby's throat with a knife. Another woman slept for seven hours one afternoon during her first week home. She had been dreaming that her baby was in the oven and she couldn't wake up to get her out. Fantasies such as these and blue periods in themselves are not indicative of a long-term depression even if they persist beyond the hospital stay. Many of us have found it essential to talk to someone about these feelings.

If you find yourself unable to cope, even after the first couple of months when the twenty-four-hour demands of the baby are clearly a major cause, you may want to

get some help. Some of the symptoms of serious depression are: early-morning waking and inability to get back to sleep; inability to concentrate; loss of appetite; loss of interest in your surroundings; or possibly an obsessive interest in housekeeping. The many possible reasons for more prolonged postpartum disturbance—physical, emotional, marital, financial, institutional, and so on—are discussed at length later in the chapter. Sorting out the causes in your particular situation can help you figure out what you want to change and how to go about it. Just because being a mother is supposed to be easy and natural, we tend to think that we should be able to handle postpartum problems ourselves. But don't hold back from seeking help from your friends, particularly from women who have children, and from professionals, if you feel you need it.*

In some instances, postpartum disturbance is acute: more than 4,000 women (one out of a thousand who give birth) are hospitalized each year in the United States because of postpartum disturbances. At least 20 percent, or 800 women, are permanently incapacitated.† Twelve and a half percent of the women admitted to a state hospital in Washington were admitted within six months of a delivery or had previously been admitted within six months of a delivery. Of this group of 47 women, 36 were first admissions. The largest number of postpartum admissions were third-time mothers.‡

This is the story of one woman who was hospitalized after the birth of her first child.

* * *

After I miscarried, I was advised to get pregnant again right away as the best way to deal with the feeling of loss. I had misgivings—I wanted some time to think it all over again. I had been spotting and bleeding on and off for five months and didn't feel ready to go through another difficult pregnancy. On one level I felt freed up and began to think of all the things I could do if I put off having a baby for a while. I was unable to articulate these ambivalent feelings and to feel legitimate about getting another prescription for birth-control pills.

I became pregnant again immediately after the mis-

---

*In one recent study, fourteen primiparas (women having first babies) who had more than the usual contact with their babies in the three days following delivery (one hour with their babies within the first three hours following birth, and five additional hours during each of the first three days) were matched with fourteen primiparas whose hospital stay followed usual hospital procedures. Twenty-eight to thirty-two days later mothers who had more contact with their infants during the hospital stay displayed more motherly behavior and more intensive interest in eye contact with their babies who in turn were more attentive. (Marshall A. Klaus *et al.*, "Maternal Attachment: Importance of the First Postpartum Days," *New England Journal of Medicine*, Vol. 286, No. 9, March 2, 1972, pp. 460–63.)

*In many communities you can find inexpensive psychiatric care or counseling in the out-patient clinic of a hospital. Because of the strong antifeminist bias in traditional psychiatry, it is a good idea to find out a therapist's views on women's issues before or during the first interview. As with any other doctor, you have a right to intelligent choice, and you can change if you are dissatisfied. If the choices open to you are limited, you may want to go ahead with therapy while continuing to talk with sympathetic woman friends for feedback and support in areas of disagreement with the therapist.

†Hugh F. Butts, "Postpartum Psychiatric Problems; A Review of the Literature Dealing with Etiological Theories."

‡Virginia L. Larsen *et al.*, "Attitudes and Stresses Affecting Perinatal Adjustment," p. 6.

carriage. Throughout the pregnancy I feared I would lose this baby too. I had had an abortion several years before and feared it had damaged my uterus and made me incapable of carrying a baby to term. To make matters worse I didn't look pregnant at all until the seventh month. People would often say to me, "Are you sure you're really pregnant?"—and I wasn't sure at all.

I was so thrilled with my perfect baby and relieved by my quick, relatively easy childbirth. I experienced childbirth as liberation from all sorts of fears and hangups. It was the first physical thing I had done well in my life!

My happiness and relief at being home intensified the high. I felt elated and wanted to share my feelings with people I felt close to, and so spent a lot of time on the phone. The need to talk became progressively more intense. I experienced a rush of insights about myself, family, friends, and society. It seemed to me that my mind was extraordinarily clear. My thoughts were racing so fast that there was hardly time to communicate or write down all the ideas that I felt were so important. Even at night I hardly stopped talking long enough for my husband or me to get any sleep. One night I began to pour out a flood of childhood memories of economic insecurity and unhappiness. I cried while my husband held me in his arms. Having a child had brought my own childhood back. I kept turning the heat way up saying the house was always so cold when I was a child and I actually felt cold.

My husband became alarmed and consulted with family, friends, obstetrician, and a doctor who had treated me twice for hyperthyroidism. The consensus was that I needed to be hospitalized. I still couldn't see that there was anything strange in my behavior though to others I appeared psychotic. I knew I was behaving differently than usual but I simply felt more freed up. I was persuaded to go to a hospital, where I believed I would quickly prove my sanity. Instead I was committed.

In the hospital I was given drugs to bring me down from the high. In therapy I was told that my "high" was a defense against depression. This made me mistrust my perceptions of myself for a long time. My psychiatrist was kind and sympathetic but knew little about women or babies. I was discharged in four weeks but continued in therapy for over a year.

When I came home my depression deepened into a profound inertia. I found it impossible to start any project, knowing that I would be interrupted by the baby's feeding schedule. Except for meeting the baby's needs I let everything else go. My image of myself as a responsible, competent adult was utterly destroyed. I hated myself for feeling depressed. (A good mother should be serene and happy.) This of course intensified

the depression in a vicious cycle. In therapy I began to learn that I had a right to my feelings whether they were acceptable to others or not. Every few months some of the depression would lift and I would feel more able to relate to people and do things.

I was lucky that my baby was very responsive to my attempts at play and this set me on the road to recovery. By the time my child was a year old I could hardly remember why I had felt so hopeless, even to the point of contemplating suicide. When I felt that way I thought my life would never change—that I would always feel that way but my life was changing. Though I continued to find it very hard, I was learning how to make being a mother a part of my life without being so overwhelmed by it that I couldn't meet my own needs as a person.

POSSIBLE CAUSES OF POSTPARTUM DISTURBANCE

Because so many of us experience some form of mild or severe postpartum depression or emotional stress, we want to discuss at some length the various reasons for postpartum disturbance and what can be done about it.

The Childbearing Year as Maturational Crisis

Most doctors treat pregnancy and postpartum from a purely physiological point of view. They dismiss most of the psychological and emotional reactions as "natural." But Grete Bibring, a psychoanalyst, in cooperation with a multidisciplinary team including obstetricians, pediatricians, and mental-health workers, has completed a ten-year longitudinal study of pregnant women which shows that some far-reaching psychological changes take place during and after pregnancy.

Despite the modern myth that pregnancy is a time of pure harmony and bliss, the social workers in the Bibring team found that pregnant women who had *not* sought psychiatric counseling consistently revealed severely disturbed dreams, thoughts, and mental imagery.* However, these women were helped by some simple suggestions or sometimes merely a display of interest from the therapist. Eventually the researchers concluded that the symptoms were characteristic of pregnancy and were not individual disturbances. They came to see pregnancy as a maturational crisis, similar to puberty and meno-

*Grete L. Bibring *et al.,* "A Study of the Psychological Processes in Pregnancy and of the Earliest Mother-Child Relationship," pp. 9–72.

pause, an "intrinsically psychosomatic developmental step"[*] in which biological and endocrine changes bring accompanying psychological disequilibrium, which, *when resolved,* results in emotional growth. The bodily and emotional changes are interdependent, and Bibring sees them as equally responsible for the successful resolution of this developmental step.[†]

The maturational crisis begun by pregnancy does not come to resolution with delivery but continues into the postpartum, and the "essential maturational changes" come well after the child is born. Thus often during the early weeks and sometimes months of the child's life we are still in a state of psychological disequilibrium.[‡] This raises the question of what effect our still unresolved emotional state has on the earliest mother-child relationship. It was suggested by the research team that instead of taking the traditional psychoanalytic route of blaming mothers for being rejecting, hostile, narcissistic or smothering, child-development specialists should turn their attention to this period of crisis and maturation in the mother's life. By doing so a vicious cycle of mutual frustration, resulting in a disturbed relationship, could be prevented.[§]

Life Changes of Becoming a Parent

Often we remain upset months after the baby's birth, because we expected at some point to get our lives and feelings back to "normal." It is important to understand that once we become mothers we will never again lead altogether the same lives. Thus deciding to become pregnant ideally involves a conscious decision to change one's life forever. For the next two decades we will have to consider the child's needs in making our own plans. (Of course the special tie and caring exists even when the child grows up and is independent.) If the experiences of the childbearing year (pregnancy, childbirth, and postpartum) are resolved in a positive way, we will have grown in strength and maturity and feel good about our new responsibilities most of the time.

It is only natural to yearn occasionally for the freedom of childlessness and to feel angry and resentful toward our kids. We have our own needs as people and at times we need to be separate from our kids. By recognizing this need we can feel freer when away from our kids and enjoy them more when we are with them. Also we need to find ways to integrate children into out life styles. This

entails emotional as well as social changes. Emotional changes (changing our self-concept) take time. The social task can be a variety of things, including challenging those social and economic institutions that do not consider the needs of women and children (such as lack of quality day care, few alternatives to the nuclear family with its isolation of mothers and infants). (See section "Proposals for Change" at the end of this chapter.)

Our freedom is drastically curtailed, because the newborn human infant is helpless to meet its own needs except by crying to signal discomfort. S/he depends on us for nourishment, affection, clean body, clean clothes, and occasionally even a change of position.

* * *

I had my first child six years ago. It was a planned pregnancy and I was terrifically excited. I had my baby by prepared childbirth. It was the most exhilarating experience of my life.

The first month was awful. I loved my baby, but felt terrifically apprehensive about my ability to satisfy this totally dependent tiny creature. Every time she cried I could feel myself tense up and panic. What should I do? Can I make her stop—can I help her? I called the pediatrician daily for advice. One day I called to ask whether it was too hot to put an undershirt on the baby. He said, "For Christ's sake, didn't they teach you anything at the hospital?"

After the first month I got the hang of it, partly because I had such an easy child. She rarely cried. She slept a lot, and when she was awake she was responsive—she'd look at me alertly and smile. Gradually my love feelings for her overcame my panic feelings, and I relaxed, stopped thinking so much about my inadequacies, and was just myself. It was pretty clear from her responses that I was doing something right.

* * *

It is very important to remember that the time the baby needs us so much is short. Every few months brings a new stage of development as babies learn to sit up,

---

[*]Grete L. Bibring, "Recognition of Psychological Stresses Often Neglected in OB Care."

[†]Bibring *et al.,* "A Study of the Psychological Processes in Pregnancy and of the Earliest Mother-Child Relationship," pp. 9–72.

[‡]*Ibid.*

[§]*Ibid.*

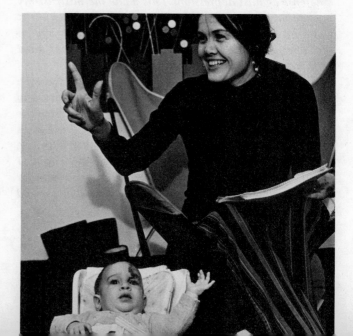

crawl, stand, hold their own bottles and begin to feed themselves solid food. Sometimes they even walk and say a few words in the first year. (Don't worry if your baby is a bit slower than your friends' babies.) As the baby develops and becomes more autonomous the total dependency on us lets up. This may mean more work for us at first. A baby's first attempts at self-feeding can be very messy. And a toddler beginning to crawl and then walk may seem to be "into everything" and does need more attention than an infant who sleeps most of the time, but the work becomes more rewarding as we see our children become more and more self-directed little people.

The Physical Context—Fatigue

(See appendix at the end of this chapter for other physical aspects of postpartum.)

In a study of childbearing stresses in which women were asked which experiences they found most stressful, fatigue was mentioned by many women, and more often during postpartum than pregnancy. Mothers of three children mentioned fatigue both before and after delivery and said that they had difficulty adjusting to the needs of their families.[*]

* * *

The first six months of my third baby's life are a blur to me. Constantly tired and irritable, I somehow got through each day, but it certainly was no fun for us all. The older children (ages six and three) suffered from not getting enough attention. Because the baby was breast-feeding six times a day, there was almost no time to take the kids out—or even get through the daily housekeeping.

Having three kids is exhausting. Time is fragmented—always punctuated by some kid's needs. I lost ten pounds. I was really short-tempered—exhausted. No time to be me.

Having three little people dependent on you is very demanding emotionally. The middle child especially needs extra attention. She came into our bed almost every night for two months and wet her bed for two weeks after the baby came home, and still has tantrums occasionally. I still feel spread thin most of the time.

* * *

Studies have shown that in the last weeks of pregnancy women experience a loss of REM (rapid-eye-movement) sleep. Rapid eye movements are associated with dreaming, which occurs in deepest sleep and, as some scientists believe, this deep sleep is needed for both physical and psychological replenishment. The loss of REM sleep and the associated disturbance in dream pat-

[*]Virginia Larsen, *et al.*, *Attitude and Stresses Affecting Perinatal Adjustment*, pp. 7 and 8.

terns may be related to the impending crisis of childbirth. Loss of sleep can and should be made up, but if the postpartum woman continues to lose sleep, she builds up a backlog of REM sleep loss, which can lead to emotional and physical disturbance.[*]

Whether one can get enough REM sleep during the time the baby is waking in the night varies with the individual. Some women feel fine even though their usual sleep pattern is segmented. If you are someone who sleeps most soundly in your sixth or seventh hour of sleep (you can tell if you feel sleepy during the day), the baby's father or someone else can feed the baby during the night, early morning, or during your afternoon nap, so that you can sleep for a longer stretch than the three or four hours between feedings. If you are breast-feeding, the baby can be given a relief bottle for one feeding each day. (See Appendix on Infant Care at the end of this chapter for more on breast-feeding.) Without sharing of family responsibilities and/or day care for older children, telling a mother of several small children to nap during the day is "little more than a sick joke."[†]

Housework should be kept to an absolute minimum during this time and shared by all family members. If

[*]Barbara Williams, "Sleep Needs During the Maternity Cycle," pp. 53–55. For more on REM sleep, see Sharon Golub, "Rapid Eye Movement Sleep," pp. 56–58 of *Nursing Outlook* (February, 1967).
[†]Beverly Jones, "The Dynamics of Marriage and Motherhood," in Robin Morgan, ed., *Sisterhood Is Powerful* (New York: Vintage, 1970), pp. 57–58.

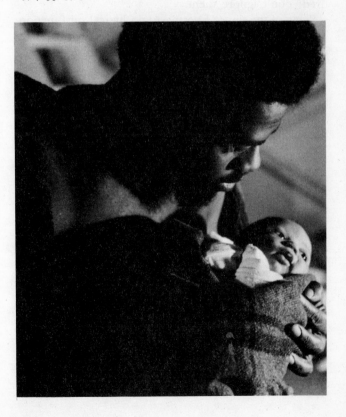

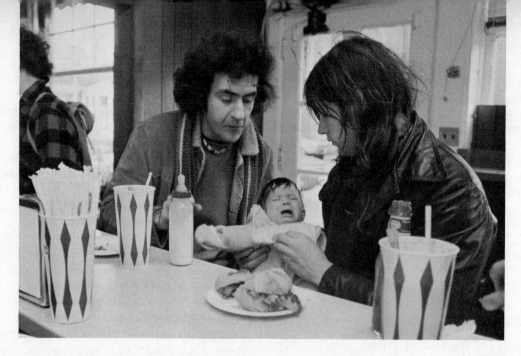

you have no help during your first week at home, plan on takeouts, frozen dinners, paper plates, and every possible shortcut. (Do not feel guilty about the legitimate use of paper products. This is industry's way of shifting the blame for pollution onto the consumer.) If you use a lot of frozen dinners and ready-prepared foods, be sure to supplement your diet with lots of fresh fruits and vegetables, cheese, and whole grains.

You may feel you want to limit stair climbing to once a day for the first week. Be careful of heavy lifting. Try to tune in to signs your body gives you to tell you it is tired; don't ignore them.

Some of the signs of postpartum physical misfunctioning are: unusually heavy bleeding, heavier than your period on any day (more details in Appendix); temperature 101° or higher; breasts feeling red, hot or painful. If you have any of these symptoms, start immediately to get more rest, and call your doctor.

The Social Context

Postpartum emotional disturbances, like many (possibly all) mental disorders, are defined by the social context in which they occur. On an Israeli kibbutz the mother who feels that she cannot leave her newborn between nursing times to contribute to the community work is regarded as in need of special counseling for anxiety. In the United States the woman who returns promptly to work after childbirth is regarded by many as cold, neurotic, and unresponsive to the needs of her baby.

We believe it is a myth that the infant will be psychologically damaged unless the mother is always present. A baby's need for stable, responsible adults can be met just as well with either parent as the primary caretaker, by both parents sharing responsibility equally, and/or in combination with day care, or by a group or community of people living together.*

Societal pressures on new mothers to drop out on most of our major interests and be with our babies constantly seem to us to be a major cause of postpartum depression. In becoming a mother for the first time we experience an abrupt social discontinuity. Although motherhood has been held up to us as a major life goal (we are considered incomplete without it), being a housewife (that is, a drudge) is generally considered pretty low status.†

The lack of quality child care and the additional shopping, cooking, laundry and housecleaning that comes with having children causes the two roles to be inseparable for most of us: motherhood and the status it

---

*Studies of stunted children who have grown up in orphanages are often cited in an attempt to prove that infants need one constant caretaker (usually construed to mean the mother) rather than several. In fact, attachment to the caretaker is a developmental step preparing the child to make additional human attachments, which usually follow soon after. It is only when mother and baby are isolated (with father often or always absent) that the baby will continue to focus exclusively on the mother. Even child-development specialists are beginning to look to other factors—especially sensory deprivation, like a lack of bright colors, mobiles, things to look at, and toys to manipulate; not enough touching and fondling; and lack of emotional warmth on the part of over-worked staff—as causes for the failure of children in institutions to thrive emotionally and intellectually. For more on this see Rochelle P. Wortis, "The Acceptance of the Concept of Maternal Role by Behavioral Scientists: Its Effects on Women," *American Journal of Orthopsychiatry*, October 1971, Vol. 41, No. 5, pp. 221–36.

†Having given up our own opportunities for accomplishment, the child becomes the mother's "product"; in keeping with the Spockian ideal that the child's character, personality, and accomplishments, reflect the quantity and quality of the mother's care (Philip Slater, *The Pursuit of Loneliness*, Beacon Press, 1971). Though we are told that as mothers we have an unparalleled opportunity to shape society, we are in fact (with only minor variations) forced to raise our children to conform to the same sexist, competitive society that relegates us as women to an ineffectual role in society by keeping us in the home.

confers on us are held out as the reward for unpaid household labor.

During those stressful first weeks when so many of us are isolated at home with the baby, there is in most cases no support group or professional person we can turn to for help. For many of us the most stressful day is the first day home from the hospital. For others of us the glow from childbirth carries us through the first months and greater stress is experienced later.

Education and Preparation for Child Care

Even the visiting nurse seems to have gone out of style as women become "better educated." That our education rarely touches on baby or child care is taken into account by no existing public or private institution.*

Although there are classes that help us to deal with the physical side of pregnancy and childbirth,† there is little readily available instruction that prepares us emotionally and experientially for parenthood. Child care is demanding and becomes more so if we expect ourselves to know instinctively things which are learned skills. We can learn how to take care of our babies through our own experiences, through watching or listening to friends or relatives and through reading or classes.

* * *

I feel ecstatic about this baby. I don't have any of the fears and trepidations I had the first time. I feel very adequate to meet my baby's needs and make him happy. I enjoy this baby so much. With my first baby I kept looking forward to the next stage even when she was going through a great stage. With this baby I appreciate each day. I find myself wishing they wouldn't go so fast. I'm acutely aware that he'll only be a baby for a short time.

* * *

A study of women who attended prenatal classes during pregnancy showed that those women who attended two extra sessions of discussion focusing on *helpful suggestions for new parents* (see chart A) took more of the recommended suggestions and had significantly less emotional upset postpartum. *When husbands attended special instruction classes, fewer than half as many of the wives developed emotional disturbances compared to the women who participated alone.* Six months later those

mothers who had attended the child-care discussions had fewer problems that still persisted. Their babies were less irritable and had fewer problems with sleeping and feeding.* The instruction emphasized that the responsibilities of mothers are learned and are not inborn. This confirms our conviction that knowing what to do with a newborn does not get into our heads by "maternal instinct."

HELPFUL SUGGESTIONS FOR NEW PARENTS

The responsibilities of motherhood are learned; hence get informed.

Get help from husband and dependable friends and relatives.

Make friends of other couples who are experienced with child rearing.

Don't overload yourself with unimportant tasks.

Don't move soon after the baby arrives.

Don't be overconcerned with keeping up appearances.

Get plenty of rest and sleep.

Don't be a nurse to relatives and others at this period.

Confer and consult with husband, family, and experienced friends, and discuss your plans and worries.

Don't give up outside interests, but cut down on responsibilities and rearrange schedules.

Arrange for baby-sitters early.

Get a family doctor early.†

The Family Context

The first child, particularly, brings completely new experiences for the parents, and each new baby brings new relationships and new family interactions. The husband and wife become mother and father as well. The stresses of the postpartum period may bring clashes of child-care ideas, unfamiliar roles, fatigue and financial strain.‡

* * *

I hadn't known what to expect—what it would be like to be a mother. I experienced watching myself take care

---

*We are by no means advocating a return to the kind of education that prepared women to be "educated companions" and mothers and little else. What we want is free education for those men and women who want to learn about becoming parents.

†Education for childbirth (prepared or "natural" childbirth) may improve the postpartum adjustment of women with stressful life histories. (See section on "Social Factors and Prevention" in this chapter.) Such women often cope better than women with more favorable histories who do not prepare for childbirth. (Leon Chertok, *Motherhood and Personality*, Lippincott, 1969.)

*Gordon, Kapostins, and Gordon, "Factors in Postpartum Emotional Adjustment," pp. 158–66.

†*Ibid.*, pp. 158–66.

‡Virginia Larsen *et al.*, "Prediction and Improvement of Postpartum Adjustment," p. 1.

of David as if I were two people. . . . Though Mark was willing to help, it took some time before I felt okay about letting him. Becoming a mother for the first time, I really felt legitimate as a person. I was threatened by sharing the responsibility. I was hard on myself too. I felt I ought to know what to do as a mother instinctively.

When my second child was born I felt lots more comfortable in knowing how to take care of her. I had wanted a girl child. There were a lot of hassles in my marriage. I really wanted her to be my child. I had a lot of anger at my husband. After she was born I was tired and depressed. It took me six months to realize what I was doing. I wasn't sharing taking care of her. With David I would often ask Mark to help with diapering, etc. When he offered to do something for Ruth I'd say, "Oh, that's okay, I'll do it." But in spite of my anger I saw that it was an unfair thing to do to Ruth. A child needs two parents.

Having a new sister was very hard on David. At first he took to biting her toes and putting pillows on her head. I had to be very firm about that.

After Ruth was born I was feeling so many strains, marriage problems, fatigue, David's needs. He needed me so much, and I had so little energy for him. It just took time to work out. When I nursed Ruth I would read to David, holding the book on my lap, or David would hold it and turn the pages. He was very interested in the nursing. I took out pictures of me nursing him and told him how much fun it had been.

* * *

In response to a postpartum questionnaire, one woman reported that her marriage had undergone so much strain that she and her husband were now seeing a marriage counselor. She felt her husband becoming distant during the pregnancy. The feeling of elation from childbirth is still with her, and she is not sure that her marital problems are related to the birth of the child.*

And another woman said of her marriage:

* * *

It was different—I knew I was guilty of putting the baby before my husband all the time. I often used the baby as an excuse for him to do a lot of things for me. (I was a bitch to him.) He really was wonderful. His sexual desire increased after the baby, and my desire was nil. This was a complete reversal of our situation before the baby.

* * *

Some new fathers feel inadequate to comfort a crying baby who is being breast-fed. Many parents feel jealous of each other's attention to the baby, and some fathers

*A study of 800 couples by Dr. Harold Feldman at Cornell University showed significantly lower levels of marital happiness among couples with children (quoted by Ellen Peck in *The Baby Trap*, Bernard Geis Associates, 1971).

even experience sexual jealousy when the baby is breast-fed. We may need mothering and support ourselves, and may find that we have little emotional reserves for being supportive to our men. We may have little energy for or interest in sex. During this time it is important to keep communication as open as possible. Talking to other couples who have had babies recently will be helpful. Other suggestions that have proved helpful for reducing the stress of early postpartum are listed in the box on page 213.

Here is the statement of a woman whose postpartum experience was affected by many of the factors we have been discussing, compounded by the fact that she had a multiple birth, two boys and a girl.

* * *

My first three postpartum days were spent in hiatus waiting to see if all three would live and be healthy.

The excitement of having triplets was continually reinforced by a lot of attention from other people. I was so engrossed in the practical realities of taking care of three babies and one nine-year-old girl that any postpartum depression I might have suffered was indistinguishable from the general struggle against being overwhelmed. My older daughter was fortunately old enough to ride out the trauma with some resources of her own. Other mothers of triplets to whom I have spoken have said that young children presented with triplet siblings "have never known what hit them."

At my six-week postpartum checkup, when my obstetrician said it was all right to resume sexual intercourse, I asked, "When am I going to find time?"

"You'll get together even if you have to meet in a phone booth," was his reply.

We found very little time to be alone, but Jonathan didn't work for the first three months, and the adjustment with three was not as great in some ways as it had been with our first. My mother came for a month when the babies came home from the hospital.

Over a period of time I noticed that my mind suffered. I dropped out on everything that had been going on before the babies were born. My recall of facts and images, especially those predating the birth, was sharply impaired. It was like becoming senile. All of my psychic energy was going into sustaining the babies and the family. We rented the large home of friends, and other friends joined us to share the rent and help with the babies.

The high wears off. The crisis orientation fades. The helpers fall away. We lost our living quarters and had great difficulty finding others we could afford, which are also temporary. Six months after the babies were born I had resumed teaching one class a week, because I had to have something else to think about. When we moved I increased my teaching schedule to as much as I felt

I could handle. When the oldest boy, who had been the sickest at birth, got bronchitis again and again and nosebleeds, a hysterical fear of leukemia rose up in me. Memories of the loss of our first son took over in full Technicolor and Panavision. It was a hook to hang my resentment on for having worked like a slave for three years. I wanted out. I wanted help. There has got to be some change in my life.

The Medical Context

Pregnancy is treated by the medical profession as merely an initiation period that must be gotten through, with birth as a climax. This focus on the delivery, with its emphasis on the doctor as specialist and performer, is a sop to the doctor's ego. The doctor is the magician, the "deliverer." With his fee paid up until the birth of our child, he is our doctor afterward only in extreme cases except for the perfunctory six-week check-up.*

The postpartum check-up is rather arbitrarily set at six weeks because by then the episiotomy will be healed (it usually heals within three weeks), and most women who are not breast-feeding will have begun to menstruate (between 3 and 8 weeks after childbirth). This is the best time to prescribe contraceptives. We believe that the time of the postpartum check-up should be decided by the woman and her doctor on the basis of her individual situation, taking into account such factors as whether the woman is breast-feeding, whether she feels her episiotomy is healed, how she feels generally and when she wants to start having intercourse again.

The pediatrician usually does not see the child after the initial check-up in the hospital until four weeks after birth. We may need to call before that if we have questions. (Some pediatricians provide a book of commonly asked questions, which may be helpful.) Since the pediatrician does see the child and parent(s) at the end of the first month, if s/he is an aware and sensitive person s/he can recognize when parents are having difficulty and refer them to classes, counselors or whatever kind of help is useful.

Why is there so little medical research on postpartum disturbances? Dr. Hugh F. Butts writes, "The paucity of adequate clinical investigations into the psychiatric ills of women in the postpartum period is amazing in the light of the gravity of these conditions and the catastrophic effect . . . upon the unfortunate family." He cites the difficulty of multidisciplinary cooperation in

medicine as a reason for the lack of research, as well as the poorly defined etiology [cause of origin] of postpartum disturbances, in explanation of the limited amount of research.*

We suspect that the general lack of interest in postpartum disturbances is due to the male orientation of the medical profession as well as the fact that research funds usually go to diseases, rather than prevention, and especially those diseases that affect the affluent middle-aged men who control the economy and thereby control medical research funds as well. Whether new mothers feel well or not does not directly affect the functioning of the economy.

THEORIES OF CONTRIBUTING FACTORS AND SOME CLINICAL RESEARCH

The "traditional" and first serious theory (thirty years ago)† was that women who suffered from severe postpartum depression had deep-seated mental illness and the birth of the baby was merely the trigger that brought the pre-existing psychic disturbance to the surface. Women suffering from psychotic postpartum disturbances used to be diagnosed as schizophrenic, manic depressive, or whatever clinical syndrome their behavior was thought to resemble. In many cases they were hospitalized for years, in some cases for life.

Today this attitude is being rejected in favor of stress-triggering theories. These can be broken down into two schools of thought: (1) The depression is caused by physical stress—that is, hormonal imbalance and the bodily shock of labor. (2) The depression is caused by social stress, including one's background and one's current environment.

Physical-Stress Theories

In 1962 a study found postpartum depression analagous to combat fatigue.‡ Women who exhibited severe symptoms were sometimes found to have thyroid difficulties, and made dramatic recoveries when treated with thyroid compounds. Hypothyroidism of itself will not cause psychosis, but may help to trigger it in combination

---

*For ways to eliminate a lot of the fragmentation of health care see the "Pregnancy" section of this chapter for the discussion of the childbearing year as a continuum and also the "Proposals for Change" at the end of the chapter, particularly the suggestion regarding midwives. See also in Chapter 15, "Women and Health Care," the section on "Choosing and Using Medical Care: Management of the Ob-Gyn."

*"Psychodynamic and Endocrine Factors in Postpartum Psychoses," pp. 224–227.

†G. Zilboorg, "Post-Partum Schizophrenias," *Journal of Nervous and Mental Disorders*, 68:370–83, 1928. Quoted in Hugh F. Butts, "Postpartum Psychiatric Problems, A Review of the Literature Dealing With Etiological Theories."

‡J. A. Hamilton, *Postpartum Psychiatric Illness* (St. Louis: C. V. Mosby Co., 1962), quoted in Butts, pp. 224–27.

with psychological factors.* It is known that there is normally a change in the amounts of 17-hydroxycorticoids—steroids related to the adrenal gland—in the blood level whenever there is a general emotional arousal. Perhaps the imbalance in the sex hormones, the dramatic reduction in estrogen and progesterone that occurs at the end of pregnancy, can help to trigger the depressed feeling so often encountered.† Those who favor the physical-stress theories emphasize hormonal treatments, drugs such as tranquilizers or antidepressants, and sometimes hospitalization in severe cases.

The incidence of recurrence of acute postpartum psychosis is high without intervention, estimated at 20-50 percent. One current and yet unpublished attempt at preventing recurrence uses hormone treatment and drugs: tapering dosages of estrogen and progesterone, as well as tapering dosages of cortisone, are given over a period of about two months following delivery, so that the hormonal changes will not be so dramatic as to trigger a psychosis. Tranquilizers are administered when necessary. The only criterion of success is that the subjects do not require hospitalization.

* * *

I agreed to participate in the hormonal study because I feared a repetition of the experience which had resulted in my hospitalization after the birth of my first baby. Whenever I expressed anxiety over this possibility I was told to put my trust in the experiment and the doctors and "not to get in a flap over it." When I asked to see the psychiatrist who was supposed to be associated with the project my obstetrician told me to call and set up the appointment myself. I called the psychiatrist and was told that I could see him only as a private fee-paying patient.

I went to a clinic and got some help from a social worker. After my baby was born I was occasionally depressed and sometimes agitated, but as long as I took the pills and didn't become sick enough to be hospitalized, I was counted as a success for the hormonal experiment.

Possible Connections Between Physical and Social Factors

A preliminary study of new mothers hospitalized for psychiatric problems showed that they had lower thyroid activity than is normal following childbirth. Interviews showed these women had more negative attitudes toward motherhood and different kinds of social stress in their lives than a control group of unhospitalized new mothers. This suggests that there may be a relationship between emotional and social stress and lowered thyroid function. Also third-time mothers had significantly lower postpartum thyroid activity than first-time mothers. The researchers recommend that thyroid activity in the postpartum months should be explored with respect to age, number of children, nutrition, and emotional stress.*

Clearly a great deal more needs to be done by the medical profession and the mental-health professions to recognize mind-body connections such as in thyroid function, and more broadly, the "psychosomatic" nature of pregnancy. They should be prepared to work with us as whole people rather than focusing on that which their limited training and fragmented medical practices make convenient, lucrative, and ego-gratifying.

Social Stress Theories and Prevention

Other reports show that the social factors, including background and current environment, can be major contributors to depression in most people.† Reports of depression in fathers‡ and adoptive mothers§ indicate that the causes are not *purely* physical.

A questionnaire developed by Richard and Katherine Gordon was successfully used to predict the likelihood of postpartum difficulties.¶

The fourteen stress factors listed by Gordon, Kapostins, and Gordon:

1. Primipara (woman having first baby).
2. No relatives available for help with baby care.
3. Complications of pregnancy in family history.
4. Husband's father dead.
5. Wife's mother dead.
6. Wife ill apart from pregnancy.
7. Wife ill during pregnancy.
8. Wife's education higher than her parents'.
9. Husband's education higher than his parents'.
10. Wife's education incomplete.
11. Husband's occupation higher than his parents'.

---

*Butts, "Psychodynamic and Endocrine Factors in Postpartum Psychosis," pp. 224–227.

†It is not known why low levels of estrogen and progesterone should be related to depression. The menopausal woman also has low estrogen, and depression in menopause has been treated successfully by giving estrogen.

*Virginia L. Larsen *et al., Attitudes and Stresses Affecting Perinatal Adjustment,* pp. 67–72, 94.

†Rita F. Stein, "Social Orientation to Mental Illness in Pregnancy and Childbirth."

‡Beatrice Liebenberg, "Expectant Fathers," presented at annual meeting of American Orthopsychiatric Association, Washington, D.C., March 1967.

§F. T. Melges, "Postpartum Psychiatric Syndromes," *Psychosomatic Medicine,* 30:95–108, January-February 1968.

¶Gordon, Kapostins, and Gordon, "Factors in Postpartum Emotional Adjustment," pp. 158–66; see also Virginia Larsen *et al., Prediction and Improvement of Postpartum Adjustment.*

12. Husband's occupation higher than wife's parents'.
13. Husband often away from home.
14. Wife has had no previous experience with babies.*

The fourteen stress factors are divided into two categories: Category 1 consists of factors that might bring a woman into "Conflict with the Motherhood Role," such as the woman's preparation for achievement outside the home, along with such upward mobility factors as the man's and woman's educations being higher than that of their respective parents, and their general desire to get ahead socially and economically. Category 1 is also associated with living far from close relatives who could provide practical help and emotional support, and a husband who was often away from home, two conditions that usually accompany moving up in our society. Category 2 is related to unfortunate past experiences of failure, fear, and loss, such as the death of the wife's mother or the husband's father, the wife's formal education being incomplete, a history of pregnancy complications in the wife's family. Inexperience with babies is included. (Is this an experience of failure or loss? Only for women, presumably.)

The Gordons found that the more stresses, past and present, the more "abnormal" the postpartum emotional reaction. Of 95 women with higher scores (five or more out of fourteen stress factors) 40 percent developed emotional difficulties at six weeks and 29 percent continued to have trouble after six months. Of the 211 women with lower scores (less than four out of fourteen) only 6 percent had emotional problems, which tended to last for fewer than six months.

The present environmental factors of Category 1, such as lack of emotional support and assistance, the husband often away from home, and other relatives not available to help, were significant in cases where problems persisted for longer than six months.†

If you are pregnant and many of the above factors are present in your life, first of all do not be alarmed. Remember, 60 percent of the 95 women with high scores did *not* develop problems. We have included this information in the hope that it may help pregnant women to sort out which aspects of our lives are likely to give rise to conflicting feelings and roles following childbirth. We want to suggest fruitful areas for discussion with the baby's father, woman friends, prenatal classes, doctor's visits, etc., and to suggest some alternatives for minimizing the stress.

Present environmental stresses could be lessened by new fathers arranging to spend more time at home during the early months and years. (See our proposal for paternity leave with full pay in the section on "Some

*Gordon, Kapostins, and Gordon, pp. 158–66.
†*Ibid.*

Proposals for Change.") Also couples or single women with infants and small children can develop a network of friends to exchange baby-sitting and share their concerns or possibly try living with other people.

The findings of the Gordon study are an invaluable advance in our understanding of the many-faceted triggers of postpartum difficulties. A questionnaire similar to that developed by the Gordons could be routinely used by obstetricians and clinics as a screening device, and women with high-stress scores could be offered whatever special help is appropriate and desired—financial aid, baby-care classes, counseling, and in some cases abortion.

Though we applaud any approach that stresses prevention and takes the social milieu into account, it is important to look carefully at the biases inherent in even the best-intentioned researchers. It would be interesting to see a list of stress factors compiled by a group of women. For example, is the category labeled "Conflict with the Motherhood Role" caused by preparation for achievement outside the home, or is it the lack of good child-care facilities and the mystique of the full-time mother that are really the causes of stress? (See "Some Proposals for Change" below for ways that childbearing and child rearing can be made less stressful—and more joyful!)

Unfortunately, our society encourages us to fuse and confuse ourselves as people with our roles as mothers. We are taught to believe that we and *only* we can best raise our children, and that it must be a twenty-four-hour-a-day commitment. We are in conflict with ourselves because our society makes it so difficult for us to pursue our own goals while providing good care for our children.

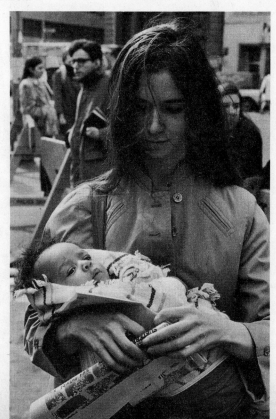

SOME PROPOSALS FOR CHANGE

We as women can begin to organize ourselves to fight those aspects of our society that make childbearing and child rearing stressful rather than fulfilling experiences: the fragmentation of medical services, the lack of education for parenthood, the mystique of the full-time mother. We need paid maternity and paternity leave and good child-care facilities so that women need not choose between family and career. We must fight the male-supremacist mystique that requires women to be responsible for the greater part of home and child care even when both parents work.

Some of the changes we need are:

1. Adequate Federal subsidies for the diet of pregnant and postpartum women. The government should also subsidize each child, so that better nutrition and a more healthful and stimulating environment would be guaranteed to each child.

2. Timely help for pregnant women who are likely to be upset postpartum. A questionnaire similar to the Gordons' could be widely distributed to obstetricians and clinics, with follow-up provided for women who showed five or more stress factors. Or women's groups could distribute these questionnaires directly to women at medical buildings, clinics, childbirth classes, and maternity shops, inviting women to come to meetings to talk about infant care, women, and the effects of social stress on pregnancy and postpartum. Group counseling could be organized for women who are already experiencing emotional upset or who just want to talk to other women. Given the findings of the study by Grete Bibring *et al.*,* it does not seem unreasonable over the

*"A Study of the Psychological Processes in Pregnancy and of the Earliest Mother-Child Relationship."

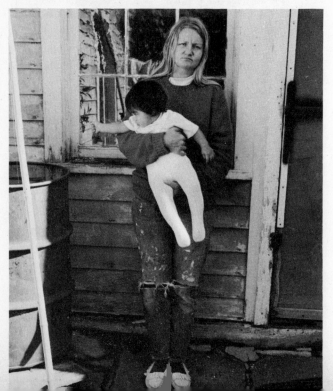

long term to expect obstetricians and clinics to provide group- and individual-counseling sessions as part of routine obstetrical care. We pay enough for it anyway.

3. Groups for expectant parents to explore feelings, fears and hopes about pregnancy, childbirth and parenthood and to provide instruction in the skills of infant care. (The groups can take many forms depending on the needs and preferences of the participants—couples' groups, women's groups, possibly other kinds of groupings.) Those who currently teach such classes (usually nurses) should get some training to be able to deal with feelings and group interaction. Midwives, as well as psychiatrists, social workers, marriage counselors and other mental-health workers should be available for consultation with individuals or couples. The government should subsidize these too, to be sure they are available at all income levels.

4. Prenatal and postnatal "hot-line" telephone services set up and staffed by women. Any woman with a problem could call for advice or just to talk. Women who wanted to be in groups could be brought together. Serious problems would be referred to qualified people.

5. New organizations of visiting laywomen to help with postnatal problems and baby care.

6. A nurse-midwife approach such as exists in England. The midwife sees the woman throughout her pregnancy, stays with her during *all* of the delivery, and helps with child care for the first few months of the child's life. She can handle all routine procedures competently and can recognize complications. Then the obstetrician would be on call for all difficult pregnancies and births, and pediatricians could be on call for all serious infant illnesses, without distinctions made for private and clinic patients.

7. More females in obstetrics-gynecology. Only six percent are women! Ob-gyn is listed as a surgical specialty and 'because there is a bias in the medical profession against female surgeons, women have a hard time if they want to be in that field.

8. Safe home delivery for those of us who want it. Mobile emergency units could be equipped as delivery rooms to stand by with whatever may be needed should complications arise. This would have the dual benefit of removing the birth process from the hospital setting with its associations of sickness and trauma and at the same time would free up hospital beds and medical personnel for sick people. Specially trained practical nurses could be provided to care for mother and baby where needed.

9. Realistic and up-to-date information in every clinic and doctor's office, where it will be readily available to patients. (The doctors should pay something toward the printing.)

10. Maternity leave for mothers and paternity leave for fathers with full pay provided by all places of em-

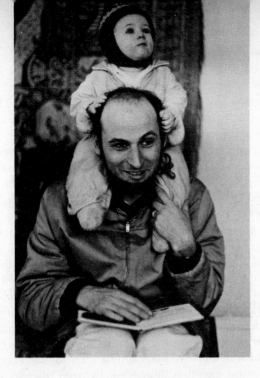

ployment, as in Sweden. Subsidized day care or baby-sitting for older children. Both parents need time to learn together to meet their baby's needs as well as to readjust their family relationships.

11. Day care to be provided by all places of employment (as well as in the community) so both parents can return to work when they feel they want to, with mothers able to nurse the child on the job if they choose to. This would have the added benefit of breaking down puritanical prejudices against public breast-feeding, a natural function of a woman's body. It is ridiculous that a woman cannot feed her child in public without breaking a law or being accused of exhibitionism. (*N.B.:* Day care must be provided by *all* places of employment, not just those that employ large numbers of women. Parents should have the option of deciding which parent will take the child to day care, and employers should not be able to claim that provision of child care makes it more expensive to hire women rather than men.)

We must free ourselves from these equations: woman-passive, man-active, woman-child-rearer, man-provider. We are all human beings, all one species. Our reproductive organs determine complementary roles in reproduction. They need not and should not determine our roles in society.

APPENDIX:
FEELINGS WHEN THE BABY DIES

There are more deaths during the first few days of life than at any subsequent time during childhood, and almost all occur in a hospital. Hospital staff have little knowledge of how to behave toward parents whose babies may die or have died. Little research has been done, and so medical personnel just follow customary medical procedures and relate to the parents according to their own personal reactions and common cultural assumptions.

In Latin America all the relatives come to mourn the death of a newborn with the parents. In the United States all traces of the baby's existence are wiped out, largely for the peace of mind of others.

Until recently mothers were not permitted to touch their premature infants because of the fear of infection and also because women were thought to have more of an emotional reaction if the baby died after they had held it. Now that aseptic techniques have reduced the risk of infection, some hospitals are letting the mother, scrubbed and gowned, handle her baby in the incubator. The authors of the Kannel study seem to feel that having held or touched the baby before it died may have increased the initial grieving to a minimal extent, but helped women in the long run to work through the mourning experience.*

In one hospital certain changes in procedure were made following a study of parents whose babies had died. Room assignments were changed so that bereaved mothers did not have to watch other women's babies brought to them. Staff communication was improved so that parents were given consistent reports as to their baby's chances. Discussions and interviews were held to inform the parents about common reactions to loss and how long they are likely to last. The couple is advised to talk freely to each other about their feelings,† and follow-up interviews are held three to four months later to help work through feelings of grief.‡

This is the experience of a woman who lost a baby for the second time. The first time the cord was wrapped around the baby's neck. The next baby died of hyaline membrane disease.

* * *

The physical recovery, even after a Caesarean, went quickly, but the emotional recovery of pulling myself together to function every day took much longer than everyone, even those closest to me, could comprehend. Such a large part of me had died, not once, but twice—all the hopes, plans, proffered love, with no one to give it to. My arms, my belly were empty. I felt like an empty

*For all the above see John H. Kannel *et al.,* "The Mourning Response of Parents to the Death of a Newborn Infant," *New England Journal of Medicine,* Vol. 283, August 13, 1970, pp. 344–349.

†Men in our society seem to need extra help in expressing feelings, and those sessions with both parents present seemed to be most valuable. Some men tended to repress their grief and bury themselves in extra work.

‡Kannel *et al.,* pp. 344–349.

shell, making only the motions required by the rest of my family.

Everyone said, "Be grateful for the two sons you do have," and I was, but they weren't the right size or shape to be the baby that my body had been preparing for. A year later at a physical exam when I got weepy talking about losing the baby—the doctor said, "Oh, you're overreacting. After all, you never held him." And all the rage and frustration rose again. I had held him, the baby, minute by minute for nine long months close inside, ready to offer him life with us as part of our family and all I could give him as a mother. And then nothing.

I wanted to adopt a baby immediately, but my husband said, and everyone said, that we had to wait until I was more rational—and that angered me. The reasons were valid. My husband said that the wanting in me was so strong that I'd devour the child emotionally, and that he wouldn't go ahead until I could truly say that if we were turned down by the agency, I could learn to be content with our two sons and let the rage and sorrow wither away. We talked and talked, did apply for a child, and received a five-month-old daughter about a year after the last loss. She is wonderful, and she speeded up the process of recovery by being a baby for us and by becoming far more important to us than what might have been.

APPENDIX: PHYSICAL ASPECTS OF POSTPARTUM

There are enormous physical changes occurring in the postpartum period. Popularly considered natural, "under no other circumstances does such marked and rapid tissue breakdown [catabolism] take place without a departure from a condition of health," says the author of a widely used textbook on obstetrics.* Under any other circumstances the drastic change in blood volume (30 percent) that takes place during the postpartum period would be felt as exhaustion, but many women feel exhilarated instead.†

A woman should be aware that such changes are taking place and that they can affect her physically as well as emotionally. It is important to note here that feelings, particularly depression, are intensified and of longer duration if the woman permits herself to get run-down physically. Some women have stubborn virus infections that may lead to depression, or substitute for it (in women who cannot acknowledge depression).

*N. Eastman, *Williams Obstetrics*, 11th edition, 1956.
†Reva Rubin, "Puerperal Change," in Nancy A. Lytle, ed., *Maternal Health Nursing.*

After a normal delivery the new mother is out of bed twenty-four to seventy-two hours postpartum. Those who get up soon after delivery feel better and stronger sooner, and have fewer bladder and bowel problems. By getting women on their feet earlier it has been possible to reduce the recommended hospital stay to four or five days (two days for clinic patients and those who are annoyed by hospital routines), as compared to the customary ten days of the recent past.

However, it should be emphasized that just because we are able to get up out of bed and move about, and because those of us who have had prepared childbirth feel better sooner, it does not mean that we should expect to reassume all of our former responsibilities immediately. It is important to get enough sleep and to set aside some time in the afternoon to make up sleep lost during night feedings. For six weeks—or longer if you find it helpful—time should be set aside for exercise (postpartum exercises suggested by your doctor) and rest. After the first six weeks see chapter on "Women in Motion" for ideas on exercise.

As with pregnancy, some women will experience a number of discomforts, while others will hardly have any at all. Some discomforts of this period are sweating (especially at night), loss of appetite, thirst (due to loss of fluids), and constipation. You may feel great, you may have few or no discomforts, you may have many; you will not know until the time comes. But when you are aware of the range of possibilities, you can probably cope with them better when they occur.

Uterus. For at least one hour after the completion of labor the physician or midwife should remain in attendance in case there are complications. If at the end of that period—up to six hours—the uterus has satisfactorily contracted, the woman may be left alone. If not, contractions should be stimulated and progress carefully watched until all danger of hemorrhage has passed.

The uterus, by a process called involution, becomes reduced to one-twentieth to one-twenty-fifth of its size at delivery. Involution is effected by autolytic (self-breakdown of cells) processes, by which the protein material of the uterine wall is broken down, absorbed, and cast off through the urine. The lining of the uterus [endometrium] is excreted as a blood-stained discharge [lochia] through the vagina. The discharge is bright red for the first few days; after three or four days it becomes paler; and usually after ten days there is merely a whitish or yellowish discharge. Unusually heavy or long-term bleeding requires rest, medical care. Though the lochia consists of waste material (substances no longer needed in the body), it is clean and should not have a bad odor. If it has an odor, it may indicate imperfect involution or retention of parts of the afterbirth, so tell your doctor.

By the end of the third week the entire endometrium has been cast off including the placental site, which means that women who bear many children do not have scar tissue in the uterus.*

Afterpains caused by contractions of the uterus are more common in women who have had more than one child. They are often accentuated while the baby is nursing. When they are severe, usually aspirin is prescribed.

Abdomen. An abdominal binder is not necessary, but many women feel more comfortable wearing one (usually a girdle that won't roll up).

The process of involution of the peritoneum (abdominal cavity) and the abdominal wall requires at least six weeks. Except for the presence of silvery lines [striae], more often called stretch marks, they gradually return to their original condition, provided the abdominal muscles have retained their tonicity. It is important to exercise during pregnancy and to do the exercises prescribed for the postpartum period, because the abdomen almost never comes back to its prepregnant condition without exercise.

Weight loss. There is usually a weight loss of about five pounds in addition to the weight loss representing the baby and the contents of the uterus. This represents water loss and other factors.

Bathing. It is okay to take showers as soon as you can get up and walk. Ask your doctor when you can begin to take tub baths (usually after six-week check-up).

Genitals. The genitals must be kept clean to prevent infection. The cervix is large after pregnancy, admitting two fingers. It is very important not to introduce anything into the vagina because of the danger of infection. The cervix returns to nearly normal condition in one week by proliferation of new cells (unlike the uterus, which first autodigests part of itself and then makes a new lining). A sterile pad should be worn until bleeding stops. The genitals are washed with an antiseptic solution each time after elimination, and the pad is changed. The author of our medical text states that the pad is useful not only to absorb the lochia but because "it makes it difficult for the patient to touch her genitalia, a practice very common among the uneducated classes."† He does not mention whether he has ever tried telling these "uneducated" women about the dangers of infection.

The vagina requires some time to recover from the distention and rarely returns to its prepregnant size. Some women feel that their genitals are more slack. The vaginal outlet is markedly distended and shows signs of laceration. The labia majora and minora become flabby as compared with their condition before childbirth. You can probably see some of the changes of your genitals if you look at yourself with a mirror. Many women have been able to correct this condition with vaginal exercises. If you are interested ask your doctor about the Kegel exercises. (See "Prepared Childbirth" section under "Exercises.")

Intercourse. The Masters and Johnson study reports that many women resume sexual intercourse within three weeks following delivery.* If the vaginal area feels okay and the bleeding (lochia) has stopped, there is no reason to avoid intercourse. The taboo period varies from one country to another even in the Western world. Many women in the United States resume sexual relations in the third week postpartum. Doctors make the six-week rule ostensibly to prevent infection, but today the rule is largely for their convenience, so that the end of the celibate period coincides with the six-week checkup. (This rule originated in the days before antibiotics.) Remember, too, that if you sleep with one person regularly, you probably already share the same germs and have a tolerance for them.

However, some women do experience discomforts and/or low sexual interest which are physically caused and certainly legitimate reason to avoid or postpone intercourse until you feel ready. Some women who are breast-feeding experience painful cramps during intercourse. In some women the stitches in the episiotomy (more about episiotomy in "Prepared Childbirth" section, p. 187) continue to be painful for several weeks. Ask your doctor about sitzbaths (*very* shallow warm baths) to help dissolve the stitches. Intercourse can be painful until the stitches dissolve.

Low sexual interest may be associated with lowered estrogen levels in your body. This is fairly common and does not mean you've become "frigid." If you do have sexual interest but find that your vagina does not lubricate easily, this again is physical (related to low estrogen levels). Just use a sterile unscented lubricant such as K-Y Jelly or ask your doctor to prescribe Estrogen Cream.

Remember too that sexual expression need not always include intercourse. (See chapter on "Sexuality.")

You must use reliable birth control from the time you begin intercourse. Your old diaphragm will not fit. You can use condoms with lots of foam or jelly. No pills while breast-feeding. Do not rely on breast-feeding or the absence of menstruation to protect you. You can get

*Ibid.
†Eastman and Hellman, *op. cit.*

*William H. Masters and Virginia Johnson, *Human Sexual Response*, p. 163.

pregnant the first time you ovulate *before* you begin to menstruate again. (See chapter on "The Anatomy and Physiology of Reproduction and Sexuality.")

Masters and Johnson examined a limited number of postpartum women during intercourse and found marked changes from the normal. The physiologic reactions of most parts of the genitals were reduced in rapidity and intensity. "Normal rugal patterns [vaginal folds] were flattened or absent and the vagina was light pink in color [usually vivid] and appeared almost senile to direct observation. Particularly was this steroid-starvation true for the three nursing mothers."[*]

Orgasm as measured by Masters and Johnson was not as strong or as intense. Interestingly enough, the feelings of sexual tension reported by participants did not correspond to the physical criteria observed by Masters and Johnson, as they usually do. "Sexual tensions frequently were described at non-pregnant levels, particularly among the nursing mothers." This may be due in part to pelvic congestion, which can be experienced as sexual arousal. But even more important, the women could not subjectively feel the difference between orgasms during this time (three to four weeks) and those of three months later when the physiologic response patterns of their orgasms became more intense.[†]

Urination. Between the second and fifth day there is a condition called diuresis. The body eliminates excess water, causing frequent urination. During pregnancy the body tends to retain water, and this diureses of the postpartum is simply a reversal of the process and a return to normal of the urination patterns. Urination may amount to over a gallon a day. Occasionally sugar is found in the urine. This is due to the presence of lactose, or milk sugar, and has no connection with diabetes. If the patient does not urinate within six hours after delivery she must be catheterized, because the bladder may become distended. A patient who has had analgesics in labor may not be aware that her bladder is full. If you experience a burning sensation when you urinate, call your doctor.

Bowels. Within the first few days the postpartum woman loses one-eighth to one-sixth of her body weight, which has accumulated gradually over nine months. This entails some displacement of internal organs and relaxation of abdominal walls, and is the reason it takes several days for bowels to function normally. Many women feel bewildered and upset by this.[‡] Getting up and walking as soon as possible seems to prevent severe constipation.

A mild cathartic may be given on the second or third day to relieve constipation. It is desirable to get the bowels moving during the hospital stay, but this is not always possible. The anus should be cleaned with an antiseptic solution after each bowel movement, and the pad changed. Some women develop small hemorrhoids during pregnancy which linger on and are annoying during postpartum. (They are usually temporary.) If you have this problem, check with your doctor.

Anemia. Most of the blood and metabolic alterations of pregnancy disappear within the first two weeks postpartum. In a study of one thousand deliveries, 20 percent of patients had anemia on the fourth day postpartum. In 15 percent it was mild, but in 5 percent it was severe. If you feel unusually weak or tired during the first two weeks, anemia may be the cause. It is very important to continue taking your prenatal iron pills through the first six weeks postpartum.

Diet. The postpartum woman may eat a normal diet. La Leche League lists foods for nursing mothers which may help to avoid colic in babies. If you are nursing, your diet should be the same as during pregnancy, with the addition of a pint of milk, bringing the milk total to a quart and a half a day. You need at least 80 to 100 grams of protein per day when nursing. There is a great deal of attention given to the pregnant woman's diet and vitamin supplements, which usually ceases with delivery. Whether you are breast-feeding or not, you need good nutrition to get *your* strength back. Good appetite may be an indication of postpartum adjustment.[*] If you are not eating well, you should try to figure out why and then try to get some help from your doctor. Remember, your diet postpartum is important in getting your strength back for *yourself* as well as for your baby. Continue taking your vitamins and iron supplements throught the first six weeks postpartum. (See chapter on "Nutrition.")

Temperature. Temperature should be carefully watched during the first two weeks, because fever is usually the first sign of infection. If it is over 101°, call your doctor right away.

Lactation. The baby's sucking reflex is fully developed at birth. When the baby is put to the breast, the sucking sets off the milk-ejection reflex (popularly called the "letting-down" reflex). When the milk comes in, it discharges oxytocin, which causes the uterus to contract—which feels like cramps—and speeds the involution of the uterus.[†]

[*]*Ibid.*, p. 151.
[†]*Ibid.*, pp. 150–51.
[‡]Rubin, "Puerperal Change."

[*]Virginia Larsen, *Attitudes and Stresses Affecting Perinatal Adjustment*, pp. 91–93.
[†]Michael Newton and Niles Newton, "The Normal Course and Management of Lactation," in Nancy A. Lytle, ed., *Maternal Health Nursing*.

See Infant Care Appendix and Further Readings for help with breast feeding. If your doctor is not helpful with nursing problems, call La Leche League.

Care of the nipples. Little attention is required beyond simple cleanliness. If the nipples become sore, a nipple shield may be used temporarily.

Menstruation. It usually returns in eight weeks in women who do not nurse. In nursing mothers, there is ordinarily no menstruation as long as the child is completely fed by nursing; but there is great variation, with menstruation occurring sometimes as early as two months postpartum, but most commonly at four months. Most women do not ovulate while nursing, but a substantial number do, so it is essential to employ reliable birth-control precautions.

APPENDIX: INFANT CARE

In our society now we are given encouragement to think of childbirth as "nothing" and of motherhood as "natural." Neither generalization is true, and both lead us into feelings of guilt and inadequacy. Many of us feel that sole responsibility for a newborn infant is more of a burden than we have been prepared for. We need to have other people around right from the start to share the work and the fun of motherhood.

The full impact of having a child often doesn't hit us until we're home from the hospital and faced with the reality of caring for that new, helpless human being. Many feelings, thoughts, and fears come to mind: I am supposed to be fulfilled because now I am a mother, but I feel ambivalent; I have to be around all the time just to care for my baby's needs, so I don't have any time for my other interests—I lose my independence; I feel scared—what if I do something wrong? I'm afraid even to bathe the baby for fear I might drop her.

All these feelings are common to so many of us. Just because we're women we don't instinctively know how to care for children. Experience is essential; we learn how to be good mothers.

Talking over our ambivalent feelings and fears with other women helps us to put those thoughts in proper perspective. We realize that we don't have to perform perfectly right from the beginning; everyone feels uneasy at first.

Once your child is born, s/he is a separate being, whom you have to get to know, and who has to get to know you. S/he's not really as fragile as s/he might seem to you, and s/he has a built-in will to live. But don't let that stop you from calling your doctor or clinic any time you have a question about the baby's health or welfare. Even if you haven't seen the pediatrician yet, s/he's there to help you. Don't feel satisfied until all your questions are answered.

We have learned that our independence and emotional well-being are as important for our children as for ourselves; we must remain people in spite of the fact that we're now mothers! Therefore, in thinking about child care we have to talk about our own needs as well as the needs of our baby.

Even though we have physically borne the baby alone, we know that we cannot for our own sakes, and must not for our children's sakes, rear them alone. Depending on our own living situations, we have to find the easiest way to share baby care from the very beginning. Sharing means to us joint responsibility, not just a division of tasks. We expect the other adults who are constantly part of our children's lives to know how to take care of the baby without having to turn to us as "the expert."

* * *

I didn't know how to change a diaper any more than my husband did. In fact, I may have been more nervous about it, since as a woman I was supposed to know how. I learned to do it because I had to learn, and my husband learned too. I always resent those fathers who pride themselves on never having changed their baby's diaper.

* * *

Our children need intimate, loving care from more than just one adult. That care can come from ourselves, the child's father, friends with whom we might be living collectively, relatives, good child-care centers, and close family friends. The important thing to remember is that if we as mothers allow ourselves to think that we are the only adults able to care for and love our children, we will almost always come to think of our children as exclusively our possessions.

We don't want to push women out of the home, but we want to leave the door wide open—both for ourselves and our children—to grow and develop as independent people.

When you decide how to feed your baby, whether to use breast or bottle, you may want to consider how that method fits in with the idea of sharing infant care. Most of us in this group who have children, breast-fed our babies. We did it because we wanted that experience, and also because we were feeling proud of our bodies and glad that as women our bodies can provide nourishment for our children. However, it is no wonder that many women in America feel ambivalent about breast-feeding. We are told that our breasts are our sexiest parts, and we are whistled at and winked at until we begin to think of ourselves as little more than sex objects for men. Conse-

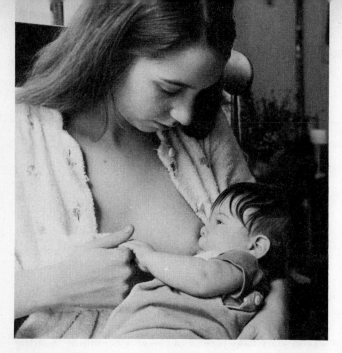

quently, many of us feel embarrassed or uncomfortable using our breasts to feed our babies.

Breast-feeding is a kind of sexual thing, but not because men tell us our breasts are sexy. Breast-feeding is sexual because it is satisfying, sensual, and fulfilling. It is a pleasant and relaxing way for both mother and baby to enjoy feedings, and it is an affirmation of our bodies.

Also, human milk is ideally suited to a baby's needs. Often babies who cannot tolerate any other food will have no trouble digesting breast milk. Furthermore, breast-feeding helps to strengthen the infant's resistance to infection and disease. Colostrum, the liquid in a new mother's breasts before the milk actually comes in, is especially high in antibodies that protect the tiny newborn against staphylococcus infections, polio virus, Coxsackie B. virus, infant diarrhea, and *E. coli* infections. These are the very germs to which infants are usually most susceptible. Breast-feeding also gives our babies a natural immunity to almost all common childhood diseases for at least six months, and usually until we stop breast-feeding completely. Moreover, the physical closeness of mother and baby during breast-feeding is important to the baby's future emotional health. If you've chosen bottle feeding, or if you find that you want to switch from breast to bottle feeding, don't feel that you can't be close to your baby. Whatever the method of feeding, babies like to be held close and cuddled by the person doing the feeding.

Child-care sharing is easier with bottle feeding, but can be very compatible with breast-feeding, especially when the baby gets a little older. It's difficult to establish a successful part-time breast-feeding arrangement, but if you want to have time for yourself away from your baby, it's worth the effort. Also, it's important for the other members of your family not to feel that you have the exclusive power to meet your baby's needs.

Don't try to impose a schedule for feeding on your newborn at first. Feed the baby whenever s/he cries for food during the early weeks. S/he will gain faster and be happier, and your milk supply will grow. Of course, after a few weeks or at most a couple of months, a modified schedule will work itself out. Then you can begin to move about more freely and leave other people in full charge more often.

Our milk supply and the baby's growth needs are perfectly coordinated. The more the baby nurses, the more milk our breasts will produce. It's just that simple. Feed the baby from both breasts at each feeding, and try to see that at least one breast is emptied each time. Be careful not to let your nipples get too sore; whenever you can, leave them exposed to the air.

During the early weeks you need a lot of rest, so it's best not to resume too many activities outside the home right away. You can, of course, have someone else give the baby an occasional bottle when you go out, but try not to miss two consecutive feedings. At this point other household members can bathe the baby, play with the baby, and change the baby. Then, after a few weeks, or a month or two, you can begin to share the feedings by missing one regularly. Try not to miss more than one feeding a day during the first two months; not only may

The baby's suckling generates impulses which reach the hypothalamus (an area of the brain believed to contain vital autonomic nervous centers) and stimulates the pituitary gland (located at the base of the brain) to release the hormone oxytocin. This hormone travels through the bloodstream and, in a matter of seconds, when it reaches the breast, the oxytocin causes the alveoli (tiny glands deep inside the breast) to contract. This in turn actually squeezes, first colostrum, and then, after a few days of nursing, milk, into the ducts. The opening of the ducts is in the nipple.

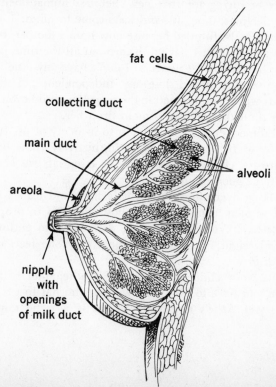

fat cells

collecting duct

main duct

alveoli

areola

nipple
with
openings
of milk duct

your milk supply suffer but your baby may find it easier to suck milk through a bottle nipple and balk at having to suck harder (even though that is better for her or him) at your nipple. We would like to emphasize that regularity, missing the same feedings every day, is the key to successful part-time breast-feeding. You may experience some problems at first, but don't give up. Good high-protein food, lots of liquid, enough sleep, and determination will see you through. (For some special hints, such as taking brewer's yeast to increase your milk supply, see Adele Davis, *Let's Have Healthy Children,* Lester Hazell, *Commonsense Childbirth,* and the La Leche League book described below.)

Many books have been written about breast-feeding. They are full of the basic information you'll need to breast-feed successfully. The La Leche League book, *The Womanly Art of Breastfeeding,* will give you facts and confidence. It will answer any specific questions you might have, but its philosophy is different from ours. We do not believe that breast-feeding has to dominate your life to the extent that you have the sole responsibility for your new baby. The baby's father, or another household member who will be sharing child care, wants to feel that s/he, too, can have a part in satisfying the baby's needs, the most prominent of which is food.

We have learned that there are no final rules to follow regarding infant care; our children are as different from each other as we are from our friends. The key thing is to try to relax and enjoy our children; they can be great fun as long as we don't have exclusive responsibility for them twenty-four hours a day.

Here are some random pointers that come to mind:

1. Very few books are adequate, because they rarely take into account the mother as an independent person. Talking to friends is more helpful. Dr. Benjamin Spock's *Baby and Child Care* can be reassuring at times with specific information.

2. Time for yourself alone is essential—awake and asleep. You'd be surprised to learn to what extent getting enough sleep determines your ability to cope. When you're away from your baby, enjoy being yourself; motherhood is only one part of you.

3. If you're planning to breast-feed, read some good, supportive books about it first. We recommend Lester Hazell, *Commonsense Childbirth,* Sheila Kitzinger, *The Experience of Childbirth,* Karen Pryor, *Nursing Your Baby,* La Leche League, *Womanly Art of Breastfeeding,* Alice Gerard, *Please Breast Feed Your Baby.* Check the bibliography for others and for the publishing information about these.

4. Check with family and friends; their experiences will give you support as well as information.

5. Here is a list of some of the products we have found helpful. (You may want to try some of these.) If you get

your baby used to these things from the start, you'll probably have less hassle.

Disposable diapers. Good for traveling especially, but lots of women use them instead of cloth diapers all the time. Ecologically, however, constant use of the product can't be defended.

Pacifiers. Some babies won't take them, and probably don't need them, but it's useful to introduce them during the first week to get your baby accustomed to them. After a while the baby may reject the pacifier completely, so don't force it on her or him at that point.

Babycarriers, infant seats, portable beds—anything that increases your mobility. A baby can sleep anywhere and under most circumstances if you teach him or her early enough. Security shouldn't come from a bed or a place, but from adult reassurance and your expectation that the child can do it.

Other equipment that gives the baby mobility and variety: jump seats, swings, jumpers, mobiles, and so on.

A baby-food grinder. You can buy a grinder for about a dollar, or a special baby food grinder for under five dollars. A blender will work too, but it's a more expensive purchase if you don't already own one. This will allow you to grind all adult food into baby food, thus almost eliminating the need to buy baby food.

We can't emphasize enough that caring for a baby is a learned skill, and one that we are continually learning. It also seems clear to us that successful infant care is as much political as it is physical and emotional. Paid maternity and paternity leaves, adequate housing, and excellent child-care facilities are nothing more than reasonable demands which we can rightfully expect to have fulfilled. We can't hope to be "naturally" good mothers without preparation, education, determination, and help.

FURTHER READINGS

I. *General Books* (Asterisk means really worth while.)

*Fitzpatrick, Elise, *et al. Maternity Nursing,* 11th ed. (There is also a 12th edition.) Philadelphia: J. B. Lippincott Co., 1966. $10.
  Interesting, readable, comprehensive textbook written for nurses. A lot of good useful information. Takes into account our feelings as well as our physiological changes.
Gray, Madeline. *The Normal Woman.* New York: Charles Scribner's Sons, 1969.
  Written by a laywoman who has an oppressively traditional attitude toward women. Not worth buying, but worth reading for some good information about childbearing.
Guttmacher, Alan F. *Pregnancy and Birth.* New York: Signet Books, 1962 (paper).
  Guttmacher is head of International Planned Parenthood, and he practiced obstetrics and gynecology for many years in New York. He has written many books for the general public. This book is adequate if you don't expect to understand topics in too great depth.

*Lytle, Nancy A., ed. *Maternal Health Nursing*. Dubuque, Iowa: William C. Brown Co., 1967 (paper).
> Interesting collection of articles connected with childbearing. Discussions of issues that interest us and that are rarely discussed, such as the pros and cons of induction of labor, and causes and diagnoses of abnormalities in babies.

Richardson, Stephen, and Alan Guttmacher, eds. *Social and Psychological Aspects of Childbearing*. Baltimore: Williams and Wilkins Co., 1967.
> A collection of articles that discuss many aspects of childbearing, useful because it includes the results of various studies we wouldn't ordinarily hear about, especially concerning childbirth in other societies.

*Shaw, Nancy. "So You're Going to Have a Baby: Institutional Processing of Maternity Patients." Doctoral thesis, Brandeis University, 1972, to be published in Spring 1973 by Pergamon Press.
> Powerful sociological analysis of how women are treated by hospitals, doctors, and nurses during pregnancy and childbirth.

GYNECOLOGY AND OBSTETRICS TEXTBOOKS

Brudenell, J. M. *Obstetrics*. London: Staples Press, 1964.

Eastman, Nicholson, and Louis Hellman. *Williams Obstetrics*. 13th ed. New York: Appleton-Century-Crofts, 1966.

Garrey, M. M., *et al. Obstetrics Illustrated*. Edinburgh and London: E. & S. Livingstone, Ltd., 1969.

McLennan, Charles E., with collaboration of Eugene C. Sandberg. *Synopsis of Obstetrics*. 8th ed. St. Louis: The C. V. Mosby Co., 1970.

Obstetrics in General Practise (British Medical Journal, 1966), British Medical Association, Tavistock Square, London WC 1, England.

Reid, D. E., and T. C. Barton, eds. *Controversy in Obstetrics and Gynecology*. Philadelphia: W. B. Saunders Co., 1969.

Tenney, B., and B. Little. *Clinical Obstetrics*. Philadelphia: W. B. Saunders Co., 1969.

Willson, J. Robert, Beecham, and Carrington. *Obstetrics and Gynecology*. 3d ed. St. Louis: C. V. Mosby Co., 1966.

II. General Pregnancy

Colman, Arthur D., and Libby L. *Pregnancy: The Psychological Experience*. New York: Herder and Herder, 1972.
> Husband-wife team examine emotional aspects of pregnancy and childbirth; has more detailed discussion of men's feelings than we usually find.

Eastman, Nicholson J. *Expectant Motherhood*. 4th ed. Boston: Little, Brown & Co., 1963.
> Very traditionally oriented, but author gives some useful information in spite of himself.

Flanagan, Geraldine L. *The First Nine Months of Life*. New York: Simon and Schuster, 1962 (paper).
> Story of conception and week-by-week progress of baby in utero. Very detailed, clear, and exciting.

Ingelman-Sundberg, Axel, Claes Wirsen, and Lennart Nillson. *A Child Is Born*. New York: Dell Pub. Co., Inc., 1969 (paper). $3.95.
> Beautiful, detailed color photographs of the growth of the fetus, and photo story of a couple during pregnancy and birth.

Kitzinger, Sheila. *An Approach to Antenatal Teaching*. Distributed in the United States by the Boston Association for Childbirth Education, Box 29, Newtonville, Mass. 02160, by the National Childbirth Trust.
> A sympathetic, knowledgeable discussion of meaningful childbirth education.

Smith, Anthony. *The Body*. New York: Avon Books, 1969 (paper).
> Many random facts about our bodies. Useful for its detailed description of the growth of the fetus, the functions of the placenta, amniotic sac, etc.

NUTRITION IN PREGNANCY

Annotated Pregnancy Nutrition Bibliography (rev. January 1972 in chronological order): 50 articles relating to nutrition and pregnancy. Distributed by Nutrition Action Group, 3414, 22nd Street, San Francisco, Cal. 94110.

Brewer, Thomas. "Human Pregnancy Nutrition: An Examination of Traditional Assumptions," *Australian and New Zealand Journal of Obstetrics and Gynecology*, Vol. 10, No. 2 (May 1970), pp. 87–92.

————. *If You Are Pregnant and Want Your Child* (1969). Pamphlet distributed by Student Research Facility, 2214 Grove Street, Berkeley, Cal. 94704.

————. *Metabolic Toxemia of Late Pregnancy: A Disease of Malnutrition*. Springfield, Ill.: Chas. C. Thomas Pub., 1966. $8.50.

Davis, Adele. *Let's Have Healthy Children*. New York: Harcourt, Brace, and World, 1959.

Matchan, Don. "Don't Risk Toxemia in Pregnancy," *Prevention* magazine (January 1972).

"Maternal Nutrition and the Course of Pregnancy." Summary report, National Academy of Sciences, Washington, D.C., 1970. Available from the U.S. Government Printing Office.

ECTOPIC PREGNANCY

Quilligan, Edward T. "Ectopic Pregnancy," *Hospital Medicine*, Vol. 5, No. 4 (March 1969).

PREGNANCY AND SEXUAL INTERCOURSE

Brecher, Ruth and Edward. *An Analysis of Human Sexual Response*. New York: Signet Books, 1966.

Israel and Rubin. *Siecus Study Guide* No. 6 (1967), Siecus Publications Office, 1855 Broadway, New York, N.Y. 10023 (Sex Information and Education Council of the U.S.)

Kitzinger, Sheila. *Intercourse During Pregnancy and in the Puerperium*, National Childbirth Trust Teacher's Broadsheet No. 2 (April 1967). Available from the Boston Association for Childbirth Education, Box 29, Newtonville, Mass. 02160.

INFERTILITY

Roland, Maxwell. *Management of the Unfertile Couple*. Springfield, Ill.: Chas. C. Thomas Pub., 1968.

DRUGS

Steinbach, Alan. "Drugs and Women's Bodies," University of California at Berkeley SESPA paper, 1972.

EXERCISE

Preparation for Childbearing. Maternity Center Association, 48 East 92nd Street, New York, N.Y. 10016 (50 cents each).
> Inexpensive, well-illustrated booklet showing how to exercise, walk, stand, sit, and function, as well as how to prepare for childbirth when you are pregnant.

III. General Childbirth Books

Bean, Constance. *Methods of Childbirth: A Complete Guide to Childbirth Classes and Maternity Care*. New York: Doubleday, 1972.
> How to choose a childbirth class, what hospital to go to, how to choose a doctor, and so on.

Bing, Elisabeth. *Six Practical Lessons for an Easier Childbirth*. New York: Bantam Books, 1969.
> One of the best step-by-step studies to the American Lamaze method, especially for people who cannot attend classes.

Bing, Elisabeth, Marjorie Karmel, and Tanz. *A Practical Course for the Psychoprophylactic Method of Childbirth.* 1961.
>   Lamaze techniques. Original ASPO manual.

Bradley, Robert A. *Husband-Coached Childbirth.* New York: Harper & Row Pub., Inc., 1965.
>   Folksy, talkative book; useful information. Childbirth is discussed in a humane way.

Chabon, Irvin. *Awake and Aware.* New York: Dell Pub. Co., Inc., 1969.
>   History of childbirth practices. Lamaze method; short, moving birth descriptions by women; exercises and good pictures. Current, easy to read.

Daly, Ann. *The Birth of a Child.* New York: Crown Pub., Inc., 1969.
>   Very graphic photographs of a birth in Holland, with a fairly good accompanying narration. Useful, because it helps us see how we look as we give birth.

Dick-Read, Grantly. *Childbirth Without Fear.* 2nd ed. New York: Harper & Row Pub., Inc., 1959.
>   Written by an English doctor who was the originator of "natural childbirth." Method more mystical than Lamaze method; more stress on relaxation, and less on activity and breathing.

————. *The Natural Childbirth Primer.* New York: Harper & Row Pub., Inc., 1956.
>   A how-to for natural childbirth, with exercises, diet, and guide to labor and delivery.

Eloesser, Leo, Edith J. Galt, and Isabel Hemingway. *A Manual for Rural Midwives* (1959). Instituto Indigenista Interamericano, Niños-Heroes 139, Mexico 7, D.F.
>   Informative, practical home-delivery guide (in English). If you use it at home, you should supplement it with lots of other information, and preferably a midwife.

Ewy, Donna and Roger, els. *Preparation for Childbirth.* Boulder, Colo.: Pruett Pub. Co., 1970.
>   Well-illustrated Lamaze guide for parents. Available from ICEA (International Childbirth Education Association) supply center.

Haire, Doris and John. *Implementing Family-Centered Maternity Care with a Central Nursery.* 3d ed. Hillside, N.J.: International Childbirth Education Association, 1971.
>   Complete guide for hospitals or anyone interested in converting a conventional maternity unit into a service where prepared mothers and fathers can participate fully in labor, delivery, and care of the baby afterward. Exhaustive documentation.

Hazell, Lester D. *Commonsense Childbirth.* New York: G. P. Putnam's Sons, 1969 (paper).
>   Written by a woman. Best over-all book for many reasons: good to read, complete, and sensible approach to childbirth. The author has had children of her own, and conveys what it feels like to give birth. She has an understanding of the source of many women's problems during childbirth (that is, the medical profession) and is very critical of it. Excellent section on why to have a baby at home; also good section on breast-feeding.

Karmel, Marjorie. *Thank You, Dr. Lamaze.* New York: Doubleday & Co., Inc. (paper).
>   Lively personal account of two experiences with prepared childbirth. Author's first child was delivered in France by Dr. Lamaze, the second in America. Comparison of practices in the two countries. Fun to read. A little outdated.

Kitzinger, Sheila. *The Experience of Childbirth.* New York: International Publications Service, 1964.
>   English woman and childbirth teacher. Method described combines Read and Lamaze. Strong psychological orientation. Has a good chapter on home delivery.

————. *Giving Birth: The Parents' Experience of Childbirth.* New York: Taplinger Pub. Co., Inc., 1971.
>   A book for all women, not just those who want natural childbirth. Encourages us to acknowledge and express our individ-uality in childbirth. Many moving personal accounts of parents' experiences.

Tanzer, Deborah, and Jean Block. *Why Natural Childbirth.* New York: Doubleday & Co., Inc., 1972.
>   A psychologist's experience working with dozens of couples who shared the event of their childbirth. Fascinating insights about childbirth and sex.

Vellay, Pierre, *et al. Childbirth Without Pain,* translated by Denise Lloyd. New York: E. P. Dutton & Co., Inc., 1959.
>   A series of lectures and exercises by an associate of Lamaze. Good; thorough in original Lamaze method. Shouldn't be the first book you read. The pictures of deliveries are very exciting—be sure to look at them.

Walzer, Stephan, and Allen Cohen. *Childbirth Is Ecstasy.* San Francisco: Aquarius Pub. Co., 1971; distributed by Book People.
>   Though the text is mystical, sentimental, and silly, the photographs of the woman in labor during and after delivery are fine.

Wessell, Helen. *Natural Childbirth and the Christian Family.* New York: Harper & Row Pub., Inc., 1963.
>   Not worth buying, but worth reading for chapters on history of childbirth, mistranslation of the Bible, and accounts of anesthetic death statistics. Also illustrates how to build a simple backrest for home delivery.

White, Gregory. *Emergency Childbirth,* rev. 1968, ICEA supply center.
>   Indispensable for people living in deep country or for anyone who might have to deliver a baby unexpectedly. If you aren't having your baby in a hospital, this is must reading.

Wright, Erna. *The New Childbirth.* New York: Hart Pub. Co., 1968.
>   Manual to prepare women for childbirth, written by a midwife who has had children. Excellent preparation in British version of Lamaze method. Less critical of the medical profession than the Hazell book. A woman could do all the physical preparation necessary with this book alone.

ARTICLES

Johnson, Wayne L. "Regionals Can Prolong Labor," *Medical World News,* October 15, 1971, p. 41.

Ullery, John C. "Obstetric Malpresentations," *Hospital Medicine,* Vol. 3, No. 12 (December 1967), pp. 22–29.

IV. Breast-feeding

Gerard, Alice. *Please Breast Feed Your Baby.* New York: New American Library, 1971.

Jelliffe, D. B., and E. F. Jelliffe. "The Significance of Human Milk" (a symposium), *American Journal of Clinical Nutrition* (August 1971).
>   Articles by many leading authorities on all aspects of lactation.

The Womanly Art of Breastfeeding. Franklin Park, Ill.: La Leche League International, 1963 (paper).
>   Some helpful information if you can get past the sickening stuff about a woman's role is to bear and raise children. Somewhat outdated in comparisons between breast and bottle milk. Does give a woman lots of support for breast-feeding.

V. Postpartum

Bibring, Grete L. "Recognition of Psychological Stresses Often Neglected in OB care," *Hospital Topics,* 44:100–3 (September 1966).

————. "Some Considerations of the Psychological Processes in Pregnancy," *The Psychoanalytic Study of the Child,* Vol. XIV (1959), pp. 113–21.

———— *et al.* "A Study of the Psychological Processes in Pregnancy and of the Earliest Mother-Child Relationship," *The Psychoanalytic Study of the Child,* Vol. XVI (1961), pp. 9–72.
>   Excellent study of "normal" pregnant women with ten-year follow-up.

Butts, Hugh F. "Postpartum Psychiatric Problems: A Review of the Literature Dealing with Etiological Theories," *Journal of the National Medical Association*, Vol. 62, No. 2 (March 1969), pp. 224–27.

Good review article.

———. "Psychodynamic and Endocrine Factors in Postpartum Psychosis," *Journal of the National Medical Association*, Vol. 60, No. 3 (May 1968), pp. 224–27.

Interesting case histories.

Chertok, Leon, *Motherhood and Personality*. Philadelphia: J. B. Lippincott Co., 1969.

Golub, Sharon, "Rapid Eye Movement Sleep", *Nursing Outlook*, February 1967, pp. 56–58.

Gordon, R. E., E. E. Kapostins, and K. K. Gordon. "Factors in Postpartum Emotional Adjustment," *Obstetrics and Gynecology*, Vol. 25, No. 2 (February 1965), pp. 158–66.

Hamilton, J. A., *Postpartum Psychiatric Illness*, St. Louis: The C. V. Mosby Co., 1962.

Jones, Beverly, "The Dynamics of Marriage and Motherhood," in Robin Morgan, ed., *Sisterhood Is Powerful*. New York: Random House, Inc. (Vintage), 1970, pp. 57–58.

Kane, F. J., Jr., *et al.*, "Emotional and Cognitive Disturbance in Early Puerperium," *British Journal of Psychiatry* (1968), pp. 99–102.

Kannel, John H., *et al.*, "The Mourning Response of Parents to the Death of a Newborn Infant," *New England Journal of Medicine*, August 13, 1970, Vol. 283, pp. 344–349.

Klaus, Marshal H., *et al.*, "Maternal Attachment" *New England Journal of Medicine*, March 2, 1972, Vol. 286, No. 9.

Larsen, Virginia, *et al. Attitudes and Stresses Affecting Perinatal Adjustment*. Final report, National Institute of Mental Health Grant MH-01381-01-02, September 1, 1963, to August 31, 1966. (Gordon questionnaire contained in appendices.)

———. *Prediction and Improvement of Postpartum Adjustment*. Final report, Children's Bureau Research Gdant A-66, September 1, 1965, to March 31, 1968.

Pages 95–99 have an excellent bibliography.

Liebenberg, Beatrice, "Expectant Fathers," presented at annual meeting of American Orthopsychiatric Association, March 1967, Washington, D.C.

Masters, William H., and Virginia E. Johnson, *Human Sexual Response*. Boston: Little, Brown and Co., 1966.

Melges, F. T. "Postpartum Psychiatric Syndromes," *Psychoanalytic Medicine*, 30:95–108, January-February 1968.

Newton, Michael and Niles. "The Normal Course and Management of Lactation," in Nancy A. Lytle, ed., *Maternal Health Nursing*. Dubuque, Iowa: William C. Brown Co., 1967.

Peck, Ellen. *The Baby Trap*. New York: Bernard Geis Associates, 1971.

Rubin, Reva. "Puerperal Change," in Nancy A. Lytle, ed., *Maternal Health Nursing*. Dubuque, Iowa: William C. Brown Co., 1967.

Stein, Rita F. "Social Orientation to Mental Illness in Pregnancy and Childbirth," *International Journal of Social Psychiatry* (Winter 1967-1968), 14:56–64.

Williams, Barbara, "Sleep Needs During the Maternity Cycle," *Nursing Outlook* (February 1967), pp. 53–55.

Wortis, Rochelle P., "The Acceptance of the Concept of Maternal Role by Behavioural Scientists: Its Effects on Women," *American Journal of Orthopsychiatry*, October 1971, Vol. 41, No. 5, pp. 221–36.

VI. Infant and Child Care

Ainsworth, Mary D., *et al. Deprivation of Maternal Care*. New York: Schocken Books, 1966.

Anthony, E. James, and Theresa Benedek, eds. *Parenthood: Its Psychology and Psychopathology*. Boston: Little, Brown & Co., 1970.

Heavy psychoanalytic and pathological bias.

Bettelheim, Bruno. *Love Is Not Enough*. New York: Avon Books, 1971 (paper).

Written about children in his special Orthogenic School in Chicago. Although the book is not about "normal" children, and Bettelheim is a very authoritarian man, he has some important things to say about all kids. Good sections on food, in-between times, and space.

Bowlby, John. *Maternal Care and Mental Health*. New York: Schocken Books, 1966. A report prepared on behalf of the World Health Organization as a contribution to the U.N. program for the welfare of homeless children.

Brazelton, T. Berry. *Infants and Mothers: Differences in Development*. New York: Delacorte Press (Dell), 1969. (Also available in paperback.)

Follows three "typical" infants from birth through the first year, with emphasis on the effects the infant can have on his/her environment, and the mother-infant interaction.

Fraiberg, Selma. *The Magic Years*. New York: Charles Scribner's Sons, 1959 (paper). $2.45.

Ilg, Francis L., and Louise Bates Ames. *Gesell Institute's Child Behavior*. New York: Dell, 1955.

It provides some information about what to expect from a child of a given age. Don't take age norms too seriously. Remember, it's a statement about children in this society ten years ago. Things are changing and need to be pushed more. (For instance, children can begin to relate to each other from the time they are only weeks old. Yet this and other books say they can't relate until age three, an assumption that the child is in the nuclear family until that age, and then goes to nursery school, which gives the child a first encounter with the outside.)

Montagu, Ashley. *Touching: The Human Significance of the Skin*. New York: Columbia University Press, 1971.

Fascinating account of human needs and emotions relating to physical contact at all ages, includes some animal studies, etc. Especially shows artificiality of society in the United States.

Nelson, Waldo E., *et al. Textbook of Pediatrics*. 9th ed. Philadelphia: W. B. Saunders Co., 1969.

Newton, Niles Anne. *The Family Book of Child Care*. New York: Harper & Row Pub., Inc., 1957.

A good book, written from a woman's viewpoint, coordinating child care with the rest of your life.

Prenatal Care, Infant and Child Care, Your Child from 6 to 17. U.S. Department of Health, Education and Welfare, Children's Bureau pamphlets.

Salk, Lee, and Rita Kramer. *How to Raise a Human Being*. New York: Random House, 1969.

Interesting, readable, and very clear approach to various developmental stages, without rigid norms. Better than Gesell.

Spock, Benjamin. *Baby and Child Care*. New York: Pocket Books, rev. ed., 1968.

Still a classic, and if you haven't read it, do. (Much misquoted.) Not good on breast-feeding or socialization, but good for basic everyday troubles.

N.B.: Also worthwhile, really helpful reading: books by psychiatrists such as R. D. Laing, Fritz Perls, David Cooper, Arthur Janov, and other modern "existential" psychiatrists; and books by educators John Holt, A. S. Neill, Sylvia Ashton-Warner, George Denison, Jonathan Kozol, and Herbert Kohl.

14
Menopause

MENOPAUSE is defined as the period of cessation of menstruation, occurring naturally between the ages of forty-five and fifty. Menopause involves the gradual decline of the working of our ovaries. Our ovaries can begin to produce less estrogen starting even in our late twenties. But most of us do not actually begin to notice *signs* of menopause until our late thirties or early forties. In other words, menopause is a long process which ends with the complete cessation of menstruation and of our ability to conceive and bear children. Our bodies have to adjust to these changes in ovarian and hormonal function. The length of time and the quality of this adjustment will vary from woman to woman. Removal of both ovaries (as in a total hysterectomy) before the age of natural menopause will bring on menopause symptoms.

A few older friends sat down and told some of us recently what their experiences of menopause had been like:

* * *

I have found life after 55 and the menopause very similar to life before 55 and the menopause.

* * *

Just beautiful not to have to worry about the damn periods. And no more birth control!

* * *

I was tired in the afternoons for a couple of years and worried that I was going into a decline, but being luckily a vigorous person, I kept going with my work. Then one day I realized it must have been the menopause.

* * *

I don't really think of telling my kids I'm in the menopause because that would be overplaying its importance.

* * *

When I was about age fifty-six I began to menstruate less often and felt mildly nervous at times. The woman gynecologist to whom I had been going yearly for Pap smears probed at some length into any possible dangers and then recommended a daily amount of Premarin, and when this brought back the periods, suggested halving the daily pill. This was six years ago and I have had no menopausal symptoms since.

* * *

Although we know that not every woman has the easy time with menopause that these particular women did, it was a relief for us to hear such positive things about menopause, because so much that we have heard and absorbed about "the change of life" has been negative and scary. The popular image of the typical menopausal woman is negative—she is exhausted, haggard, irritable, bitchy, unsexy, impossible to live with, driving her husband to seek other women's company, irrationally depressed, unwillingly suffering a "change" that marks the end of her active (re)productive life. Our idea of menopause has been shaped by ads like the one in a current medical magazine that pictures a harassed middle-aged man standing by a drab and tired-looking woman. The drug advertised is "For the menopausal symptoms that bother him most." Menopause is presented as an affliction to us that makes us an affliction to our friends and families.

In our youth-oriented culture, menopause for many people marks a descent into un-cool middle and old age. In a society that equates our sexuality with our ability to have children, menopause is wrongly thought to mean the end of our sexuality, of our responsiveness to men, of pleasure in bed. In a society that considers babies to be our major contribution, menopause, often coinciding with our children's leaving home, marks the end of our only important job, the end of our reason for existing. Menopause is called "the change" and all the implications are that life goes downhill from there. ("The words 'change of life' must have had a catastrophically destructive effect on countless women," writes one friend. "I'm not willing to suspect it's such a change.")

These views are being changed by women like those who spoke above—who value themselves as more than baby machines, who move into middle age as a welcome time in which they can pursue other kinds of work, who make careful use of the drugs available to minimize menopausal discomforts, who learn about ways that good diet, rest and exercise can help to prevent problems with menopause. Not everyone finds menopause physically easy, but we are learning that if we feel good about ourselves and what we are doing at that time in our lives, we will tend not to be so depressed and bothered during menopause. And if we know what menopause is and what to expect, we will be less mystified and alarmed by our body changes. And for many of us, the freedom to talk openly with our family or friends about what we are experiencing promises to make menopause a less trying, tense and difficult time. It also seems important that our awareness of how men feel about themselves during their forties and fifties will help to prevent possible difficulties in our relationships with the men in our lives. (As they reevaluate their own lives during middle age, many men are faced with the fact that they will not "advance" further in their careers or that their lives will not be as they had hoped, and many fear a loss of virility and the approach of old age.)

Because almost all of us at some point during menopause will go to a doctor about physical symptoms, it will be really important to us to insist on good medical care and advice. Many women up until now have been adversely affected by their doctors' own ignorance and carelessness. One woman told us that she went from doctor to doctor asking why she was so tired all the time—not one of them suggested she was going through menopause. Another woman, feeling tired, went to her doctor and complained that she couldn't do as much as she was accustomed to doing. Her doctor said, "Well, after all, you *are* getting old." Used to bowing to his authority, she accepted his verdict and resigned herself to her loss of energy. Pitifully little research has been done into symptoms and cures for symptoms of a physical experience more universally shared by women even than childbirth.

WHAT IS MENOPAUSE?

In order to understand how menstruation eventually ceases, it is helpful to know what causes it. (See the section on menstruation in the "Anatomy" chapter, and the Appendix to that chapter, for a full description of the hormonal process involved.) The following is a simplified explanation of how the normal hormonal process of menstruation changes as menopause occurs.

As we get older, our ovaries become less and less able to respond to the ovary-stimulating hormones from our pituitary, which formerly caused the regular maturing and releasing of ova. Since progressively fewer ova are being released, the cyclic production of progesterone is interrupted, and this in turn causes estrogen levels to fall below the amount necessary to start endometrial bleeding (menstruation). The pituitary, without the usual cyclic feedback of estrogen and progesterone, generally overreacts, producing excessive amounts of those hormones that stimulate the ovaries. The result is a

hormone imbalance, occurring to different degrees in different women. The most important feature of this hormone imbalance is a decrease in the amount of estrogen to which a woman's system has been accustomed.

This estrogen decrease is thought to be the major factor in many of the problems we might experience during menopause. However, the interrelation of all the hormones, and their relation to our physical and mental health, are extremely complex, and to say that all symptoms of menopause are caused by a lack of sufficient estrogen would be inaccurate. Some doctors have gone so far as to declare menopause "an estrogen-deficiency disease," which they claim can be "cured." Most others are more conservative but agree that many of the symptoms can be alleviated in some women by readjusting the body's estrogen level.

If your estrogen level is low, your whole endocrine system is affected. Depending on your individual hormonal and glandular make-up you might have symptoms that may be alleviated by estrogen-replacement therapy. However, if for any reason your doctor feels it would be better to keep your estrogen level low (for example, to permit the shrinkage of any possible tumors stimulated by estrogen), you may feel that taking estrogen is a bad idea. In any event, there is some estrogen secreted by some other glands—the adrenals, for example—and a woman's body may produce enough estrogen from sources other than the ovaries so that she will not experience low-estrogen symptoms, even though her estrogen production is lower than her original level.

An average natural menopause occurs around age forty-seven, although natural menopause may start as early as thirty-five or as late as sixty. The following factors can cause early onset of menopause: removal of ovaries, or infection destroying them or interfering with their blood supply; excessive exposure to radiation; very poor health; prolonged nursing of a baby; disorders of the endocrine glands; hypothyroidism, with serious obesity; having babies too close together; frequent abortions or miscarriages; very cold climates; hard manual labor or excessive output of energy. The claim that the earlier menstruation starts the later it will stop is apparently not substantiated by fact. Women who have late menopause are generally very healthy, although perfectly healthy women can experience menopause any time between thirty-five and sixty.

Ovarian function starts to taper off at age twenty-seven or thirty, but you probably won't notice anything happening until you are in your forties, at which time menstrual bleeding may become shorter and then longer; then this stage may be followed by irregular skipping or lengthening of periods. In a few cases menstruation occurs regularly until one month when it just stops forever. Most women, however, will taper off in both amount and duration of flow, and will experience irregular and progressively more widely spaced periods for a time of two to three years. Some excessive bleeding is quite common during this time and need not be a cause for worry. However, if you have extremely profuse or prolonged bleeding, or if you bleed between the dates when you think your periods should be coming, you should see a doctor, because you may have a benign or malignant growth. Your breasts may increase in size or become tender, and at this time cystic mastitis (nonmalignant breast growths) or similar conditions may develop or become more serious. It is a good idea to keep a record of exactly what happens after you first notice irregularity in your menses; the information can be useful in determining treatment, if you should need it.

The removal of ovaries by themselves or in combination with other parts of the reproductive system, as in a hysterectomy, will cause early menopause. When ovaries are removed, your body must adjust to a lower level of estrogen, and this brings on all the low-estrogen symptoms associated with menopause. If you have any choice in the matter, hang onto your ovaries as long as you can—don't let anyone remove them as part and parcel of a hysterectomy unless s/he has proved to you that it is absolutely necessary for your health. One ovary is better than none. Ovaries continue to secrete small amounts of estrogen after menopause, and this is useful for strong bones and other parts of your body, as we will discuss later.

* * *

I had one ovary and tube removed about three years ago when I was twenty-eight. Since then I have had hot flushes and backaches, and I wondered if I was going through menopause. But my period still comes regularly, and the hot flushes don't come so often now.

* * *

Sometimes a complete removal of the uterus, tubes, and ovaries, often called a complete hysterectomy, is unavoidable.

* * *

One of my friends recently had a complete hysterectomy, and after a week began to have the hot flushes associated with the drop in estrogen. Her doctor prescribed Premarin, a form of estrogen, and she is now functioning well, working, feeling better than before.

* * *

WHAT ARE THE SYMPTOMS?

The symptoms that occur because of the new balance of hormones are chiefly the result of your body's reaction to a drop in estrogen after it has been used to lots of it. Some symptoms usually associated with menopause may occur very early.

The most commonly reported symptom is the hot flush, or the hot flash, with sweating. This is called a vasomotor disturbance, and although the hormonal process causing it is not totally understood, hot flushes are often relieved by estrogen therapy. A typical hot flush is usually a sudden wave of heat from the waist up; you may get red and perspire a lot; then when the flush goes away, you feel very cold and chilled and sometimes shiver. It lasts from a few seconds to a half hour and may occur several or many times a day. When hot flushes occur at night, they can cause insomnia, and sometimes perspiration may be heavy enough to require a change of bedclothes.

* * *

Suddenly, without warning my temperature seemed to skyrocket about a hundred degrees. It wasn't the sensation of standing in front of an open oven, as some have described it, but the breathless feeling of having stayed too long in a hot shower or a steam bath. I was hot, I was wet, and I was breathless. Charging across the room I slammed up the window and began to gulp down the cool, comforting fresh air.

The book said "hot flashes" were named by woman. Right on. They had to be, the name is so accurate. How to describe them—like a wash of wet heat; unexpected, unwanted and uncontrollable.

* * *

Lack of estrogen allows the usually acidic vaginal secretions to become less acidic, thus increasing the likelihood of vaginal infection. Some women have a heavy discharge as a result. Without as much estrogen, the skin and mucous membranes atrophy somewhat, particularly those of the genitourinary tissues. The vagina starts to become narrow, shorter, and less elastic, and the surface of the vagina is easily eroded and may bleed and become ulcerated. This condition can make intercourse painful and may be responsible for so-called emotional problems such as "frigidity" or irritability during and after menopause. Lack of skin and muscle tone often leads to frequency of urination, pain on voiding, and incontinence. After menopause there is often a loss of fat and shrinkage of tissues; breasts usually shrink and droop.

Estrogen, besides being necessary for your general skin tone, is apparently needed for bone tone. Osteoporosis (porous and brittle bones) is related to the long-term metabolic effects of declining estrogen, and estrogen therapy has been shown to arrest mineral loss from osteoporotic bones. Low backache in menopausal women may be the beginning of osteoporosis; as postmenopause advances, women often lose height and develop "dowager's hump" as their spines compress.

The lower estrogen level of postmenopause is now thought also to be related to an increase in coronary heart disease (atherosclerosis) and cancers in postmenopausal women. Some doctors feel that after their estrogen level drops, women become as vulnerable as men to heart disease and more vulnerable to cancer.

A whole range of other physical complaints—common

ones are insomnia, headache, fast-beating heart and palpitations, vertigo, vague abdominal pains, constipation or diarrhea, nausea and vomiting, gas, tiredness, loss of appetite or weight gain, and back or other muscle aches—are not always so clearly related to the lower estrogen level. We feel that these very common symptoms, so often dismissed by doctors as psychosomatic, deserve thorough medical research to find causes and cures. If every male doctor went through menopause, no doubt this research would already be well on its way.

Emotional symptoms of menopause include irritability, nervousness, depression, frigidity, lack of memory, difficulty in concentrating, and temporary distortions in close personal relationships. These emotional symptoms can be caused or aggravated by a feeling of ill health due to some of the physical symptoms of menopause. We feel that they can often be minimized when a woman feels generally happy about herself and involved in what she is doing.

WHAT YOU CAN DO ABOUT IT

Since so many of the physical discomforts of menopause are caused by insufficient estrogen, estrogen-replacement hormone therapy is a solution that many women can turn to, being careful to consult a knowledgeable doctor about its possible side effects and dangers. Before talking about hormone therapy, however, we want to emphasize that there are other important ways of dealing with and preventing some of menopause's discomforts. Good diet, exercise, enough rest, where these are possible, can give our bodies enough physical vigor and good health to minimize menopause's physical effects, just as work that is meaningful to us either in or outside our home can help tremendously to minimize the emotional effects often associated with menopause.

If you are having uncomfortable physical symptoms you might want to discuss estrogen therapy with your doctor. Estrogen may relieve low-estrogen symptoms like hot flushes, sweating, cold hands and feet, osteoporosis, and discharges from the vagina. Sometimes relieving low-estrogen symptoms brings general relief from irritability or depression. Estrogen is commonly given in the natural form, Premarin, or in synthetic forms, Stilbestrol, Progynon, and Meprane. Stilbestrol, however, has been mentioned as a carcinogen (cancer-causing agent) in some research. A natural form is usually well tolerated; side effects from the synthetics include nausea, allergies and pain in the breasts, but they are more powerful and cheaper and you and your doctor may feel they're worth trying. The Maturation Index test is done to determine how much estrogen you should take; it simply involves examining a sample of your vaginal secretions or cells. Estrogen is not generally prescribed for women with severe kidney or liver disease, some heart problems, or a history of breast or uterine cancer. (*It is important to take estrogen or any prescription drug only under the guidance of a doctor.*)

* * *

Aunt Sarah has not had any estrogen prescribed because she has fibroid tumors in her uterus that should shrink when the estrogen level goes down. She still is having some very heavy menstrual flows, but it usually is on the alternate months. She gets what she calls "fluid headaches," which seem to be period-related—not every month, they vary somewhat. Her doctor was not at all concerned about the tumors, and did not recommend surgery at all.

* * *

The majority of those receiving estrogen at menopause are being given it in cycles: they take a pill daily for three weeks, then stop for a week. This is very similar to many birth-control pill regimes, and similar to the timing of the estrogen a woman's own body produced.

* * *

Here I am, one of the lucky females, taking Premarin since August, a little yellow pill every day for three weeks, then none for a week. I guess this is the answer for me. The gynecologist did not routinely prescribe it until I complained about the depression, the spilling over with tears at very slight provocation, and then I realized that intercourse was really painful. This must have justified his decision, along with the Maturation Index from the Pap smear, to prescribe the hormone.

* * *

Bleeding is a common effect of estrogen, especially on the week you don't take it. For this reason some regimes include progesterone, which brings the total hormone situation closer to the premenopause state in that it promotes a predictable endometrial bleeding—an induced period in effect. You have a menstrual-type flow and feel very much as though you had a regular period but the flow is not as heavy nor for as many days. This "medical curettage" avoids protracted bleeding, which can occur when estrogen only is taken. Relief of menopause symptoms, however, can usually be obtained with estrogen doses small enough so that no bleeding occurs. Mid-cycle bleeding on an estrogen-induced cycle should be checked immediately by a doctor. In fact, any bleeding at all that occurs in a postmenopausal woman, whether or not she is taking estrogen, should be carefully investigated by a doctor; it may be a first sign of endometrial or cervical cancer. In about one-third of the cases reaching surgery the bleeding proves to be of malignant origin.

Possible side effects from too much estrogen are gastrointestinal disturbances, fluid retention and weight gain, breast and pelvic pains due to swollen tissues, headache, high blood pressure, vaginal discharge, and skin pigmentation. As with birth-control pills—most of which also contain estrogen—sensitivities vary enormously. It looks as though you're damned if you do, damned if you don't take estrogen—the trick is to find the right amount, if any, for you, to get regular check-ups twice a year if you are taking estrogen, and to find a doctor who is aware of both the positive uses and the potential risks of estrogen, who will be very careful about what s/he prescribes.

What can you do about weight gain? Eat less, especially refined carbohydrates, and exercise more. Estrogen relief of some of your other physical symptoms may improve your general feeling of health enough so that this will be easier for you. If the extra weight bothers you, it is probably worth losing; thinner people live longer, according to insurance statistics—and they've got money on it. Excessive weight can also make activity difficult. A good diet and sensible exercise have done a lot to help many women feel better through menopause. (See the chapters on diet and exercise, "Nutrition" and "Women in Motion.") Not nearly enough research has been done on diet and menopause. One woman wrote to us:

* * *

Perhaps I have been fortunate in the matter of diet, which may eventually be found to be important. I had been drinking a concoction of brewer's yeast and wheat germ known as "tiger's milk" for about five years before the onset of menopause. I am sorry that I was not also taking three grams of Vitamin C daily and some Vitamin E at that time, for I might have been spared the recurring bouts of cystitis. The cystitis has disappeared since I have taken Vitamin C, but this may of course be unrelated.

* * *

Another woman, a vegetarian who practices yoga, writes:

* * *

To you younger sisters, vegetables and headstands may not seem to be the pot of gold at the end of the rainbow, but if you haven't tried it, don't knock it!*

DEPRESSION AND MENOPAUSE†

About one in ten women experience severe depression during menopause. Though physical changes do play a part in these depressions, Pauline Bart feels that we often become depressed simply because we are middle-aged. We have no clear or important role to play in our society.‡ Very little if anything is expected of us. We have no status. But at the same time, our life span has lengthened, we have twenty or thirty good years ahead of us. If we have had children, we end our childbearing years

* Irene Davall, National Coordinator of the Feminist Party.

†For some of the ideas in this section we are especially grateful to Marliese Wior, who let us use her unpublished paper, "The Menopausal Woman" (see "Further Readings").

‡Bart, Pauline Bernice, Ph.D., *UCLA Dissertations: Depression in Middle-aged Woman: Some Sociocultural Factors.* December 1967.

sooner than we did in the past, and we are left with a lot of time on our hands and space in our lives. For there are no clear societal norms which give us a useful place in our children's lives. Often we are in their way after they leave home. If we have overprotected them or expected them to live out and fulfil our own lives for us, we are both angered by their leave-taking and saddened by our loss. Often, not understanding that we feel anger, unable to direct it toward our children or unable to express it in any way, we turn it inward onto ourselves and become severely and heavily depressed.

We are faced with other real losses. Some of us feel deeply saddened by the end of our ability to bear children. We are losing our youth. And if in general we feel unfulfilled personally, we may be bitter about not having achieved happiness yet.

If we are already working during menopause and middle age, we are less likely to suffer certain forms of depression, though heavy work can take its physical toll on us.

There are many legitimate reasons for our depression. We have to recognize that its causes are not so much personal as social; that is, our society does not recognize us as necessary or valuable members. More research needs to be done on both the physical and social causes of our depression. And we must try to provide discussion and work groups for ourselves and others to understand better our own feelings and capabilities, to share them, and to move out of depression into new and worthwhile lives.

The following is an excerpt from a letter by a woman in her fifties, previously depressed and now taking estrogen and feeling much better.

* * *

Menopause itself is no longer a period to fear and wonder about. It is simply a time when menstruation stops and you can no longer become pregnant. As far as I could tell, from interviewing all the women around, this was a redeeming feature for all but one person, who had had a hysterectomy at thirty-three. Of course, it coincides with the aging process, and as much as we look forward

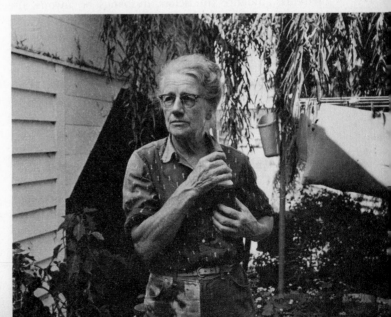

to growing older, it is quite an adjustment to accept yourself with the wrinkles, the sagging, and the aches and pains that may follow. In my case, however, I really feel better. My back doesn't hurt any more, I have more energy than before, I no longer have the premenstrual tension to as great a degree. I still am getting headaches periodically that feel as if my skull is too small for the amount of pressure inside.

I have come to terms with me, though, and that's the most important adjustment. I like what I'm doing. I feel worthwhile; my marriage is better than during the period when my children were all at home. I am looking forward to perfecting some more skills, reading so many books I've never had time for, and sharing thoughts and feelings with more people.

I was always very shy in my younger days, and somehow was afraid to expose myself. It was very hard to trust a relationship. Now, after all these years, I realize that I'm just another human being, a woman with many of the same feelings that my friends have. Building a wall around me was keeping me isolated and terribly lonely. There is a solution to every problem if you stay with it and prepare to make any changes in the present that will improve the situation in the future.

* * *

It makes sense for each of us to try to prevent emotional problems at menopause by doing what we can to keep not only our bodies but our minds healthy. Our psychological state, how we cope with stress and maintain our security, is going to affect how we feel physically all the rest of our lives. Remember, the stress of menopause can often magnify already existing mental problems.

We must make sure that society does not make our later lives miserable by denying us rewarding roles in addition to motherhood. For many of us, dilettante interests are not enough to prevent the feeling of worthlessness that many older women experience. Many of us need to be employed and to be paid fairly by society for work that it values. We must at no time in our lives allow parents, guidance counselors, husbands or anyone else to talk us out of starting or continuing to pursue our interests and careers. It is our present and future mental health that is at stake, not theirs! (See the "Childbearing" chapter for some discussion of the problems of combining motherhood with outside work so that we don't reach 45 with one job all over with and no other work begun.)

PREGNANCY AND MENOPAUSE

It is a very rare thing to become pregnant after menstruation has stopped for a year. Some doctors think that the odds are good enough so that you can do without birth control six months after your menses stop. In an extremely small number of cases eggs have been released without any sign of bleeding, and they have been fertilized and been born as healthy children of sixty- or seventy-year-old mothers whose menstruation had stopped decades ago. But more often menstruation can occur around menopause, with no egg being shed—it is called an anovulatory cycle.

For all practical purposes you can assume you are infertile a year after your last period. To be extra safe, some doctors recommend two years. If you are that extremely rare bird who has a fertilized egg after menopause, you should certainly consider an abortion if you don't want a child at that time, because the odds of producing a deformed child or mongoloid child are high. If you become pregnant after the age of forty, the incidence of mongolism is one in seven. However, if you want to have the child, there is a test that can determine whether the child is a mongoloid. The test involves taking some amniotic fluid from the womb by needle (amniocentesis), and you should discuss it with your doctor. For women who have not had earlier pregnancies, a late first pregnancy is likely to be a difficult birth.

SEX AND MENOPAUSE

Many of us have feared that menopause would bring an end to our sex lives. But Masters and Johnson tell us, "There is no time limit drawn by the advancing years to female sexuality."[*] And an older friend says, "I was curious to see if my sexual life would be the same after menopause and am delighted to find that it is." Many women report that they enjoy sex even more after menopause because they no longer have to worry about getting pregnant.

There *can* be problems with sex for us as we grow older:

Our sex organs gradually atrophy (deteriorate) with the lowering of estrogen, and vaginal lubrication can become scarce, so intercourse can become painful in menopause or post menopause. A lubricant like saliva or K-Y Jelly may help, and estrogen therapy might correct it.

Other non–sexually related symptoms of menopause—tiredness, emotional irritability, nervousness, hot flashes, headaches, and so on—can do a lot to lessen our sexual drive and pleasure. Once we are past these symptoms, through time or hormone therapy, our sexual life can be as good as ever.

Sometimes in going through menopause we may feel that we have "lost our womanhood." It is true that we can no longer offer our partner the chance to produce a child, but the odds are good that our partner wouldn't want one anyway.

Many of us as we get older get fewer chances for heterosexual sex. Middle-aged men often go through a change of life in which they are impotent for anywhere

[*]William H. Masters, M.D., and Virginia E. Johnson, *Human Sexual Response* (Boston: Little, Brown & Co., 1966), pp. 223–38.

from two months to a couple of years. Divorce, death, and a cultural norm which pushes men to seek younger sex partners, leave many middle-aged women without partners, and in the past it seems that many of them resigned themselves to a life without sex. But an increasing number of women are breaking the silly convention that women should pair up only with men older than they are. We are enjoying male company without insisting on marriage, so that the male-female numbers ratio is not so important. And there are many good kinds of sexual expression that don't involve men: we can enjoy fantasies, masturbation or sex with women.

Here is one woman's experience with sex in middle age:

* * *

Sex was great—probably—until I had a hysterectomy for fibroid tumors five years ago. After the surgery I was sore and rather dead for a long time. Foreplay was less good because there was a broken link—no visceral response when he played with my breasts, and this had been very nice to feel before.

Sex became less joyful. Coincidentally, my husband became ill and was prescribed a tranquilizer which overdosed him to near impotence. My frustration was total, and for the first time in my life, at forty, I masturbated to orgasm. Out loud, in wonder, I said, "So that's what it is!"

I spent about three and a half years trying to reconcile the two very different experiences, very different pleasures, of intense masturbatory orgasm and intense shared love-making with little increments of sensation which make me rest and relax before returning for more sharing. By now I just figure I have two great goods for my pleasure. My husband doesn't thrive on thinking about the vibrator, and I don't have as good an orgasm with it if he's there, so it's a private pleasure. I recommend it to everyone (not person-to-person or door-to-door, but here, anonymously).

* * *

The writer Simone de Beauvoir talks about sex and older people. She points out that for some the joy of sex lies in their own physical beauty, and as this fades from youthful prime, they derive less and less joy from sex. They may even be unwilling to participate at all. However, she says, those for whom sex is a joyous, friendly act will frequently continue to enjoy it into the seventies and later.

FURTHER READINGS

A Clinical Guide to the Menopause and the Post Menopause. New York: Agenst Laboratories Information Publishing Company, 1968.
   A very clear book.

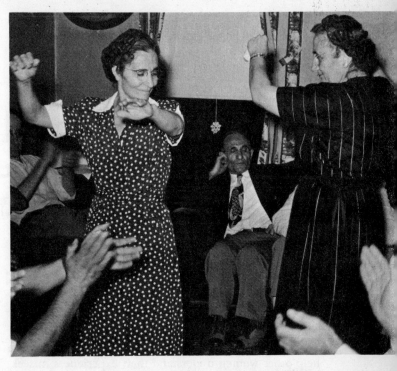

Dodge, Eva F., M.D. *The Doctor Talks About Menopause.* American Medical Women's Association, New York, 1968.
Gilbert, C. R. A., M.D. *Better Health for Women.* New York: Doubleday & Co., Inc., 1957.
Gray, Madeline, *The Changing Years: The Menopause Without Fear.* New York: Doubleday & Co., Inc., rev. ed. 1967.
Kelly, G. L., M.D. *A Doctor Discusses Menopause,* Chicago: Budlong Press Co., 1959.
   This is written in a very optimistic style, mostly leveled at women who are married and at home. "There are many things that might interest you for the first time and many activities that might benefit others, charity and civic enterprises, PTA or Girl Scout activities, writing, painting, sewing, entering business, no end of worthwhile and engrossing activities."
"The Menopause and the Role of Estrogens" (transcript of conference in Amsterdam), Excerpta, Medica Foundation, New York, 1967.
Stopes, Marie, M.D. *Change of Life in Men and Women.* New York: G. P. Putnam's Sons, 1936.
   A sensible book though out of date in some areas.
Wilson, Robert A., M.D. *Feminine Forever.* New York: M. Evans & Co., Inc., 1966.
   This is a medically radical view of menopause: "menopause is curable," "menopause is completely preventable," and "Every woman alive today has the option of remaining feminine forever." Later in the book the author tells you what "feminine" is: "I believe that such matters as dress, grooming, manners and style of language are as much related to a woman's femininity as her physical attributes. . . . I am often disturbed at the crassness and blatancy with which women themselves proclaim their sexual liberation. Feminine fashion, for instance, appears to have abandoned the ancient wisdom that concealment is the secret of allure." In spite of all this the man has done a lot of research on estrogen, and his medical opinions are interesting.
Wior, Marliese. "The Menopausal Woman." Unpublished paper written for a biology course at the University of Southern California at Los Angeles, 1971.
   This extensive and careful study of menopause from the perspectives of biology, developmental psychology, social psychology, and social work is an excellent example of the kind of research and analysis that needs to be done in the area of women and menopause.

15
Women and Health Care

SECTION ONE: THE AMERICAN HEALTH-CARE SYSTEM

INTRODUCTION

THIS SECTION represents the efforts of several of us to help other women understand their experiences in seeking and receiving health care. We have focused not only on the general and political context in which the system operates in the United States but specifically on how women may deal personally with doctors and hospitals, and what they can expect from routine examinations and treatment for common illnesses.

Hundreds of books have been written on various aspects of medicine and medical care, although only a few appear in our bibliography. And many books have been written about women and their health problems, but almost all by men. We have tried to give some basic facts, to discuss the issues that affect women, and to meet the need for support that has been expressed by so many women.

We hope that women will come to feel entitled to more information about their medical care, will demand better care for themselves, and will work for better care for all women. This is a beginning in trying to spare other women the confusion and frustration we have known.

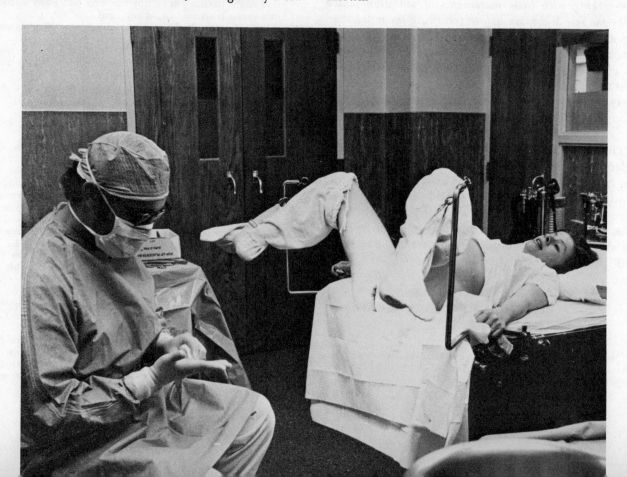

PROBLEMS OF INADEQUATE CARE FOR WOMEN

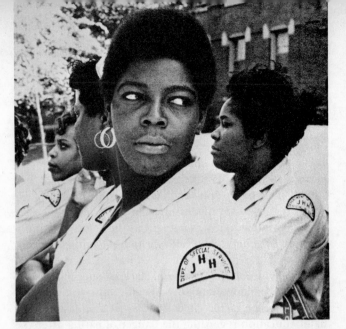

We cannot hope to discuss fully all the failures of the present health system and the reasons for them. The focus on women's relationship to health care, however, is especially appropriate, because we consume the largest proportion of health services, average 25 percent more visits each year to the doctor than men (100 percent more if visits of mothers with children are counted), take 50 percent more prescription drugs than men, and are admitted to hospitals much more frequently than men.[*] Not only are we the largest consumers but we make up 70 percent of all health workers in the United States, 75 percent of all hospital workers, and three-fifths of all the medical workers in the world.[†]

In stark contrast to women's numerical superiority as workers and consumers is the fact that only about 7 percent of the physicians in the United States are women. Only three countries have a lower percentage of female doctors—South Vietnam, Madagascar, and Spain.[‡] Given the extraordinary status, wealth, power, and prestige that physicians have, it is evident that women as workers and patients occupy the wide base of a pyramid, with white male doctors at the narrow top controlling everything and everyone below them for their own interests.

Naturally, some women fare better than others, but all of us suffer as a group from the effects of male-dominated medicine. We have listened to our black, brown, and yellow sisters tell us that for them health care is in addition often pervaded by racism—in the poor quality of care, the unavailability of services, and the alienation of the largely white medical personnel they have to deal with, who have little comprehension of their situation or of the community from which their needs arise.

Critics have lately commented on the frequency with which nonwhite people seem to be chosen as experimental populations. A graphic example of this was a study reported in *Medical World News,* in which seventy-eight multiparous chicano women were given placebos or "dummy" pills in a Texas birth-control pill experiment without their knowledge, with the result that ten of the women became pregnant in the first four months of the experiment.[§]

If you are a woman and also happen to be poor, your health problems are likely to be greater and your access to proper health-care services more difficult than that of the rest of the population.[*] In a sense, poverty, with its attendant problem of malnutrition, is the greatest health problem in the nation. This was illustrated by what happened when Tufts University started its health program in Mississippi. It was discovered that the greatest community health need was for adequate food. The health center pharmacy that had been set up proceeded to stock and distribute food the way drugs are usually supplied. Eventually the project became involved in a farm co-op in order to help solve the food needs. As one doctor pointed out, "The last time we looked in the books, the specific therapy for malnutrition was food."[†]

Even though this country spends billions of dollars a year on health care, we do not compare well with other Western nations in some health statistics. For instance, our maternal mortality rate in 1968 was twelfth in the world, and both Hong Kong and Bulgaria had fewer maternal deaths per 100,000 births than the United States. The cost of inadequate health services can be counted in part in a needless loss of life. A nationally prominent male gynecologist claimed that 50 percent of all maternal deaths associated with childbirth are potentially avoidable, and nearly half the women delivered in city and county hospitals in this country have no prenatal care.[‡] And if we are to believe the predictions of yet another prominent gynecologist, things will be getting worse not better. He predicts that by 1980, "40 percent of babies will be born on wards of municipal and

Health Policy Advisory Center Bulletin (March 1970), p. 1.
†"Woman Power Under-Used Though More Mothers Work," *American Journal of Nursing,* Vol. 71, No. 4 (April 1971), p. 664.
‡*Ibid.*
§Report cited in "Aiding the Poor," *Health Policy Advisory Center Bulletin,* No. 40 (April 1972), p. 11.

*William Richardson, "Poverty, Illness and the Use of Health Services in the U.S.," *Hospitals,* Vol. 43, No. 13 (July 1, 1969), pp. 34-40.
†H. Jack Geiger, "Community Control—or Community Conflict?" *NTDRA Bulletin* (November 1969).
‡Robert J. Wilson, "Health Care for Women: Present Deficiencies and Future Needs," *Obstetrics and Gynecology,* Vol. 36, No. 2 (August 1970), p. 178.

community hospitals in which there are not and will not be enough physicians to deliver the babies or even enough to provide adequate supervision.*

The following information with regard to maternal mortality associated with the administration of general anesthesia may help make clear how the shortages of personnel and skills take their toll in the lives of our sisters. In a study done in North Carolina from 1946–1960 on the causes of deaths from maternal anesthesia during childbirth, it was noted that the errors in administration of general anesthesia (which accounted for 90.6 percent of the deaths over the duration of the study) were attributable in part to a "lack of specialized personnel and inadequate coverage for obstetric anesthesia."† Another factor cited was the lack of careful prenatal education regarding the danger of eating after the onset of labor and preceding general anesthesia. A further cause was that many doctors were not trained well enough in administering anesthesia.

The lack of adequate free birth-control information, and even of education about reproduction, goes side by side with the moralistic and punitive attitude of many gynecologists toward unmarried and even married women who seek birth control. These factors often result in the anguish of unwanted pregnancies and suffering and death through illegal or self-induced abortions, since it is difficult and expensive to obtain legal, safe abortions in most parts of the country. The opposition of segments of the medical establishment to providing low-cost abortion on demand is famous. (The chapters on "Birth Control" and "Abortion" discuss this in some detail.)

Women are also extremely vulnerable to needless hysterectomies. One study of the quality of care in a community hospital found that only 30 percent, or slightly less than one-third, of the hysterectomies done were considered medically justified.‡ Perhaps this kind of operation should be called a "remunerectomy," since the main indicator is the doctor's fee. It has long been the judgment of many people in the nonwhite community that unnecessary hysterectomies, as well as other operations that result in sterility, have been performed on nonwhite women without their consent.§ On the other hand, when a woman wants to be sterilized, it is sometimes difficult to get a physician to perform a tubal ligation if he thinks she doesn't have enough children, or isn't stable, or doesn't have her husband's permission.*

THE ORGANIZATION AND CONTROL OF HEALTH CARE

Some of these problems, and many others, can be traced to the lack of emphasis on preventive medicine and inadequate public health programs. Instead, our present health system relies mainly on geographically centralized, crisis-oriented, expensive hospital-based facilities for dispensing many health services. Thus the present system is disease- rather than health-oriented and doctor- and hospital-dominated. The recent organization of medical power into urban empires based around university teaching hospitals, where the priorities of profit, research, and medical education all come before patient care, is an important development of the last two decades, and is described in the Health Pac book, *The American Health Empire.*

THE CAPITALIST THEORY OF DISEASE CAUSATION

The basic idea of health care with which the public at large and women in particular have been indoctrinated by the medical profession, and the media cluster around it, is what we will call the "capitalist theory of disease." This model of illness centers around the private relationship between an individual and her physician. The economic basis immediately underlying this model is the fee-for-service system.

The emphasis is on treatment of the symptom, isolated both from the rest of the mind and body and from the social context of the illness. The glamorous image of the doctor in the laboratory making discoveries, or the heroic male surgeon doing technical and difficult operations surrounded by elaborate machines, is a common one. The ideas behind it are that most diseases are exclusively caused by germs, viruses, and bacteria—specific identifiable agents—and that the main problem of health care is to combat the enemy microbe with chemicals, or repair the damage done to parts of the body, which is conceived of as a machine. In a book published by the American Medical Association in 1961, *The Wonderful Human Machine,* this analogy is carried to absurdity with the chapters on nerves, "Nature's Radar and Computer Networks," on the heart, "The Perpetual Motion Pump," and on the digestive system, "Fuel Refinery for a Chemi-

---

*Louis Hellman, quoted in Donna M. Ledney, "Nurse Midwives: Can They Fill the OB Gap?" *RN,* Vol. 33, No. 1 (January 1970), p. 38.

†Stephen Anderson, Frank C. Greiss, *et al.,* "Maternal Deaths from Anesthesia in North Carolina, 1946-1960," *North Carolina Medical Journal,* Vol. 29, No. 1 (November 1968), p. 459.

‡Paul Lembke, "Medical Auditing," *Journal of the American Medical Association,* (October 13, 1956), p. 653.

§See also *Boston Globe* (April 29, 1972), p. 10. "Students Charge BCH's Obstetrics Unit with Excessive Surgery," by Carl M. Cobb.

*P. C. Steptoe, "Female Sterilization," *Nursing Times,* December 9, 1971, pp. 1529-30.

cal Engine." It is also interesting to speculate on the effect on doctors of their first contact with the human body in medical school—a corpse, the ultimate, passive object.

We feel that a very different model of disease causation should be developed. On one hand, we must realize the social context of illness and admit that certain diseases seem to be occupational hazards arising from conditions that impair the health of large numbers of workers, and that the responsibility for these conditions rests with those corporations and industries whose manufacturing processes or products are at fault. Some of the disease-causing substances used in industry are cancer-causing, or carcinogenic. It is interesting to note that insurance figures show that "death from cancer is 39 percent greater among 'industrial' policy holders [chiefly lower paid wage earners] than for holders of standard policies [chiefly middle-class salary earners]."*

Another social cause of disease is the enormous impact of automobile accidents on the nation's health. No matter how much the emergency room facilities of the nation are improved to cope with the results of accidents, this health problem ultimately has to be controlled by policies that strive for safer automobiles, reduction in the rate of alcoholism, and more mass transportation.

The need to control the activities and change the profit-above-all policies of some American corporations in the interest of public health is illustrated again by iatrogenic diseases—those caused by the practice of medicine. The American drug industry has marketed worthless and dangerous drugs that have caused many serious side effects.† Critics have pointed out that there are so many different kinds of drugs on the market under so many different names that it is next to impossible for doctors to be knowledgeable enough about them all to prescribe them with safety. In that sense the marketing practices of drug companies are in themselves a health hazard.

We would like to look more thoroughly at one example of the cost of inadequate preventive health care for women: 12,000 annual deaths of women as a result of undetected cervical cancer. The treatment and cure of cervical cancer in its early stages has been known for roughly fifteen years. The Pap smear test involves a relatively simple procedure: the doctor or other health worker takes a sample of cells from the cervix, and a cytologist looks at them under the microscope to see if there are any abnormal changes in the cells. These small changes in cells usually show up well before an actual danger develops. Yet only a small percentage, estimated

to be 20 percent,* of American women have one each year.

There is also a test you can give yourself, which was tried out in Rhode Island by health aides going from door to door. This test is called a Davis Pipet and is self-administered according to simple directions. Some medical sources consider it almost as good at detecting precancer signs as the Pap smear. If abnormal cells showed up from the tests in this investigation, the women received further tests. The test apparatus, which was invented by an American and costs 25 cents, was unavailable in the United States in 1967 and had to be imported from Denmark. While conducting this study the researchers met with good acceptance, but remarked that 53 percent of the women approached had never had a Pap smear previously.†

Even though these simple diagnostic procedures are known, thousands of women have this kind of cancer, which goes unnoticed until it has spread to other parts of the body, when it is much less treatable and in many cases is fatal. There are many contributing factors to this situation, and we can only point out some of them.

THE POWER AND ROLE OF MALE DOCTORS

Since the Depression, when the incomes of many doctors decreased, the medical profession has practiced what Rick Kunes has called "professional birth control." The result is that we have fewer doctors per person than we had fifty years ago. This alone might not be such a disaster if doctors were willing as a profession to share their skills widely and train paramedical personnel or give more responsibility to nurses for routine procedures. The facts seem to be to the contrary. One doctor in a community south of Boston, told a friend of mine he objected even to public-health nurses giving free Pap smears. Instead of sharing their skills, the medical profession has kept its knowledge restricted, and only very recently has it permitted other health workers to assume roles that alleviate the crisis of the doctor shortage.

Another result of this imperialism of knowledge is that many women have not learned enough about their health needs to demand Pap smears as a public service. This kind of ignorance about our bodies, and particularly those parts related to reproduction and sexuality, is connected with the alienation and shame and fear that have been imposed on us as women. Some people feel that this is an internalization of male values, of the male

*John A. H. Lee, "Prevention of Cancer," *Postgraduate Medicine*, Vol. 51, No. 1 (January 1972), p. 86.
†Morton Mintz, *By Prescription Only*.

*Richard W. Telinde and Richard F. Mattingly, *Operative Gynecology*, 4th ed. (Philadelphia: Lippincott, 1970), p. 704.
†Jean Maynard, John Tierney, *et al.*, "Cervical Screening with the Davis-Pipet on a Door to Door Basis," *Public Health Reports*, Vol. 84, No. 6 (June 1969), p. 556.

fear and envy of the generative and sexual powers of women.

There are economic reasons why many of us don't have Pap smears regularly. We may not have the twenty-five dollars or more for an annual checkup with a gynecologist. The usual alternative is the humiliating and time-consuming ritual of the public hospital clinic, where you see a new doctor each time you go. The attitudes of many gynecologists—their condescension, their technical manner, their assumption of women's ignorance, and their stereotyped view of us—do not usually make going to see them a pleasant experience, and so we put it off or avoid it. A related cause is the insidious myth that women's "complaints" are psychosomatic and neurotic in origin, combined with the doctors' myth of their own importance. After all, we wouldn't want to bother such a busy and important man with a silly problem; so we don't go to see him. For all these reasons and many more, thousands of women die needlessly because cervical cancer has not been detected early enough.

The American doctor has claimed for himself unusually broad powers. It is he who decides which patients are treated and where, the cost of treatment, who goes to the hospital, which treatment is given and for how long, and which drugs are administered and in what quantities. In fact, all health care has become equated in the public mind with the practice of medicine by physicians. This has enormous implications. One result has been that the roles of other health workers—nurses, for example—have been unnecessarily limited by licensing and tradition.* Through its organizational representatives, chiefly the AMA, the medical profession has jealously

*For a provocative historical study of the rise of male medical professionals, the suppression and decline of women healers, and the resulting decline in the quantity and quality of health care, see Barbara Ehrenreich and Deirdre English, *Witches, Midwives, and Nurses—A History of Women Healers.*

guarded the prerogative of being the exclusive access route for health care by the threat of legal punishment of paramedical people and nurses who practice medicine.

One of the sacred privileges of being a doctor seems to be the right to make a lot of money.

> The physician is the gatekeeper of the health-care system. . . . not only does he control the entry into the health-care system, he provides the only pathway through the system. Other health professionals who might offer great relief or meaningful benefits to the patient may never see him because, from the doctor's perspective, he is not sick or his health needs are not the kind the doctor recognizes or understands. No matter how many other professionals are available, patients must wait until the doctor screens, refers, or "writes orders."*

WOMEN AS WORKERS IN THE HEALTH SYSTEM

Restricting the roles of women in health care to the most menial and lowest-paying status seems to be further evidence of the dominance of male doctors. The financial rewards of being a doctor are on a high level, while the salaries of other health workers, nurses, and hospital workers in general—predominantly female—have been notoriously low. One nurse told me that, having had several years of experience as an R.N., she went back to school, and after receiving her college degree her salary was increased by about four dollars a week.

The fact that nursing has been an overwhelmingly female profession, with little autonomy and molded to serving the needs of the mostly male medical profession, has probably frustrated many talented nurses and deprived the people at large of the benefits of skilled independent nursing care.

*Catherine M. Norris, "Direct Access to the Patient," *American Journal of Nursing*, Vol. 70, No. 5 (May 1970), pp. 1006-1007.

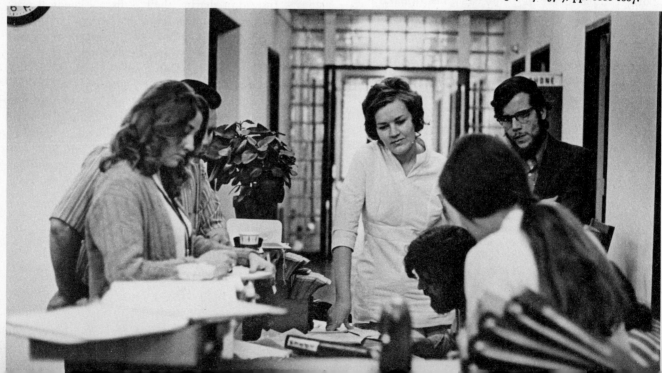

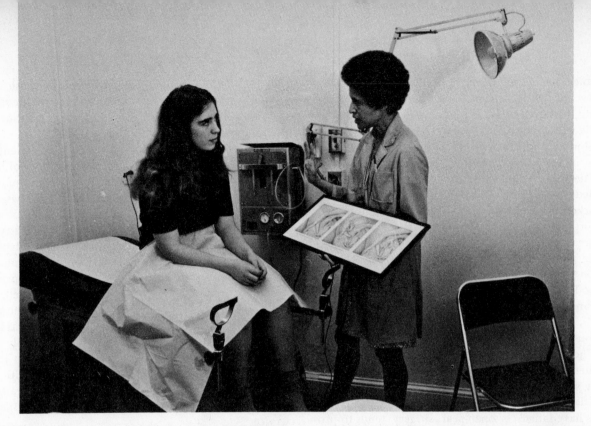

Recently feminist voices are being heard in the nursing profession, challenging the traditional subordination of women in our system of male medicine. In the *American Journal of Medicine* Virginia Cleland stated:

There is no doubt in my mind that our most fundamental problem in nursing is that we are members of a women's occupation in a male-dominated culture.

She goes on to point out the lack of overall administrative power that plagues nursing.

I am appalled every time I recognize that the vast majority of directors of nursing do not control their departmental budget even though the nursing department frequently spends 80 to 85% of the total personnel budget of the institution. I cannot imagine a man accepting a similar title with such absence of corresponding authority.*

Nursing is a profession in which the sex role is confused with the occupational role in a particularly profound way. The general image of the nurse involves so many of the traditional female virtues. Dr. Cleland points out further evidence of sex-role confusion in the advertisements that hospitals use to recruit nursing personnel. After looking at ads obviously designed to make getting a man the most attractive aspect of working at certain hospitals, Dr. Cleland says, "I can only conclude that they would rather entice nurses by cheap sexual inducement than pay an honest salary. Could this common practice be called 'procuring'?"†

*Virginia Cleland, "Sex Discrimination: Nursing's Most Pervasive Problem," *American Journal of Nursing*, Vol. 71, No. 8 (August 1970), pp. 1542, 1545.
†*Ibid.*, p. 1545.

Women have usually been excluded from the elite institution of medical school on the grounds that they are not strong enough to survive the rigors of training, or that they will drop out of the profession to marry and have families. Many women never even consider going to medical school because of the generally prevalent idea that they are not good at science and couldn't compete intellectually with men in male professions. So they are channeled into nursing or other fields by counselors.

Once inside the sacred circle, women are encouraged to specialize in areas in which they are thought to have, as one doctor said recently, "intuitive understanding."* Thirty-three point six percent of the female graduates of medical school from 1931 to 1956 who passed specialty board requirements were in pediatrics.† Once again we are presented with our biological and predetermined nature. After all, women care for children, so pediatrics is a good place for them. Surgery, which occupies the opposite level of the medical status ladder from pediatrics or obstetrics and gynecology, has very few women in it.

THE PROFIT MOTIVE IN HEALTH CARE

Over the last two decades, and especially since government funding of Medicare and Medicaid, the health business has become a huge growth industry involving drugs, hospital supplies, and construction and insurance

*"Women MD's: An Extraordinary Accomplishment," *MGH News* (Bulletin of Massachusetts General Hospital), Vol. 31, No. 3 (March 1972), p. 7.
†*Ibid.*

companies. In the decade of the sixties the total dollars spent for all health care in the United States doubled, reaching the figure of $62 billion in 1969. It is expected that this will climb to $94 billion by 1975, and that the health industry will then be the nation's largest in dollar volume and number of people employed.

It is not simply that there are profits of millions each year made out of our illnesses* but that the impact of the marketing, advertising, and product development of large corporations on our health-care system as it is presently organized tends to get in the way of effective general and preventive health care for those of us who depend on the system for our survival.

A good way to become aware of the influence of marketing and advertising in medicine is to scan the medical journals, in which the results of the most recent research in various fields are made available to the medical profession. The aggressive marketing of expensive electronic instruments and complex equipment for use in crisis care in such unusual and sophisticated treatments as kidney dialysis (a process of cleaning the blood when the kidneys have failed), or open-heart surgery, tends to produce a wasteful duplication of facilities, many of which are underused. The market dynamic is to sell as many machines as possible, not to encourage the careful centralization of complex equipment for maximum use. Pouring money into therapeutic medical instruments related to the care of uncommon conditions diverts funds

*Harold B. Myers, "The Medical Industrial Complex," *Fortune* (January 1970), pp. 90–95.

and attention from much more common but basic needs for preventive care. Some of the machines are life-saving, but many lives are lost because resources are sacrificed to the interests of the marketplace.

The medical-supply industry, geared to in-patient care in hospitals, benefits from an increased number of hospital stays. And although it would be more reasonable to deliver some health services on an out-patient basis, the influence of this industry causes too many people to be treated as in-patients. The construction industry has benefited from building many modern hospital plants, which in some cases have resulted in an edifice complex, producing as a by-product increasing transportation problems for women with children and the aged, who have to travel long distances to get to a large hospital. Accessibility to service is an important concept that is not necessarily served by making the hospital the only place to go for care. Another reason many people go to the hospital when their problems could be dealt with in a well-equipped out-patient clinic is that their health insurance is hospital-oriented and won't pay for out-patient services.

Perhaps we have to rethink the idea that health is a commodity to be bought like any other item in the marketplace. We feel it is time to assert that the health of all the people in the broadest sense is a basic right and a highest social priority and that we should work to eliminate the profit motive from the health-care system and develop a planned, decentralized system that is responsible to the community and funded by public money.

SECTION TWO: CHOOSING AND USING MEDICAL CARE

INTRODUCTION

Are there any good doctors? There is a tremendous bitterness about doctors and medical care in our group, which in many ways parallels a more widespread bitterness at many levels in our society.

To explain why things are so bad and how they might be changed is partly the purpose of the preceding section, "The American Health-Care System." While the legislative process will clearly be bringing some changes in the delivery of basic health care within the next few years, from the patient's viewpoint, and especially the woman's, the problems of attitude, communication, information and continuity when dealing with physicians will probably remain for a long time to come. For women who need medical care and doctor care today, who can't wait

for the revolution to get here, we've tried to bring together some thoughts and experiences that may be helpful.

The idea of "choosing" medical care is in itself a myth. For a number of important reasons most of us do not have unlimited choices, and many of us have no choice at all. First, we are limited by our economic status. If we are at the bottom of the ladder, or on welfare, there are only certain clinics and certain doctors that will accept the Medicaid or Medicare fees as adequate reimbursement. If you are not on welfare you may still be able to afford only clinic care. If you have some form of health insurance you will probably discover that it will pay only a portion of any hospitalization costs associated with clinic care and still may not include the cost of the out-patient care itself. If you are a private patient seeking private care, these same insurance terms may apply. In fact, there are hardly any health-insurance programs in existence that will pay for office visits to a doctor. Only if you are a private patient with a health-insurance policy and a considerable amount of additional money to spare are you in the "right" income bracket to get good care. But even this is not a guarantee.

Second, apart from the fact that there is a doctor shortage, there is a severe maldistribution of doctors and hospitals, so your choice of both is determined by where you live. It limits both the number of doctors and hospitals that you may choose, and it also defines their quality. If you live in the deep country, only one doctor may be available, with a hospital even farther away. If you live in the big cities, on the other hand, the number of hospitals and doctors is so great that it may be a matter of pure chance that you get satisfactory care.

Third, you are limited by your education and social class, which also determine how well informed you are about the health-care nonsystem—the training and qualifications of doctors and nurses, the drugs and procedures they use, the settings in which this care is given, and the state of the art and science in general. There is no other area of American life in which so little consumer information is available in proportion to the amount spent for services. Discrimination according to social class is also more widespread than in other areas of consumer spending.

Fourth, you are limited by your own personal values and value system. If you insist on having only doctors and hospitals associated with academic medicine, or if you refuse to go to a large, busy hospital, then these kinds of convictions will in themselves affect the quality and often the attitude with which you are treated. The fact that some doctors have large, busy practices may convince you that they are superior, and if some doctors charge less and seem to have more time for you, you may feel you are getting a bargain. Many people, including the doctors themselves, can be influenced by the fact that a certain doctor or hospital cares for prominent local or national citizens. All of these ideas are all true and all false, for different reasons at different times. Some of the least able doctors have the highest incomes.*

Fifth, you are limited by time. Because there is no plan of preventive care, most of our contacts with the nonsystem are emergency contacts, made when a problem or even a crisis is already apparent. This is the most difficult time to try to negotiate, to argue, to ask questions and demand answers. Paradoxically, however, it is when you are sickest that you may get the very best possible care and service from people in the medical world. You can almost get real love from them if you are sick enough. But if you are basically healthy and need their services to maintain your health or simply prevent dis-

ease, the treatment can be very different. Somehow, your wanting information and answers to questions and your wanting to feel a sense of cooperation in developing a philosophy of preventive care for yourself can inspire outright hostility. Medical people, especially in hospitals, are simply not trained to deal with normal people who have a sense of entitlement and have expectations of give-and-take about their care. Often they label healthy curiosity or determination "uptight" or "making waves." If we want to have what seems to us a normal and reasonable amount of control, we are categorized as aggressive or difficult patients, and of course we are wasting their time. While there has always been great emphasis on getting medical information from only the most authoritative sources, very sharp limits have been set on both the length of time we spend with the doctor and what we have a right to know, so time becomes one of the limiting factors in our ability to negotiate the system. Also, most of us don't have time to "shop" for care.

Finally, even if you are in an ideal position with respect to all the above limitations, you are limited irrevocably in what you can get from the system because you are a woman. The value placed on your health, the respect given your complaints or requests, the general way in which treatment is prescribed and administered differs from that of male patients, and a United States Health Education and Welfare report has documented this. Complaints are even labeled "neurotic" and dismissed, "sometimes until physical diseases are beyond treatment."*

In other words, if you live in a sizable city that has many hospitals and doctors, are a man, have health insurance and can also pay for the inevitable extra costs, are well educated and somewhat informed about health care, are flexible in your values and have time to develop a relationship before a crisis by interviewing doctors and hospitals, you are in the best position to choose good care. Only if you are a doctor or are related or married to someone who is a health professional could you have a greater advantage. But the most that can be said is that all this would help you to avoid the worst; it still doesn't guarantee you the very best.†

The following is an attempt to give a brief guide to some of the background information every woman consumer should have when making health decisions. We hope that women who read this book will share with us their own personal experiences, such as those that have been so helpful in the preparation of this chapter, and will also guide us in defining the areas in which more information is needed.

*Fred Cook, *The Plot Against the Patient*, p. 24.

*Beth Fallon, "Feminists in a Fever over Medical Care," New York *Daily News* (April 25, 1972), p. 48. See under "Further Readings" for information on the HEW report.

†Edward Kennedy, *In Critical Condition* (New York: Simon and Schuster, 1972), pp. 168-69.

CHOOSING THE DOCTOR

The Doctor*

A doctor is any person who has completed four years of medical school and has received an M.D. degree from a recognized institution. In order to practice medicine, a license is required for each specific state. Once the license is acquired, an M.D. is an M.D. for life unless he commits an act that causes the license to be revoked (extremely rare). "A license to practice permits any M.D. to prescribe for any case. He may also perform any operation (short of an illegal abortion)."† Only hospitals, and only a few of them, have limited the procedures that doctors may perform, usually on the basis of training and occasionally experience. Therefore, all any doctor needs is your willingness to have his care.

Basically there are two types of physicians available to the consumer: (1) the general practitioner and (2) the specialist.

The general practitioner. The general practitioner, or G.P., is a doctor who has completed four years of medical school and a year of internship and then has set up a "solo" practice, much the way a businessman sets up a small self-operated business. He sets his own hours, hangs out his shingle, and collects his own fees, which are usually set after conferring with other colleagues in his own county medical society (a practice that would be called price-fixing in any other industry). Thus, since the amount of money a G.P. makes depends on the number of patients he sees in a day and the number of surgical procedures he performs (as for any non-salaried doctor in "fee-for-service" practice), there is tremendous pressure to see too many patients too briefly, to prescribe tranquilizers, antibiotics, and barbiturates too readily, and to perform unnecessarily too many operations for which he may not even be fully qualified.

This pressure, plus the shortage of available doctors and the higher prices charged by the specialist, make the G.P. among the most overworked of all doctors. The medical scandals concerning unnecessary surgery and drug addiction caused by medication given in obesity-control "clubs" and in general prescriptions for "nerves," which have been sensationalized in the media in recent

years, are largely excesses of the G.P., though not entirely. G.P.s also form the backbone of the AMA, which has been so conspicuous in opposing medical reform and Medicare/Medicaid, and National Health Insurance. Taken together, all these problems have done a great deal to tarnish the image of American medicine.

Fortunately or unfortunately, G.P.s are a declining group in medicine as the rise of the specialist and subspecialist has continued, and fewer and fewer medical-school graduates choose general practice. For these reasons G.P.s tend to be found in small towns or in private home offices in city and suburb. They are held in ill-concealed contempt by the specialists, and it has been estimated that probably only a quarter of G.P.s are really giving good-quality care; an equally large percentage are probably totally incompetent through overwork, old age, or a general failure to keep themselves informed about the latest medical developments. These last are the ones who never open a journal and are the darlings of the drug detail men. Members of the American Academy of Family Practice, on the other hand, have high standards and are expected to spend a certain amount of time on a regular basis studying, attending postgraduate courses, and otherwise keeping up, something that is a voluntary matter even among specialists.* For these reasons members of the AAFP are sometimes quicker to make appropriate referrals to a specialist than the specialists themselves, because they try to know and respect the limitations of their own competence, whereas the specialist sometimes is tempted to play psychiatrist or endocrinologist or surgeon himself, rather than pass the patient on for another opinion. However, both groups are guilty of this tendency.

The loss of the G.P. has meant the loss of an easily accessible doctor with whom a family and all its members could have a relationship over time, and also the loss of a general outlook on health rather than a narrow, isolated focus on a single part or system. These are factors you need to weigh in terms of your own value system, and all of the other factors listed in the introduction, when you consider going to a G.P.

The specialist. One tremendous problem confronting the laywoman today is the complicated and disorganized way in which the medical specialties have developed. It is estimated that there are now over fifty medical specialties and subspecialties, and not only is there a doctor shortage and a maldistribution of doctors but there are not enough of some specialists and too many of others.†

*Elsewhere in this book we have tried to be consistent in referring to a doctor as "he or she," or "s/he." In many other countries the "s/he" would be accurate; in the United States it is a dream that we are on our way to making into a reality. Because this section of the book deals with how things *are,* and with choices we can make today in the existing health-care system, we have referred to the doctor as "he."

†Cook, *The Plot Against the Patient,* p. 24.

*"Education for Family Practice," Commission on Education, AAFP, January 1972, pp. 1-3. Also AAFP Reprints, Nos. 101, 104.
†*The Graduate Education of Physicians,* report of the Citizen's Commission on Graduate Medical Education, Council on Medical Education of the AMA, p. 111.

As might be expected, there are far too many surgeons altogether, and in some communities too many psychiatrists,† while other areas go without the type of doctor needed most.

In a big city, where there are practically no G.P.s, and sometimes even no hospitals with which they are allowed to affiliate, patients are literally forced into making their own diagnoses in order to get care—something the doctors are adamant about not wanting patients to do. But the system forces us all into it.* Where to go with a serious, persistent sore throat, for example? If you go to the emergency ward of a suburban hospital you will be asked who your family physician is. In the emergency room of a big-city hospital you will often be asked if you are a patient of the hospital, or who your doctor is, or whether you are a resident of the city, and what means you have to pay for your care. Not that there is anything inappropriate about these questions—only that the wrong answers can be a barrier to care.

If you try to see an eye, ear, nose, and throat specialist, you may have to wait a week or more, especially if you are not already a patient. Ditto for the internist. For a sore throat you just might give up after all this. One young woman we know did just that, but apparently she had a strep infection, which finally involved her kidneys. But now that she is past prevention and really ill, of course she is getting excellent care. We know of doctors who have made diagnoses and ordered prescriptions over the telephone under these conditions. While this can be a saving in time and money, it can also be a risk. In a case like the one cited, advice might easily have been bed rest and aspirin, when what would have been more appropriate would be a culture of the throat and possibly penicillin or another antibiotic administered in case it turned out to be "strep." But there is controversy among doctors even on this procedure.

When trying to choose a specialist, then, it might seem somewhat reasonable to assume that one man is as good as another who has passed the same specialty Board examination. Much depends on the quality of the residency training, which is very uneven;† but the examination is expected to be the standard. Some experts feel that the hospital a man works in afterward has more to do with this continuing quality, partly because of the contact and stimulation of other specialists and partly because of his use of the technology available in it. But keeping up with developments elsewhere through the literature can also be important, and in some teaching centers a dangerous competitive smugness develops, which is based on the assumption that only what is done "right here" is really top quality or worth doing. Even more alarming is the fact that any doctor can announce himself as a specialist of any type even though he has not passed the Boards.*

It has been said that in no other profession do so many graduates resent the system that trained them.† There is a particular kind of town-gown split in medicine which is dangerous for the patient on both sides. Sometimes men who are isolated from the active teaching centers are extremely conscientious about keeping up with the literature and taking postgraduate programs, viewing their continuing education more seriously than many of their colleagues on the fringes of or even in the thick of academe. The latter sometimes feel more entitled to be intellectually dishonest or irresponsible in their refusal or unwillingness to apply the findings of their peers elsewhere. And a number of them are even surprisingly anti-intellectual. Of course, a great many specialists also subspecialize, and it's worth taking an interest early in what your specialist is especially interested in so you will also have some idea whether you really do have the best medical advice available for your particular problem(s).

All other things being equal, choose a man who is in group practice rather than in solo practice. You won't get that sense of luxurious intimacy that you might have gotten from a solo man, but it's probably not good for you anyway, and you won't be quite so hopelessly dependent on him, either. In some ways and in some places now group practice is almost as rushed and crowded as a clinic, where you may never see the same doctor twice, and so much more is charged for group-practice care than for clinic care that it may not seem much more desirable; but it is. The whole attitude and approach in private care is still class-oriented. You are seen as having the money if you seek private care, whether you really can afford it or not, and this does define to a large extent the attitude with which you are treated.

There are two kinds of group practice, with important differences. One kind is simply a group of the same type of specialists who have banded together to share the load and better manage their time and finances through seeing many more patients. The other is a collection of different specialists who are trying to offer families and individuals a more comprehensive view through both general and specific perspectives, such as internal medicine, pediatrics, and so on. Quite new and somewhat rare, this latter type seems to offer the best hope of working one's way through the specialist maze, usually through prepaid systems. Both types are still specialty medicine for those who can afford the fees or prepayment plan supporting it, though multispecialty, prepaid groups have shown substantial cost reductions. One reason for these lower costs is the avoidance of unnecessary tests and repeated visits. Salaried doctors gain no finan-

*Ibid., p. 34.
†Ibid., pp. 57-59.

*Edward Kennedy, *In Critical Condition*, pp. 160-61.
†J. Knowles, "Views of Medical Education and Medical Care," (Lowell Lectures, Boston, February 1966), pp. 87-89.

cial rewards from extra, unneeded services. But people below this income bracket are still forced to deal with the clinic.

Two other important new developments are worth looking into when you are choosing a physician. The first is the recent creation of an approved residency-training program in Family Practice. These doctors are members of the AAFP, just as the G.P.s may be (as we mentioned earlier), but unlike the AAFP G.P.'s, who commit themselves to keeping abreast of medical developments after their internships, these doctors go on to a full, approved residency training, which is followed by Board examinations and certification. In other words, they are specialists like other specialists, but their training is in so-called family medicine. This term, incidentally, does not mean that a doctor sees only families; it means that he is able to give basic, comprehensive care to any person of any age, who may or may not be a member of a nuclear family. In medical circles this kind of doctor is frequently called a "primary-care" physician, someone you would turn to first with any kind of problem, who would then refer you to a specific type of specialist if that became necessary.

A few medical schools in the country have recently established whole new medical curricula designed to train from scratch the kind of doctor who will become a "primary-care" physician. There seems to be a high possibility that some of these doctors will provide more satisfactory medical care for many people than the self-selected specialist method or even clinic care. Ask at local clinics and look up newer doctors in the community with this idea in mind.

What to Look For

Once you know what your doctor's qualifications are, you at least know how competent he is supposed to be. However, we cannot really rate a doctor's performance, because we have almost no frame of reference—nor has anyone else really. Doctors admit that even they are not sure how to find out how really competent a man is if they do not work with him every day. Asking a medical man's peers for an opinion, however, is like asking a blood relative for an objective opinion of a member of his family. Unless he is medically dangerous or behaving in a way that his colleagues find politically threatening, the recommendations will unvaryingly be enthusiastic. In most cases doctors make referrals the way they give other kinds of nonmedical opinions; they select on the basis of their friends and their own experiences, or because an exchange of referrals has become profitable. The competitiveness of big-city, university-linked specialists should work in the consumer's favor, but most of the time it doesn't, because these doctors often behave like small boys on rival football teams.

Again, your value system plays a part here. If you are impressed with a friend's report, or by your doctor's fees or academic affiliations, you may be disappointed. Most specialists in academic medicine are much too busy to listen to your problems, and the vast majority are not interested in the relation of your life situation to the state of your health. If they are "interested" in us, it is because we are medically or scientifically interesting, which usually indicates the presence of something specifically physical, preferably something "wrong," or pathological. Only if a doctor cannot find any physical cause for a complaint will he become interested in the possible emotional causes. Then he will probably refer you to a psychiatrist. Either way, he doesn't see himself as providing any time for listening or taking a personal interest in you, except at the very top prices, and often not even then. What you are looking for is an exceptional man, and they do exist here and there, but finding them is strictly a matter of luck.

In a strange way, a doctor often feels personally attacked or threatened when he cannot find any physical cause for the symptoms you report, and this can cause him to become hostile and use a label of "neurotic" or "psychosomatic" as a weapon, when in fact he has no evidence of psychological symptoms and isn't qualified to diagnose them anyway. In other words, it is false reasoning to diagnose a psychological problem merely by ruling out other physical causes. It becomes a weapon of convenience, used whenever the doctor cannot deal with the situation in his accustomed way, and frees him from taking the complaints seriously any longer.

It is worth remembering that psychiatrists in many medical-education programs do try to help other specialists to see the "emotional component" in the patient's problems and illnesses, but in far too many cases the result is a fine example of "A little knowledge is a dangerous thing." Only a small handful of medical students can really make appropriate use of these insights, and almost all use them as a weapon at some time or other.

What about "shopping" for doctors? Doctors don't like it, of course, and neither do clinics. Some psychiatric clinics even have a blackball system whereby they will not give you treatment in their setting once you admit that you have been to another system even for a preliminary intake. Thus you either have to go back to the first clinic or do without help. However, private "shopping" for doctors is becoming more common, and to some extent the profession is learning to live with it. The AMA has always given lip-service support to the practice, because it upholds the myth that only by retaining the present "fee-for-service," private-enterprise system does the consumer truly have a "choice." Actually, there is some truth in this, but the myth is that all people have a choice, and that you know what you are choosing. In fact, only private patients, never clinic patients, have such a possibility of choice.

Some doctors charge for an exploratory talking interview, others do not. Some will answer a few basic questions about their practice and how they handle patients in a phone call, without charge, but not all. "Shopping" takes a lot of time and may even cost a lot of money, but some people feel it's worth it. They track down every lead they have, try to get some feeling for the reputation of the hospital in which the doctor practices, and have some trial interviews. They ask questions about the decision-making process; they ask about honest answers to straight questions in the future, and about the sharing of information generally. They sometimes also ask how the doctor would feel if his advice were not followed on some occasion; because unless the doctor recognizes a patient's right to disagree, he may not recognize a patient's right to know.

When you are actually in the process of trying to get information from a doctor about your functioning, you can discover just how willing he is to spend time making sure you have the information you want, need, and have a right to know, and whether you really understand what he is saying. In other words, is the doctor willing to make you a partner in the process of caring for yourself, or does he prefer to do it all? Apart from the tests he performs himself, however, with which most of us are reasonably familiar, the modern doctor depends for much of his information on increasingly sophisticated laboratory work. Some doctors are overly dependent on laboratory tests when they should be taking more careful histories and examinations. Others dismiss symptoms without testing to check their judgment.

Some doctors obviously prefer to control all of the information they have about you; others let you know in subtle or not so subtle ways that they think you are not bright enough to understand it, or they may present it in such a way that you couldn't anyway, thus fulfilling their own estimate of you. If you question the doctor in a matter-of-fact and not threatening way, conveying your feeling that you are entitled to know, he should be able and willing to tell you what he is looking for, and what are the norms of the tests he is ordering, so that when the results come in, you will understand their significance. One doctor we know sends at least some of his patients Xerox copies of all their test results, and discusses these openly with them. While this may seem generous and unusual (and in some ways it is), it also points up an issue that deserves some discussion.

It is difficult to think of any other area in American life where we pay such high prices for information to which we are denied access. When a doctor orders tests from a laboratory or special office outside his own office, he expects you to pay for these tests. Yet if you ever try to learn the results of such tests directly from the laboratory, you are told that only the doctor can release the information, because he ordered the test. One woman was asked by her husband's physician to wait two weeks to learn the results of a biopsy on her husband's prostate gland, because the doctor "didn't have the test handy" and was in a rush to get out of town for a vacation. Very upset, convinced that the results must be malignant and that the doctor wanted to break the news during an office visit with both of them, the woman agonized for ten days before she finally gathered courage to force the reluctant office nurse to read her the simple word "benign" over the telephone. Probably someday there will be a legal test to determine who owns this information; in the meantime we can try to get both laboratories and doctors to be quicker and more open about test results and any other kind of information.

Information about risk-taking is even harder to get. Many people thought that the object of the hearings that were held in 1969 on oral contraceptive risks was to determine once again the safety of the pill. But the hearings were rather an effort to discover for the first time whether or not women were being adequately informed about the *risks* of oral contraceptives. No more direct challenge has ever been presented to the sanctity of the doctor-patient relationship and, as might be expected, there was indignation and outrage from the doctors, particularly obstetrician-gynecologists, who were among those most frequently prescribing the pill. But the hearings concluded with a recommendation that women had a guaranteed right to knowledge from the manufacturers that there were side effects and possible risks in some cases.

The hearings did establish that a woman need not be dependent exclusively on her doctor for this knowledge, even though the final package insert was much watered down from the original proposed by the Food and Drug Administration. It contained repeated warnings to report any unusual signs to the doctor and to take the pills only under a doctor's care, and stated that a woman had to go to her doctor in order to obtain the information booklet. To the last the society of specialists in ob-gyn opposed *any* package insert, later falling back to the position that they wanted to be involved in planning the wording (which they ultimately were). The reasons they gave were the usual: that the patient might become unduly alarmed over reading about the hazards; that she might not take the pill even though it was indicated, and so on, and so on.* The essential principle of the patient's

*"Statement on 'Pill' Insert," ACOG (American College of Obstetricians and Gynecologists) *Bulletin*, Vol. 14, No. 5 (May 1970), p. 12.

right to know and even decide against a certain procedure if she chooses escaped them right to the end. The paternalistic mode still prevails in their thinking, and the concept of patient as partner in her own health care remains a threatening and unacceptable one.

Another example of the difficulty of getting information on risk-taking concerns obstetric analgesia and anesthesia, and inductions. (See chapter on "Childbirth.") It is clear that few if any women are told of the risks to themselves or their babies from particular drugs and anesthestics, particularly the most common ones that are used routinely in the majority of normal deliveries though not really necessary. Most often doctors have given them instead completely positive, glowing descriptions of the drugs' benefits.

At the upper limit of this issue, many doctors still do not recognize a patient's right to refuse any procedure, life-giving or otherwise. On a recent TV show a young doctor argued with distinguished senior men that an old woman in a city hospital had the right to refuse to take advantage of a possibly life-extending approach he offered her. The older doctors insisted that the decision was a medical decision that the patient was not equipped to make, and that therefore she did not have the privilege of deciding. The young man saw, however, that there was a consumer right, a human right, for the patient to know the chance and the risks of the treatment, and then refuse it if she wished.* Actually, in hospital practice it has been legally established that a patient's informed consent must be secured before any drug is given or procedure carried out. The familiar "ether permit" of the past still exists in some places, but it does not stand up legally. Similarly, a nurse can no longer hide behind "doctor's orders." She herself can be held liable if she administers a drug without the patient's consent, even if a doctor did order it.†

However, many doctors, hospitals, and patients are apparently still unaware of all this in its practical, everyday application, and it is still common to hear reports of women who refused drugs, for example, and then were told, "You're going to get it anyway." There is also increasing evidence that patients frequently do not understand what they are agreeing to when they do give consent or sign a permission form. There are even reports of procedures that were carried out without the patient's knowledge.‡ It is essential to read very carefully

any consent form and to inquire about any vague or technical terms you don't clearly understand. For example, when you are asked to accept "possible risks," find out what they are and how often they occur. If you have any questions about the need for a procedure which requires signing a consent form, or for the need for the removal of an organ or tissue, get another opinion from someone with no financial interest in performing the procedure. It could be "cheaper" in the long run!

What about women doctors? It would be wonderful and simple to believe that just being a woman made a doctor more compassionate, more flexible, more sympathetic to women and easier to deal with than male doctors. To be sure, the sexual undercurrents that sometimes cloud the communication between a male doctor and a female patient may be absent, but there are other factors present. Most mature women in active practice today came of age in medicine during a time when prejudice against career women at all levels in our society, and especially against women in medicine, was at an all-time high. They had to "outman the men," so to speak—to be more conservative, more rigid, "better" in every way than their male colleagues, or even renounce the mother-wife role altogether, just to survive. It has also been suggested that as women they had problems with their sexuality, and perhaps in that day in the United States they did, having absorbed so much contempt for their sex from doctors and from society and yet still wanting to be doctors. At any rate, young women doctors today stand a far better chance of being at least liberal (that now dirty word), if not liberated, radical and innovative, and feeling more entitled to be women and doctors too than their senior counterparts ever did. However, don't choose a doctor just because she is a woman, but rate her just as you would any other doctor—for skill, honesty, quality of communication, flexibility, intellectual curiosity, ability to really listen, and respect for you as a person.

THE DOCTOR-PATIENT RELATIONSHIP

In the private setting, or even in the clinic setting, the fact that a woman asks for or even begs for advice and guidance with nonphysiological problems may be seen by either the woman or the doctor as a sufficient excuse for giving it. But it is very hard to measure the impact that this advice sometimes has on a woman, given as it is in the name of medical care, with all of the authority that seems implicit in the process. Often a woman ends up being utterly dependent on her doctor, and then is freed from neither her problems nor her dependency. It is this kind of relationship that doctors are eventually

*"For Women Today," Group W, WBZ-TV, Boston, week of March 1, 1972. See also "Toward a Better Death," *Time*, June 5, 1972, pp. 60-61.

†John Haire, "Consumerism in Maternity Care," address at convention of International Childbirth Education Association, Inc., Milwaukee, Wis., May 23, 1972. (To be published in ICEA Convention report.)

‡Carl Cobb, "Students Charge BCH's Obstetrics Unit with Excessive Surgery," *The Boston Globe* (April 29, 1972), p. 1.

tempted to resolve through the use of barbiturates and tranquilizers, and much of the so-called housewife drug addiction syndrome sometimes begins this way.*

For many medical specialists the development of this special kind of dependency, or "transference," as it is called by psychiatrists, is seen as a deliberate goal of the so-called doctor-patient relationship, about which so much romantic nonsense has been written. Eliciting this transference is specially taught as a technique in many medical schools—with a few vague cautions thrown in—as a useful tool for "managing" patients. When the doctor refers to this dependency, or transference, however, he calls it trust, at least when speaking to the patient (especially a woman). The parent-child relationship seems to be the model. Whenever there are real, matter-of-fact questions raised by the patient, a doctor is apt to say, "What's the matter, don't you trust me?" Also, for most doctors the fact that the transference develops is its own justification—that is, if a woman becomes overly dependent it's because she "needs" or wants to be. It is this expectation that accounts for the reflex behavior of so many doctors who constantly try to play a paternalistic role by calling patients by their first names from the first visit or telling them, "Don't worry your pretty head, my dear. Just leave everything to me." In the past, or perhaps even today at some levels of our society, there may be women who find this treatment appropriate and reassuring, but their numbers are fast dwindling.

Especially in regard to sexual problems, most doctors are dangerously ignorant, even though the public continues to see them as knowledgeable.† Until very recently most medical schools did not even have any courses on human sexuality, and the majority of schools still do not require such courses, merely offering them as optional.‡ There is nothing like making a course optional to convey to a medical student that it is not important. The courses that do exist have often been designed by urologists or gynecologists rather than by behavioral scientists and reflect a mechanistic rather than a humanistic bias. Many patients whom these future doctors will meet will have read more widely and have a far deeper knowledge of the subject. This same discussion applies to nutrition as well.§

Managing the Obstetrician-Gynecologist

While doing the research for this book several of us came upon certain sections in major medical texts—the kind that medical students study and doctors use as references—which offer medical opinions about the character of female patients. In one text on gynecology there is a long section on the psychology of women in which the doctor is advised to interview the woman patient when he first sees her and to measure what might be called her "femininity" quotient. He is told to pay attention to how the patient responds to his questions, whether "in a feminine way or whether she is domineering, demanding, masculine, aggressive or passive in her attitude."* What these value-laden terms mean exactly is not clear. Is being demanding the same as asking the doctor to explain what he is doing?

This essay goes on to more generalizations about the female character, listing basic, or core, traits of the female personality—which turn out to be "narcissism, masochism, and passivity." The doctor's approach to our health, if he follows this advice, would be influenced by whether we concur in the definition of our femininity as defined by male experts.

A more elaborate portrait of the ideal process of female socialization appears in one of the most widely used texts in obstetrics.

Having been taught and instructed in feminine ways of behavior and dress since infancy; having imitated (with encouragement) the appearance and behavior of adult women in her family circle since childhood; having indulged, when a younger girl, in fantasies of care (encouraged by loving parents who supplied dolls) for doll houses, and doll carriages; having received love and approval from her parents and other adults in the family circle when, in her early adolescence, she manifested an intense interest in improving her physical appearance, the neatness of her dress and grooming, and changed her behavior to be more like that of a "lady"; and having become aware of the increased attention paid to her by boys when she looked, dressed and behaved in a feminine manner, it is reasonable that she should accept her feminine gender role in adolescence. However, in future years, she will continue feminine attitudes and behavior as long as she receives the attention, affection and love from those whom she loves. Feeling loved, and wanted by her husband, she will take pride in keeping attractive and give him her love and devotion, encouraging him in his accomplishments. As a mother, she will give love and affectionate care to her children, taking pride in their successes in childhood and later as adults.†

The author goes on to point out that the only real way to happiness for women is marriage: "The full po-

*Roland Berg, "The Over-Medicated Woman," *McCall's* (September 1972), p. 67 ff.; also, Davidson, Muriel, "How 'Nice' Drugs Killed My Sister," *Good Housekeeping* (September 1970), pp. 96–97; also, Blum, Sam, "Pills That Make You Feel Good," *Redbook* (August 1969), p. 70 ff.

†Harold Leif, "What Your Doctor Probably Doesn't Know About Sex," *Harper's Magazine* (December 1964), pp. 92–96.

‡J. D. Cade and W. F. Jessee, "Sex Education in American Medical Schools," *Journal of Medical Education*, Vol. 46 (January 1971), pp. 64-68.

§M. G. Phillips, "The Nutrition Knowledge of Medical Students," *Ibid.*, pp. 86-90.

*Robert J. Willson *et al.*, *Obstetrics and Gynecology*, 2d ed. (St. Louis: The C. V. Mosby Co., 1963), p. 46.

†Sprague Gardiner, "The Psychosomatic Aspects of Obstetrics," in Nicholson Eastman and Louis Hellman, *Williams Obstetrics*, 13th ed. (New York: Appleton Century Crofts, 1966), p. 341.

tentialities of feminine psychosexual maturity are seldom achieved except in a marriage relationship based upon love." What follows from this line of reasoning is that other settings are not considered appropriate for the expression of female sexuality.

> Coital participation and experimentation by the adolescent or adult woman in settings other than marriage not only seldom resolves her personal problems, but more often results in guilt, shame and loss of self-respect. Few unwed pregnant women have extolled the pleasures of the event or events which led to the conception.*

The moralistic, puritanical, and judgmental tone of this comment only encourages our doctors to think that they have the obligation and right to be our moral guardians.

There is great irony in the fact that doctors are socially sanctioned as sexual counselors and advisors, and yet are astoundingly ignorant of female sexuality. In one obstetrics book, in discussing female orgasm, the author-doctor avers that "it is as variegated as thumbprints and not at all contingent on mechanical and muscular stimuli but rather on how a woman feels about her husband." He goes on to say that the only important question to ask a woman with regard to her lack of sexual satisfaction is, "Does she really love her husband?"† That certainly simplifies the counseling process for the doctor.

These attitudes toward women remind us again that many male doctors, like many other men, have created myths about the female character and personality which blind them to us as a group and as individuals. What is frightening is how much power male doctors hold over many aspects of our lives, and how their *official* ideas about women affect the medical care we get and thus our very survival.

We must not forget, however, that many of these ideas and characteristics are taken from the language of psychiatry, and psychoanalysis in particular, to which some obstetrician-gynecologists have turned as a kind of final authority. It is not possible in this book to discuss in detail the impact that psychoanalytic ideas and psychiatric care have upon women, but hopefully at a later date we can deal with this in depth.

So the notion that there are some ob-gyn specialists who are greatly superior to others is often a myth. The fact that many of us have a need to believe that we are in the hands of superior physicians is one of the problems we need to be liberated from.

* * *

I knew that my doctor had a reputation for being one of the best in the city, and it made me feel good when I said his name and other people would say, "Oh, right, I've heard of him." I felt he was great and I was one of his

*Ibid, p. 335.
†J. P. Greenhill, *Obstetrics,* 13th ed. (Philadelphia: Saunders & Co., 1965), p. 481.

lucky patients, even though I was rarely comfortable with him and always felt belittled when I went to him: I'd have to wait a very long time, or he wouldn't answer my questions, or I'd feel sometimes too timid to even ask any questions.

* * *

While I was learning a lot of things about my body I went to see a gynecologist for my yearly check-up. I thought, This time I won't feel intimidated. But it happened anyway. One of the things I remember really clearly is when he asked me how long my menstrual cycle was, and I told him, he looked surprised and just said, "That's interesting." I asked him if it was unusually long (I've since found out it is), if my hormones were out of whack, if he could even tell anything at all. He just sidestepped or didn't answer my questions. I wouldn't have cared so much if he had said he couldn't tell, or didn't know, or even if he just wasn't interested in menstrual problems. But he talked to me as if I shouldn't know. It's my body, and I felt defeated in trying to learn about it. I decided that the next time I would go with another woman, who could help me ask questions and also see what the doctor was doing during the actual examination.

* * *

Remember too: The doctor is no longer a god-figure; that's the price we pay for our developing independence. A too close doctor-patient relationship during pregnancy, for example, may actually retard or disrupt your own growth and/or developing relationship with the man in your life at a time when it needs all the strengthening it can get.

* * *

I'd had a lot of trouble conceiving and my doctor had operated to remove ovarian cysts. Four months after the operation I became pregnant. My doctor was very happy too. I remember we both felt he had been responsible for my pregnancy, and my husband had merely been the vehicle for my doctor's success. My husband felt excluded. I know I played along with that whole game, not really aware of what I was doing or why.

* * *

The first time I met him I thought he was so cold, clinical, and businesslike. Then all his "charm" made me feel dependent on him. I respected that he was going to do the best job he could possibly do. If he criticized me, I shrank inside. Sometimes I'd be annoyed that I had to travel so far for him to look at my stomach. But the mysteries still held: He was going to give me the baby. Once he confused me with someone else and I was very depressed.

* * *

Remember: Obstetricians don't provide continuity. Don't choose them to depend on emotionally. During

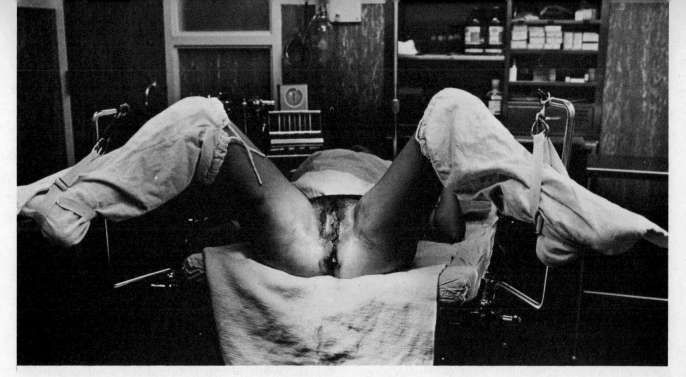

pregnancy you really need to lean on someone who will also be there after the baby is born. Find someone else to share the whole experience with, for the doctor disappears from the scene right after your baby is born, and you don't see him again for six weeks or so.

Many of us are still looking for an authoritarian figure, for a father in our doctor. And doctors foster our dependency. One well-known medical textbook discusses a woman's "strong need" for an emotional attachment to her obstetrician, speaking of this dependence as "healthy and therapeutically beneficial" (to whom?). The author speaks of a woman's need to be recognized and accepted and approved of by "an authoritarian figure into whose care she has placed *completely* herself and her baby-to-be." The obstetrician, he says, will advise her regarding her every activity, and he adds that it's little wonder that he becomes identified in her mind with other masculine figures of her life. In other cases he "may fulfill an idealized image in [her] mind when authoritarian . . . male figures in her past life were disappointing, inadequate or absent altogether."*

The fact that the specialized field of obstetrics-gynecology is now claiming that it wishes to be identified as *the* resource for all of the health needs of women needs to be looked at closely. It implies that women can expect to have all of their needs for psychological as well as physical care met by the obstetrician-gynecologist. Yet there are no standing requirements either in the residencies or as part of the specialty Board examinations for an ob-gyn to demonstrate any competence in any aspect of behavioral science, human development, psychology of women, or even psychology in general. Every woman should understand that what this means is that

*Sprague Gardiner, *op. cit.*, p. 342.

just because a doctor is a certified ob-gyn doesn't mean that he is qualified or trained or prepared in any way to give advice or counsel or any other sort of help in any human-relations area of a woman's life. He is only competent to assess the state of our organs and treat them if necessary, or prescribe contraceptives and fit them. If he does more than that he is simply guessing, or worse, answering out of his own beliefs and experience. Occasionally, of course, he may have taken some human-behavior courses or, rarely, a psychiatric residency, but these are simply not enough to qualify him for the delicate work of therapy or counseling about sexual adjustments except in the purely physical realm. Many college-educated liberal-arts majors know as much, sometimes more. Even here, however, psychological and physiological factors are so closely interwoven that even the most skilled and knowledgeable people are reluctant to separate them. In the light of these facts it is shocking to realize that some 93 percent of physicians are treating the marital and sexual problems of their patients and only about 15 percent *felt* that their medical training had prepared them; 90–95 percent felt that additional training was needed.*

At one level it is possible to think of the ob-gyn as a friend who is helping to protect you against unwanted pregnancy or venereal disease or death and disaster in childbirth. But at another level it's possible to see him as someone whose main concern is to keep you healthy and maintain you in your place as a sex object for your man, or for men: "clean," the right size, in good working order, and free from fear of disease or pregnancy; or pregnant, but to be returned to the prepregnant state

*Ethel M. Nash, "Divorce, Marriage Counseling," in Allan C. Barnes, ed., *The Social Responsibility of Obstetrics and Gynecology*, pp. 117-18.

"as good as new" and as quickly as possible, almost as if the pregnancy had never happened. Sometimes it seems as if one reason why many ob-gyn men are negative (subtly or not so subtly) about breast-feeding, for example, is that they have identified with a man's sense of sexual possessiveness about the breasts and want to preserve these exclusively for him and in nearly virginal condition for as much of the time as possible. The same may be true for the use of forceps and the practice of routine episiotomies, or the oft-repeated caution that a woman should not get overtired, which can—on the surface—seem so solicitous.

Certainly, we may want all of these things, too, for our own reasons. When we want sex we want to feel ready for it in every way and protected against pregnancy if we choose to be, but not because we see this as our exclusive or even our primary function as women, and especially not because our first "duty" is to be in shape for a man whenever he might want us. Similarly, we know that children have needs too, but especially we as women have many other needs. The doctor, and the ob-gyn in particular, can be viewed as society's representative in identifying us to ourselves and to others as creatures whose only needs appear to be meeting the needs of others. Our medical care thus sometimes seems directed toward those purposes.

The other problem for women, however, is that we have been taught to assume that the ob-gyn can at least meet all of our needs for basic medical care, even if we do finally realize that he isn't competent to help with feelings or sexual matters. Since a woman's first need for medical help these days often tends to be for contraception, she may be seeing a gynecologist even before she is at an age when her own pediatrician would consider her too old to be seen by him anymore, or when an internist would think her too young. Thus she could go for years, or even for life, without ever having a thorough adult check-up by a competent specialist in internal medicine. While the ob-gyn does give routine check-ups, they are usually very sketchy affairs, as any woman can testify, and the possibility is always present that he will not look for or will ignore certain problems that might result from treatment that he himself has given or is giving, such as the effects of the pill or other drugs, or the after-effects of surgery or childbirth.

With the kind of sophisticated tinkering going on today with our female endocrine systems before half the knowledge is even available, and with the heavily operative, manipulative interference that is routine even in normal childbirth, all of us should be a lot more careful. A once-a-year check-up with a good internist is a bit of insurance against any pet biases or enthusiasms of the ob-gyn or any other narrow specialist, and you may find that some of the complaints and symptoms that are being brushed aside or dismissed in one office may be listened to with great care and respect in another. Internists, by the way, will also do Pap smears and prescribe and fit contraceptives if you ask them to.

In other words, a woman's habit of seeing herself exclusively in terms of her genital or reproductive functioning may prevent her from seeking medical care from other specialists for her other problems, and may also make her feel uncomfortably dependent on this particular specialist for the very essence of her liberation, her conception control, as well as basic medical care. By default, the ob-gyn may become the "primary-care" physician for women, a role for which he is not trained.

On the other hand, many ob-gyn specialists get involved with the diagnosis and treatment of breast lumps, including mastectomy, and other cancer and surgery problems, when these procedures should ideally be carried out by full surgeons or in consultation with cancer experts. While ob-gyn is considered a subspecialty of surgery, it is not synonymous with the surgical specialty. Again, be sure to ask about the special interests or subspecialty of any doctor you see.

If all of this sounds like a warning against the obstetrician-gynecologist, it isn't meant to be. This specialist has many valuable skills which we as women should feel free to take advantage of, if we can afford to, whenever we need them. Our commentary is meant to be a clarification to help us as women and as consumers of health care to understand what we should reasonably expect from the ob-gyn in the way of services, and where and why to go elsewhere for other kinds of help.

Doctors: Summary

From many a doctor's point of view he is being a "good" doctor when he is best able to shut out human considerations and can focus narrowly on technical, scientific, or pathological factors. At the other extreme, some doctors use their position to allow them to give a lot of purely personal advice. The image and myth of the doctor as humanitarian, which has been so assiduously sold to the American public for the last fifty years, is out of date. If there ever were such doctors, they are mostly all gone now. A few with such leanings do get into medical school occasionally, but oftentimes they get out fairly quickly or finally end up in psychiatry. There are reports that there is a new breed of doctor now coming into medicine, but the psychological profile of most men in practice today more closely resembles the American businessman: repressed, compulsive, and more interested in money (and the disease process) than in people. Medical students are usually very carefully selected by men who are attempting to reproduce themselves, and usually succeed. After four years of training they have almost invariably become somewhat cynical and even more detached and mechanistic than they were to start with. As a group they are also more immature emotionally and sexually than their peers or the rest of the population of contemporaries, who have taken the time to do the living and loving that brings them closer to maturity. Most doctors finishing their training are in late adolescence, psychologically speaking.*

The purpose of this section is not to single out the doctor as essentially malevolent. He is only one representative of a number of largely male professions. The point is to understand better what it is we are dealing with when we try to work with doctors or get them to work with us. It takes considerable maturity to see clearly enough or feel free to identify with the person of the opposite sex in any given situation, unless it is a habitual perspective. In medicine there is scarcely any woman's viewpoint, and very little—if any—language for that viewpoint as yet. But given the personalities and the prejudices they have to work with, it is particularly difficult for doctors to develop this viewpoint, and nothing in the system they work with motivates them to do so.

We can be angry about this, and we should be, but it is a mistake perhaps to look for confirmation from the doctor of our feelings and identity as women in the first place. That is where only a group of women, being honest with themselves and one another, can hope to sort it all out. But just sharing horror stories is not enough, even though it is usually helpful. Learning about why things are the way they are, and why things that have happened to us did happen, and getting the facts so that perhaps we can change our understanding of what actually did happen, are equally important. Over and over again women who were miserably treated, just on the evidence, defend their doctors and even glorify them, saying, "He was so *good* to me. He was just marvelous." Only slowly, after a long time and gradually looking at the facts, can we face what really happened. People, and perhaps especially women, have a way of being very loyal to their concept of whatever happened to them in a medical context, and to the people who were there. When we do finally face the reality of an experience, we get very angry, of course, or even totally disillusioned for a time. We expected too much, we looked for something that perhaps never existed in American society—a "good" doctor.

If the picture of things as they are is discouraging, we mean it to be. Doctors are not gods, but human beings with serious problems, both as people and as professionals. But so, of course, are we all. The uncomfortable difference is that the system has taught the doctor never to reveal his problems and weaknesses to us, to present himself as perfect and all-wise, whereas the essence of patienthood is that we must reveal all of our doubts and vulnerabilities to him. Not to aggravate or take advantage of that essential inequality should be seen as an ethical challenge to the physician just as severe as all of the other points in the Hippocratic oath now going out of fashion. But it is rarely even recognized as an issue by most doctors, or understood if it is pointed out. The myth still persists that we meet one another as parent and child, and that you as patient must both obey and pay money for the privilege. How long it will take and how possible it will be to fully convey to both parties the sense of consumer-employee, which is the reality of the relationship, is hard to imagine. If you cannot present yourself with conviction as an adult, and if you don't really feel fully entitled to argue or protest or get information and open communication, you will probably be treated accordingly. Maybe there will always be something about the "laying on of hands" that triggers the sense of the child in us. And when pain and fear are added, perhaps it is inevitable.

If you find all this disillusioning, then we are glad if we have helped you to lose some illusions. We want you to be more alert to your responsibility in the relationship, just as you would in any other adult relationship where you are purchasing services. This book is a start, but we've only been able to touch briefly on the simplest aspects, the common medical events of a woman's life. The real toughies—the complicated diseases, the rare surgeries, death and dying—will have to be coped with and worked out individually over a longer time. But everything we've said here applies: Don't let yourself be stampeded into any sudden decisions or forced to accept any medications or procedures you don't understand or want. It's your body.

THE CLINIC

The poorest people still on the receiving end of the medical system, at the clinic level, while they may be quicker to know when they are being ill-treated as human beings, have so little health and medical information that they are almost completely at the mercy of their so-called providers of health care. They can only feel enraged and helpless at their dependency, their ill-treatment, and their ignorance. It is this combination of emotions that armchair medical experts are fond of referring to as the "apathy" of the lower classes. Not to seek medical care under these conditions can thus be seen as an act of integrity and dignity, even if not to do so ultimately risks health or even life.* This position is incomprehensi-

*Leif, "What Your Doctor Probably Doesn't Know About Sex."

*Michael Halberstam, "The M.D. Should Not Try to Cure Society," *The New York Times Magazine* (November 9, 1969), p. 32 ff.

ble to large numbers of doctors and health workers. Most of them even find it contemptible that there are some people who will not accept health care under any and all conditions.

Poorer women who demand their right to be as much in control as possible of their pregnancy, labor and childbirth, for example, run risks that richer women don't run, and can be threatened on the level of dehumanization and of safety to themselves and their babies, whereas a private patient might suffer, at the worst, minor personal degradation. Unmarried pregnant white women who want to keep their babies are often treated as immoral people.

However, a recent study of maternal care made in the hospitals and clinics of some major United States cities states in a formal way the things that many poor women learn from bitter experience. The quality of medical and personal attention we get in hospitals and clinics is determined by the following factors and various combinations of them: our background, race, religion, marital status, education, income level and source, number of times we have become pregnant, and number of children we have. If we are rich, married, white, and Protestant, we obviously get better care than if we are poor, black and unmarried.* While a well-off woman in a private labor room can "get away" with rightful demands to know what medication she is being given, a poor woman rightfully voicing these same demands might end up ignored or maltreated.

The word "doctor" to middle-class or private patients often means something drastically different from what it means to most clinic patients. Only in some settings does the clinic patient see anything but residents or house officers, those incredibly bright but dangerously insensitive young men who try their wings here as doctors before becoming full-fledged, practicing specialists.

The clinic is also the place where residents and some of the nurses, too, can act on the stereotyped thinking and prejudices they have acquired in relation to whatever population they work with.† Trained not to see them as people to begin with, but rather as whatever part of the body they may be presenting, they add to this peculiar perspective whatever fantasies they may have about blacks, unwed mothers, Spanish-speaking people, or any other group. There is nothing in their training that has required them to recognize these people as human beings like themselves, whose need for respect and help is as great, or greater, than their own.

It's hard to know whether things are better or worse

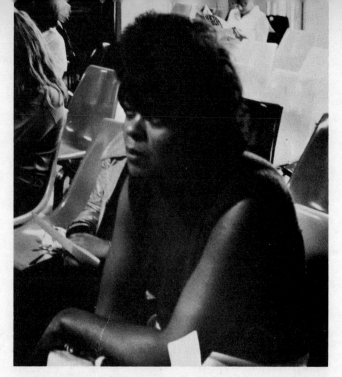

for patients in clinics staffed by "regular" men (doctors whose training is finished and who give time to staff clinics for those who cannot afford private care), because often such clinics are the settings for perhaps the most moralistic kind of charity, which confirms the doctor in his wish to believe that we are still living in the nineteenth century, and helps to keep him, in many cases, a Republican. Here he can tell himself, "Why, they are damn lucky to get me," and in exchange for the donated care, he can feel entitled to give paternalistic advice about how to manage one's life, or make decisions that infringe on a patient's human rights.

Not having a choice of doctor and not feeling entitled to make demands or ask questions even if they did know what to ask, clinic patients seem to feel doubly impotent if the funds that pay the clinic fees are derived from welfare or other assistance programs. If, to save money, you feel you must go to a clinic, do some homework first. Some clinic care is more expensive than private care from either a G.P. or a specialist who is at a smaller hospital. While there are many private doctors—maybe most—who are very outspoken and not at all defensive about not taking welfare patients, there are doctors who will accept and care for welfare patients for whatever fee welfare will pay, just as if they were private patients. It's worthwhile to try to hunt out the doctors who will take people on welfare and at least make some comparisons about fees, travel, hours, and attitudes.

Sociologists have found plenty of evidence that if you are white, college-educated, and not noticeably ethnic, you will get the best possible care from your attendants in the clinic setting. Terrible as it sounds, if you are all these things, you can try to save money by trying to get good care from a clinic, at the same time keeping yourself well informed on your own about the condition you are seeking treatment for, and asking stiff questions in

*N. Shaw, "So You're Going to Have a Baby," doctoral dissertation (Brandeis University, 1972), to be published in spring 1973 by Pergamon Press.

†"Prelude to Action," Maternity Center Association (50th anniversary seminar report, Princeton, 1968), 48 E. 92nd Street, New York, N.Y. 10025, 1969, pp. 5–7.

your very sweetest way. In other words, if you can get them to treat you as a sort of displaced equal, you can probably do well. If you do not have most of these advantages, do whatever you can to get private care, or accept your clinic care with some awareness that you are also doing them a favor. Don't ever forget that teaching hospital clinics "need" their patients. They need you and your medical problems in order to teach doctors and nurses in training and to give them experience that would otherwise be hard to get, since a private doctor does not usually allow his own patients to be "used" for teaching purposes. In spite of the fact that you may be seen by many different doctors in a clinic setting you do have a right to insist on the identity of one doctor who is primarily responsible for you and to talk with him about your overall care (See Appendix). From him as from any other doctors you have a right to expect certain kinds of information (See Box).

WHAT TO EXPECT FROM YOUR DOCTOR

1. An accurate diagnosis of your condition, healthy or otherwise, at your request.

2. Results and meaning of any tests or examinations performed by him or by others at his direction, as soon as they are available.

3. Indications for treatment, varieties and alternatives, pros and cons of particular treatments in the opinion of other experts, as well as the doctor's own preference and the reasons for it.

4. Answers to your questions about any examination or procedure he may perform, in advance of or at any time during the performance of it. Stopping any examination or procedure at any moment, at your request.

5. Complete information about purpose, content and known effects of all drugs prescribed or administered, including possible risks, side-effects and contra-indications, especially of any combination of drugs.

6. Willingness to accept and wait for a second medical opinion before performing any elective surgery which involves alteration or removal of any organ or body part.

7. Answers to your questions about your body or your general physical health and functioning, in addition to any particular condition. Or, encouragement to seek these answers from another source.

THE HOSPITAL

Whenever you decide to accept treatment from a particu-

lar doctor or clinic, it is important to realize that you are at the same time choosing potential hospital care. In other words, the doctor or clinic is your key, your "entry point" to the system. If something comes up that requires hospitalization, you may be upset to discover, if you have not thought about it beforehand, that you are in a big, impersonal place that will not permit you to visit your sick child when you can, or that there is no facility or personnel to help with an emotional crisis if one should develop for you or someone you love. Most hospital rules are not made for the benefit of the patients or families but for the staff's convenience, and some of these rules are not only arbitrary and unreasonable, they may actually be dangerous to mental or physical health.

Hospitals are rated in a number of ways, differently by different people. First of all, there are 858 so-called private proprietary hospitals, which are owned and operated for private profit.* Some people feel that they should not be allowed to exist, while others feel it is a perfectly appropriate expression of the American Way. In any case, all such institutions need only fill their beds with patients who present themselves in order to stay in business; and there is clearly no shortage of patients.

Second, there are the so-called private voluntary hospitals, run by a board of trustees, which are usually nonprofit, and therefore eligible for various state and Federal benefits (although some of them may actually make a small margin of profit). They usually practice a kind of Robin Hood socialism, through which the payments by affluent patients actually are used in part toward the costs of low-paying or nonpaying patients.† Within the voluntary, private group are the small community hospitals, the big teaching centers, and some religious-affiliated institutions. Some of these institutions are ruthless in their pursuit of unpaid bills, even to the point of causing families actual bankruptcy.‡

Third, there are the public hospitals—city, state, or county—which usually operate at a loss of some kind because of the large numbers of nonpaying citizens they handle, for which they are inadequately reimbursed by the various governmental budgets.

Doctors usually rate a hospital by the caliber and training of the men who are affiliated there and by its technological facilities—that is, modern, expensive equipment for treatment, anesthesia, or life saving, and the sophisticated laboratories that back them up. The presence of this kind of technology is one of the factors driving up the price at such hospitals, even though sometimes it is acquired just for the purpose of attracting prestigious physicians and not because it is really needed. Most specialists prefer not to be associated with a hospi-

*Kennedy, *In Critical Condition*, pp. 182-83.
†Cook, *The Plot Against the Patient*, pp. 17-25.
‡Kennedy, *In Critical Condition*, pp. 91-93.

tal that permits general practitioners to perform surgery or obstetrics there. Some hospitals are therefore specialty hospitals, and only specialists practice there.

Beyond this, most hospitals want to be "accredited," that is, meet the minimal standards set by the Joint Commission on Accreditation of Hospitals. It is important to remember that this does mean *minimum,* and is not a badge of excellence.

Most health experts believe that the "best" hospitals today are the larger, private, voluntary, accredited, specialty hospitals that are affiliated with medical schools, that is, the "teaching" hospitals. We have already mentioned many of the reasons for this. It needs to be borne in mind that the distortions of specialization have helped create the distorted structure and services of the hospital. Paradoxical as it may appear, however, it seems to be the large teaching hospitals devoted to a single specialty that are the least interested in the patient's emotional needs. Where there are so many doctors, almost all of the same mind and very narrowly oriented, it is extremely difficult for an administration to become powerful enough to make rules of its own and be sufficiently responsive to the community.

Most hospital administrators do not have very much power to begin with, but the single-specialty hospital administrator sometimes seems to have even less in this area. Patients who come to these centers usually come either because they have an unusual problem or because they fear that one might arise, and that particular fear and anxiety makes them less willing to argue. Teaching hospitals depend on large, trusting patient populations to stay in business, and they are usually willing to make only the token concessions that will assure them this steady flow.

The general hospital, on the other hand, usually offers a whole range of services, some of them interlocking, and no one specialty voice is usually given precedence over another. Some administrators of such hospitals are very cognizant of the importance of the atmosphere and emotional tone of the hospital, and can make rules or take leadership steps to ensure that the hospital remains responsive to the consumer and the community. If you have a choice, consider a general hospital, teaching or otherwise, rather than a single-specialty hospital. This can also be a basis for selecting a physician. Look the hospitals over, talk with friends who have been to different places, and then ask for a staff list from your choices. If you have never been in a hospital, or if it's a long time since you've been in one, or even if you have expectations based on a very recent experience somewhere else, you really have no frame of reference for assessing another institution. It pays to investigate in advance, if possible.

Hospital Maternity Care

Some obstetricians have affiliations with only one hospital; others may have one or more additional affiliations. There are a number of ways to rate hospital maternity care. You want to be sure they are equipped to handle an emergency. If Board-certified obstetrician-gynecologists are willing to go there, the chances are good that it is equipped to handle an emergency. But remember, many more obstetrical emergencies are preventable than is commonly believed. And remember also that complications still occur only in at most 5–7 percent of all maternity cases. Chances are good that if you have had prenatal care you will be among the roughly 95 percent who deliver normally without complications.

Another way to rate a hospital is to find out how babies are cared for there after they arrive. Most of us are so used to the central nursery system that keeps babies segregated from their mothers except for four-hour feedings that we tend to suspect any other system of being unsafe. In fact, the new Massachusetts code for medical-care practice specifically provides that it is medically safe for mothers and fathers to care for their own babies at the bedside whenever they wish, provided certain simple precautions are taken.* Most hospitals, in spite of their best efforts, and even in spite of the liberal use of pHisoHex (in the years before the use of it was restricted in hospital nurseries), have recurrent outbreaks of staphylococcus infections. Though rarely fatal, the infection can make babies very sick, and can infect a whole family or even a whole community once the baby and mother are at home. The incubation period is such that the infection sometimes does not show up until they are home. A mother caring for her own baby in the hospital more or less continuously (and breast-feeding) offers the only preventive that has ever been shown to work consistently. This procedure is routine in most military hospitals, where the luxury of an epidemic is something they don't feel they can afford.

Staph is a hospital disease for the most part, carried mainly by hospital workers. While it is possible to treat staph, most of the current strains are highly resistant to antibiotics, and for a newborn infant both the treatment and the illness are better prevented.† It is a tragic fact that some of the largest and "best" maternity hospitals have constant problems with staph. Because they are large, they are believed to be safer, but the risks of epidemic are actually greater.

*"Regulations Concerning Newborn Care in Hospitals," Department of Public Health, Commonwealth of Massachusetts, January 12, 1971.

†Doris and John Haire, *Implementing Family-Centered Maternity Care with a Central Nursery,* 3rd ed. (1971), International Childbirth Education Association, Box 22, Hillside, N.J. 07205. Pp. IV-12.

The same questions about emergencies regarding the newborn also are involved when evaluating a hospital. Selecting a pediatrician in advance of birth really helps, and while many of the larger hospitals may not permit local G.P.s or pediatricians to come into a big hospital to examine your baby, most of the smaller hospitals will allow a pediatrician to do so. Most important is early and accurate diagnosis of any difficulties, so that the baby can either be treated or moved for treatment immediately.

If you go to a teaching hospital you must assume—particularly if you are a clinic patient—that some tests or experimental treatment may be given either to you or your newborn baby.* Ethical medical rules require your informed consent, but as we said earlier, you may not always be informed in an unbiased way.

People in academic medicine insist that they are the best in medicine because they have access to all the latest knowledge and equipment. While this may mean that you become one in a trial series of experimental cases involving something new that is later abandoned because of complications or side-effects, it may also mean that certain improvements and discoveries may not be used on you. Doctors in academe may read the study or know about the new method as reported by highly reputable colleagues in another setting, but they are under no obligation to apply this knowledge, and sometimes they even refuse.

For instance it has been known for a long, long time that there are risks to both mother and baby if labor and delivery goes on for many hours while the mother is lying flat on her back.† Several confirmatory studies have recently been carried out demonstrating more clearly than ever via the fetal monitors that the back position in labor is a distinct hazard.‡ Yet most United States Women are still required to labor and deliver on their backs in hospitals for the doctors' and nurses' convenience. One doctor we know insists on this practice to such an extent that his patients may not change their positions in labor even when they ask to do so, although the dangers have been directly and repeatedly brought to his attention! (For alternatives, see the chapter on "Childbirth.")

Continue to find out about the hospital. Does it give a really adequate tour of the maternity unit, including labor and delivery area? Is it willing to discuss its practices regarding care of the baby, the presence of a friend or father in the labor room, delivery room, and after-

ward? Does it provide adequate referrals to good classes, and to physicians who work with prepared couples? A hospital should have enough links with the community to be knowledgeable in these areas.

Hospitals: Summary

Because large teaching hospitals are so crowded and so busy, they are often dehumanizing. Many of us who live in big cities have had a lot of experience with them, both as private and clinic patients and it is part of the reason why some of us have sought out smaller community hospitals, sometimes with religious affiliations. In some of these places the atmosphere is warm and quite different from other hospitals even on a casual visit, and the way you are treated during your stay becomes an identifiable and central part of your whole medical care. For some of us this is more important than the prestige of the big, impersonal centers, and often we find here a respect for our feelings, or our ideas about food, or our different life styles. Many establishment hospitals seem to be filled with people who are hostile to all differences, and can be warm and accepting only to people exactly like themselves or what they would like to be.

There are unusually fine community hospitals, but there are still others that really should be closed, in which the procedures, the medical care, and the rules are hopelessly antiquated, and the administration is merely a figurehead, without any sense of responsibility to the community and its needs, acting as housekeeper to a group of physicians who are responsible to no one. It takes looking into.

Nursing care in big-city hospitals today, even in the "best" places, is often very disappointing, and it is tempting to believe, as we are so often told, that "It's the same everywhere." There is so much transience in most places, especially in the academic centers, that it's hard to keep any program of patient care alive and in the same hands for more than a year or two at most; and transience also leads to errors in care and medication. Six-month turnovers are common. When they feel it is safe to talk, some nurses are frank about their frustrations in working with uncommunicative, unappreciative, and rigid doctors, who handle relationships poorly with everyone, especially patients. These nurses sometimes have a tremendous idealism, which drives them to make proposals and create programs to improve things, only to have them voted down, underbudgeted or summarily scrapped by a group of doctors or even one doctor with the power to do so. The best way to describe the problem is as an absentee-landlord situation in which the doctor has all of the authority but none of the ongoing responsibility, is rarely available to the patient, and is only to be con-

---

*See Appendix A (p. 271 of this book): Preamble to 1970 edition of the *Accreditation Manual for Hospitals*.

†Doris Haire, "The Cultural Warping of Childbirth," International Childbirth Education Association special report (May 1972), references 61, 68-71 on pp. 21-22 of the report.

‡L. D. Longo and G. D. Power (Loma Linda Medical School), paper presented at the Society of Gynecologic Investigation, April 1970.

WHAT TO EXPECT FROM YOUR HOSPITAL

1. Clear explanations about all charges and fees, as much in advance as possible, item by item. Also, explanations of what your hospital understands about the coverage offered by your particular insurance policy (if any).

2. Answers to your questions about any tests and procedures performed in the hospital, their purpose and nature, costs and possible risks.

3. Acceptance of your refusal to sign waivers and permission forms, whether or not you understand them.

4. Explanation of any anesthesia services being anticipated: the purpose or necessity, the type of anesthesia used, the relative cost of this and other types, and by whom the anesthesia will be administered (the doctor himself, or another colleague; a nurse-anesthetist; or an anesthesiologist).

5. Answers to your questions about the content, purpose, known effects, possible risks and side-effects of any drugs ordered for you (either orally or by injection). Acceptance of your refusal to take any drug or medication, with or without an explanation.

6. Acceptance of your refusal to accept any procedure, at any time.

7. Clear explanations of the hospital's policies on visitors and family participation in care and companionship for the patient, including any reasons and sources of authority for exclusion of family members or any other helping person of the patient's choice.

8. Acceptance of your right to leave the hospital at any time you wish to do so, whether or not you have medical permission to do so, and whether or not all bills and charges have been paid.

tacted in a crisis by the nurse. The nurse, on the other hand, has all of the ongoing responsibility and virtually no authority. She sees real needs, but has no authority to establish ways to meet them.* Under these conditions it is not surprising that she often becomes cynical or takes on the closed, nonresponsive style of the doctors or the older nurses she works with, finally becoming shut off altogether.

Nursing is undergoing a revolution of its own that will hopefully take its place as part of the revolution of

*Constance Bean, "Hospital Administration and Implications for Patient Education: A Proposed Program for Maternity Patients," unpublished report (Harvard School of Health, January 1966).

women, but thus far the patient feels very little of its impact, and new "technicians" are being created each day to supplant nurses.

Physicians in smaller hospitals often have more stable relationships with their nurses, depend on them more, and therefore sometimes treat them better, even (occasionally) listening to their advice. But the quality is still uneven, and a lot of "shopping" is required to find out. Don't hesitate to ask for a tour of the hospital, or for a chance to discuss the nursing care with the Nursing Director or head nurse. They don't get many such investigative interviews, but they should be prepared to receive many more and to answer questions about how their programs for patient care are planned. Hospitals in which nurses have little or no domain of their own where they can make decisions or have a budget with which to improve things are much less likely to be satisfactory to patients.

There are doctors and hospitals that do not give good care both inside and outside the "establishment" of the university-linked or accredited system. Until all hospitals and all medical practitioners have consumer ratings and systems of consumer evaluation readily available to other potential consumers, the most dangerous assumption you can make is that you will automatically receive the "best" care in a particular place or from a particular man just because all the right credentials seem to be there.

The trend today is toward bigger and bigger hospitals, and academic medicine has worked hard to sell this notion to the public. It is easy to get the feeling that they are talking about a manufacturing plant, or perhaps, more appropriately, a meat-processing plant. What they are saying is that the industrialization of human care is a more "efficient" way of using the resources we have, such as providing ultra-expensive technology and the ultra-specialist, and they are suggesting that this efficiency will also produce better care for patients, because only people who exercise their skills on a regular basis can perform adequately, utilizing the best and latest equipment. They are also saying that hospital care should be regionalized, that modern transportation makes many small local units unnecessary duplications.*

What they have not considered, and may not plan to if they aren't obliged to, is that human services do not always work best if they are bigger, and in fact may only be able to reach a certain size before their very bigness becomes counterproductive, tending more to compound and increase errors than reduce them, while communication begins to break down altogether. Especially in the realm of family health or family medicine or health maintenance there is reason to believe that the bigger hospitals are more of a hindrance, to say nothing of ex-

*Richard Knox, "Hospital Beds," Boston *Globe*, October 10, 1971, p. 1.

posing people unnecessarily to the risks of such special, hospital-based infections as, for example, staphylococcus. Until there is better coordination among the specialists and better conditions for nurses—and even then—there will be a definite place for the small, high-quality community hospital. These are all factors that we as women and as consumers should consider carefully when making decisions about a doctor.

SECTION THREE:
COMMON MEDICAL PROBLEMS AND PROCEDURES

In order to keep ourselves healthy we need to know about common female diseases and disorders: what they are called, how to prevent them, how to detect them before they get serious, and how they are usually treated. In this way we can be less mystified by our doctors and know what to expect and require from them.

GLOSSARY OF COMMON MEDICAL TERMS

acute: Sudden and short-lived.

benign: Noncancerous.

biopsy: The removal of tissue for laboratory analysis. To diagnose cancer, tissue from a tumor is removed, by using a needle, by cutting the whole tumor out or by cutting into the tumor and removing part of it. The tissue may be frozen and examined under a microscope immediately or prepared for later examination. Benign and malignant tumors can be distinguished in this way.

chronic: Long-term, frequently recurrent.

culture: A sample from a discharge or other body fluid, such as urine, that is incubated in a laboratory to allow any organisms in it to multiply and be identified.

generic prescription: A prescription given using the general name for a drug or product instead of the brand name, e.g., tampons instead of Tampax. Many drugs are cheaper when a generic prescription is given. Sometimes the properties, or quality, of a specific brand are desired, so the brand name is used.

infection: An invasion by bacteria or other small animals (microorganisms).

inflammation: An area that is red, hot, and possibly painful. The blood vessels enlarge, allowing more blood to flow to the area to combat a disease and help heal the damaged tissue.

malignant: Cancerous.

morbid: Diseased.

Pap smear: Short for Papanicolaou smear. Tissue is gently scraped from the cervix and tested in a laboratory for cancer. You should not douche on the day a Pap smear is taken or on the day before. You should not have a Pap smear taken when you have a vaginal infection; treat it first. Since menstrual blood makes the cervical cells unanalyzable, doctors won't do a Pap smear when you have your period. Pap smears also test for conditions other than cancer.

pH: A measure of acidity and alkalinity. A pH of 7.0 is neutral. The stronger the acid, the lower the pH; the stronger the base (alkaline), the higher the pH. Tap water is very slightly acid.

pus: An accumulation of white blood cells (one of the body's weapons in fighting infections), bacteria, and dead cells.

tumor: An abnormal mass of tissue without inflammation.

HYGIENE

In females the anus, vagina, and urethra are located very close to one another. Because of this, bacteria and other microorganisms normally found in the intestine or vagina can easily contaminate another area. Both vaginitis and cystitis (described in this chapter) are often caused by organisms that normally inhabit other parts of the body.

In order to prevent vaginal and urinary infections you should follow several rules of hygiene:

1. Wash your vulva and bottom regularly.

2. Wear clean underpants every day.

3. Always wipe your bottom from front to back!

4. Avoid irritating soaps and sprays.

5. Use disposable tissue to cover the seats of public toilets.

6. Make sure your sexual partners are clean.

7. Use a sterile, water-soluble jelly if lubrication is needed during intercourse (something like K-Y Jelly, for example—not Vaseline).

8. "Don't put anything in your vagina you wouldn't put in your mouth," as the McGill *Birth Control Handbook* says.

Douches

The role douches should play in routine hygiene is not generally agreed upon. You do not have to douche ordinarily, but douching is often recommended in the treatment of vaginal infections. *Pregnant women should never douche.* Keep your douche bag and syringe clean. Don't use them for enemas or lend them to anyone else. Letting someone else use them may give you an infection.

To take a douche, fill a container with two quarts of quite warm—not hot—water and two tablespoons of vinegar, hang the container a foot or two above the floor of a bathtub or shower, and lie down. Insert the nozzle about one and a half inches into your vagina. Slowly release the clamp, so that the water doesn't rush into your vagina, then let the water run in and drain out. A stream of water that is too forceful can push water from the uterus through the fallopian tubes and into the abdominal cavity. Be gentle. Baking soda (1 tbs. per quart) is sometimes suggested instead of vinegar. Fancy additions are totally unnecessary. Don't use harsh substances that can irritate the tissues.

VAGINAL INFECTIONS (VAGINITIS)

All women secrete moisture and mucus from the membranes that line the vagina. This discharge is transparent or slightly milky and may be somewhat slimy. When dry, it may be yellowish. When a woman is sexually aroused, this secretion increases. It normally causes no irritation or inflammation of the vagina or vulva. If you want to examine your own discharge, collect a sample from inside your vagina—with a washed finger of course. It is easiest to see if you smear it on glass.

Many bacteria grow in the vagina of a normal, healthy woman. They help keep the vagina acid, which kills yeasts, fungi, and other harmful organisms. Anything that upsets this balance may cause some organisms to multiply all out of proportion. Like all living things, bacteria give off waste products. Excesses of these waste products may irritate the nearby tissues. An abnormal discharge, mild or severe itching and burning of the vulva, chafing of the thighs, and frequency in urination often result. Unusual conditions in the vagina that can lead to an infection may result from a general lowered resistance (from another infection or disease in your body, a bad diet, lack of sleep, or other such factors); antibiotics (eating yogurt while taking antibiotics may help prevent an infection); excessive douching; pregnancy; birth-control pills and other hormones; diabetes; cuts, abrasions, and other irritations in the vagina (from childbirth, frequent infections, intercourse without enough

lubrication, or the use of an instrument medically or for masturbation).

In order to prevent vaginal infection you should follow the recommendations in regard to hygiene given above. When treating a vaginal infection you should:

1. Avoid scratching! It will irritate the tissue and cause the infection to spread.

2. Check with your doctor about taking mildly acid douches. Some women find that packing the vagina with yogurt works even better.

3. Pat your vulva dry after bathing, and keep it dry.

4. Wear cotton underpants or none at all. Nylon underwear or pantyhose retain moisture and heat, which help the infecting organisms to grow.

5. Avoid pants that are tight in the crotch and thighs.

6. Abstain from sex. Sexual activity can irritate the already fragile tissues and can force the infecting organisms up into the uterus and fallopian tubes.

7. If you don't want to give up sex, use a condom during treatment, and possibly some time afterward, to prevent infecting the man, who might then reinfect you or infect someone else.

8. Warn your sexual partners that they, too, may have gotten infected.

9. Do not stop following your doctor's directions as soon as the symptoms disappear; further treatment is often needed to really cure vaginitis.

If you get vaginitis, discuss this list with your doctor, since various points are not extensively discussed in the following sections.

Yeast Infection (also called Candidiasis or Moniliasis)

Candida albicans (monilia), called yeast (a fungus), grows normally in harmless quantities in your rectum and vagina. When your system is out of balance the yeastlike organisms may grow profusely and cause a vaginal discharge that is thick and white, and may look like cottage cheese and smell like baking bread. If a woman has a yeast infection when she gives birth, the baby will get yeasts in its digestive tract. This is called thrush and is treated orally with nystatin drops.

Yeast infections can sometimes be stopped with a mildly acid douche taken at the first signs. If a yeast infection does not go away, oral doses or vaginal suppositories of nystatin are prescribed for about three weeks. There are no side-effects from the suppositories, and they can be used when you are pregnant. Other methods of treating yeast infections include various prescription creams, or painting the vagina, cervix, and vulva with gentian violet. This is bright purple and stains, so wear a sanitary pad. It is messy, but really helps, except in occasional cases when there is a severe reaction to gentian violet. Yeast infections recur often! Even if you are checked a week after treatment and your infection has gone, you may find it back after your next period.

Trichomoniasis

Trichomonas vaginalis, called Trich, is a one-celled parasite that can be found in both men and women who have no symptoms. Generally, though, women with Trich have a vaginal discharge that is thin and foamy, is yellowish-green or gray in color, and has a foul odor. If other organisms are also causing the infection, the discharge may be thicker and whiter. Trich can also cause a urinary infection. Trich is most often contracted through intercourse (the man must be treated too), but can be passed on by moist objects such as towels, bathing suits, underwear, and washcloths.

Trich is usually treated with oral doses of metronidazole (Flagyl) for ten days—an expensive (only one company makes it!) and potent drug. Flagyl should not be used if you have a history of blood diseases, a disease of the central nervous system, or another infection at the same time. Since Flagyl kills some white blood cells, you should wait about six weeks before taking it again. Have a white-blood-cell count done before, during, and after taking it a second time. You can have only one glass a day of beer or wine while on Flagyl. You may notice darkening of your urine, nausea, diarrhea, cramps, or dizziness, and you may develop a yeast infection. If you are pregnant or nursing you should only use Flagyl suppositories.

Nonspecific Vaginitis

Other vaginal infections are often called nonspecific vaginitis. The discharge may be white or yellow and streaked with blood. The walls of the vagina can be cloudy, puffy with fluid, and covered by a thick, heavy coat of pus. The first sign of an infection may be appearance of cystitislike symptoms. There may be lower back pain, cramps, and swollen glands in the abdomen and thighs. It is usually treated with sulfa creams or suppositories (Vagitrol, Sultrin, AVC Cream). Other treatments are available for people allergic to sulfa.

One kind of vaginitis, formerly diagnosed as nonspecific, is now believed to be caused by *Hemophilus vaginalis.* The symptoms are similar to those in Trich. A sulfa cream is likely to be prescribed.

Atrophy, or Senile Vaginitis

See chapter on "Menopause" (especially "Sex and Menopause") for the effects of a menopausal lack of estrogen on a woman's vagina, and for possible treatments.

CRABS, OR PUBIC LICE

Phthirus pubis is a roundish, crablike body louse that lives in pubic hair, and occasionally in the hair of the chest, armpits, eyelashes, and eyebrows. You can "catch" them by intimate physical contact with someone else who has them, or from bedding or clothes which that person has used. They are bloodsuckers and can carry such diseases as typhus. The main symptom of crabs is an intolerable itching in the genital area; they are easily diagnosed, because crabs are visible without a microscope. The cure is a simple but very expensive white cream (Kwell), which works very quickly and effectively.

ENDOMETRIOSIS

The endometrium is a special kind of tissue that grows in the lining of the uterus each month for the nourishment of a fertilized egg. If no egg gets implanted, the endometrium is sloughed off. This is menstruation. Endometriosis results when endometrial tissue grows somewhere other than in the lining of the uterus, usually in the genital, urinary, or intestinal organs. Doctors disagree about why this happens. Endometriosis is quite common during the childbearing years, particularly during the thirties.

The symptoms of endometriosis vary, depending on the location of the extra endometrium. Menstrual pain is the most common symptom, although other pains may occur. Diagnosis is hard in the early stages and the condition is not usually suspected without menstrual pain or an endometrial cyst large enough to feel.

If endometriosis is diagnosed and you are planning to have children, you may want to have them as soon as possible, since some doctors believe that the ovaries or tubes may become blocked, depending on the location of the extra tissue. Usually infertility is the most serious consequence of endometriosis.

Endometriosis will go away by itself at menopause or when the ovaries are removed if no estrogen compounds are taken. Estrogen, produced by the ovaries during the childbearing years, is responsible for the building of the endometrial tissue. Treatment of endometriosis may involve removal of the endometrial cyst or some part of the affected organ; sometimes hormones are given. If the only symptom is severe pain with your period, certain pelvic nerves may be removed (presacral neurectomy).

CERVICAL EROSION

Sometimes a woman may develop a large or small sore on the cervix beside the cervical opening. This is called cervical erosion and may produce a heavy vaginal discharge. Treatment for cervical erosion is called cauterizing (burning the open flesh in order to seal it), but doctors disagree as to whether or not this treatment is really necessary. Some feel that cauterizing does no good and that the erosion does no harm. Others believe that cauterizing lowers the incidence of cervical cancer. Properly done cauterizing is painless. If you develop cervical erosion, you must decide along with your doctor whether or not treatment would be best for you.

CYSTITIS

Cystitis is an inflammation of the bladder. Sometime in her life nearly every woman gets it, and it can be hard to eradicate permanently. It usually means that intestinal bacteria, such as *Escherichia coli* (*E. coli*), useful in the digestive tract, have gotten into the urine. Trich can also cause cystitis. The symptoms can be really frightening, but it is not a serious condition. If you suddenly have to urinate every few minutes, and it burns like crazy even though almost nothing comes out, you probably have cystitis. There may also be blood in the urine (hematuria) and pus in the urine (pyuria). You may have pain just above your pubic bone, and sometimes there is a peculiar, heavy urine odor when you first urinate in the morning.

If these symptoms develop, you should see a doctor, although the infection may disappear without treatment. You can help relieve the symptoms before you see the doctor:

1. Drink *lots* of water, enough to pour out a good stream of urine every hour. It really helps!
2. Avoid coffee and tea; they irritate the bladder.
3. Soak in a hot tub two or three times a day.
4. Try a hot-water bottle or heating pad on your abdomen and back.

If you have chronic cystitis and expect to be distant from medical help, you can get a prescription for Pyridium. It relieves the symptoms, but does not affect the bacteria. It makes your urine bright orange, and a stain is permanent, so guard against drips.

The doctor will ask for a urine sample, so drink before your visit. If it is during your period, you may be catheterized (have a tube inserted in your urethra) to get a clean specimen. Treatment may begin immediately with Gantrisin (a sulfa drug), although it is often delayed a couple of days until the offending bacteria and the drugs they are sensitive to can be identified. Tetracycline, nitrofurantoin (get a generic prescription), or ampicillin are also commonly used.

Full treatment may take two weeks, but the symptoms should disappear in a day or so. If they don't, return to the doctor. Some bacteria are resistant to and even thrive

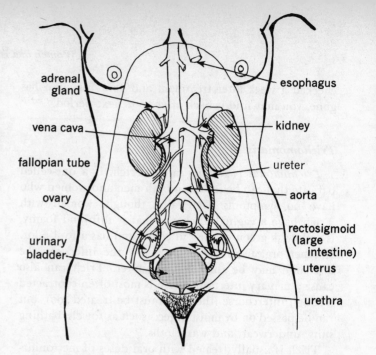

on some of the drugs. You may be asked to control the pH of your urine by drinking cranberry juice or taking vitamin C (both are acid). This is important, since some drugs do not work well when the urine pH is not in the right range. Vaginitis and some digestive upset are common side-effects. Nausea may be decreased by taking the medication with meals.

Like vaginitis, cystitis is more likely to occur when your resistance is low. Damage to the urethra from nearby surgery, childbirth, or intercourse may also make you more susceptible to infection. Women who urinate infrequently or people who are catheterized for a long period or frequently (such as diabetics) often develop cystitis. If your cystitis recurs frequently, consult a urologist, as a serious abnormality may be present.

Cystitis is sometimes, though not always, sex-related. The first time you have intercourse with a particular man or have intercourse after a long period of abstinence, you may get a sudden attack of urethritis (inflammation of the urethra), often called "honeymoon cystitis." In some cases, this can lead to true cystitis.

Women sometimes have bacteria in their urine (bacteriuria) without any symptoms, so you should have a urine test with your gynecological exam. An ordinary urine analysis is not sufficient to test for cystitis—make sure your doctor takes a clean voided specimen. If cystitis and bacteriuria are not treated, kidney infection and such complications as high blood pressure or premature birth may result.

For prevention, follow the general hygiene rules given on page 259 and drink enough to urinate several times throughout the day. If you have a chronic problem, there are several things you can do that doctors don't always mention.

* * *

After several months of nearly continuous cystitis attacks, my urologist slit a narrowed area in my urethra to help drainage (internal urethrotemy). I had only one infection in the next three years; then the same story began all over. My second operation did not help at all.

I consulted another doctor, who, while recognizing the importance of checking for serious abnormalities, also stressed the benefits of drinking lots of water. I now drink enough to urinate every hour or two (ten glasses a day, sometimes more). Ten glasses! Impossible, I thought. But it is better than drugs and not too hard if you work up to it. Take a drink whenever you urinate. I also wash my vulva every day and keep my urine pH at about 5.0 to 5.5 to inhibit bacterial growth. (Use phenaphthazine paper to check it.) In the year since I began this program I have had only two infections (when I slipped up on precautions) and nipped a minor one by using these tactics.

* * *

If you suffer from chronic cystitis, you should also make sure the hands and penis of your sexual partners are clean, and avoid stretching or traumatizing the urethra during intercourse. Finally, get a urine culture every three to six months.

One form of cystitis (interstitial cystitis, or Hunner's ulcer) is not associated with bacteriuria. It is found mostly in postmenopausal women and may be psychosomatic, but may be related to genital and hormonal changes that alter the mucus of the lower urinary tract. It is very difficult to treat.

CANCER

The thought of any kind of cancer is terrifying to most of us. As women we are particularly concerned with cancer of the breasts or reproductive organs. If we get one of these cancers, not only do we have to face our own mortality, but even when we recover, the treatment may mean the loss of a part of us that has played an important role in our definition of ourselves. The prospect of a prolonged, painful illness is also brought to mind. It is foolish to avoid these thoughts; in facing them we face life and its meaning. But we should not let them overpower us..

Cancer is now a leading cause of death in women. Cancer occurs when cells in some part of the body become abnormal and reproduce rapidly. Eventually they invade the bloodstream and lymphatic system and travel to other parts of the body. This is called metastasis. To be cured, cancer must be caught early while it is still localized. Routine breast and pelvic examinations, including a Pap smear, are the best way to do this.

The exact causes of cancer are still unknown. Viruses are the nearly unanimous suspects, although certain cell

irritants, or carcinogens, increase the likelihood of cancer. For example, tobacco tars may produce lung cancer. Prolonged exposure to X rays may lead to cancer. Psychological factors may also be important. The breasts, cervix, and dark moles develop cancer more often than other parts of a woman's body.

Breast Cancer

One-fifth of all cancer in women is breast cancer. It is the most common cancer women get. If breast cancer is caught *early*, however, it is rarely fatal. In nine cases out of ten when the disease is treated before metastasis into the nearby lymph nodes occurs, there is no recurrence. The real bugaboo here is that in six out of every ten breast cancers this metastasis occurs within a *month* after the tumor is detected. There is rarely any pain in the early stages, so all women should *examine their breasts regularly*. Treatment can then begin as soon as possible. If treatment is delayed until after metastasis occurs, only five out of every ten women have no recurrence. And the longer you wait, the grimmer the picture gets. Early treatment also ensures fairly fast recovery.

Women who suspect they have breast cancer are often afraid to face it and delay seeking medical help. These fears are quite real and understandable, but the delay in action is foolish. Only one breast tumor in four is malignant. But if you have that one, you should know right away and get treatment immediately.

Don't touch a suspected tumor repeatedly, as this may cause the cancer to spread.

A lot of research is being done into possible causes of breast cancer. Some of the many factors under investigation are:

1. Breast-feeding. Seems to lower a woman's chances of getting breast cancer. Certain societies where breast-feeding is the norm (like Japan) have a lower incidence of breast cancer.

2. Diet. The high iodine intake of Japanese women (fish eaters) may be a reason for their lower rate of breast cancer.

3. Woman's age at first childbirth. Earlier childbirth may lower breast cancer rate.

4. Heredity. Tendency to get breast cancer seems to be inherited.

5. Hormone levels. Specific types of estrogen and their levels in a given woman's body or in a given female population are being investigated as possible influential factors in the development of breast cancer.

Breast self-examination. The first principle in examining your breasts is to do it regularly—once a month is usually suggested. Thinking you have to do it more often can make you obsessed with the disease. Since your

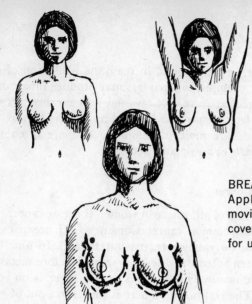

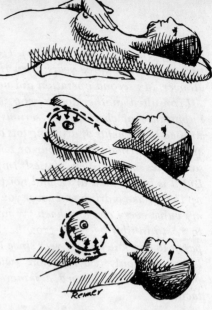

BREAST SELF-EXAM.
Applying pressure with fingers,
moving in direction of arrows and
covering one section at a time. Feel
for unusual lumps or hardness.

breasts will be different at different times in your menstrual cycle, examine them at the same time each month. A few days after menstruation is good, since they will then be at a minimum of fullness, and it will be easier to detect any unusual lumps. After a few examinations you will become quite familiar with the shape and texture of your own breasts, and will probably be able to detect an abnormality better than many doctors, who have to take into account the wide variation in the breasts of different women. For films and literature on breast self-examination write the American Cancer Society. (National office: 219 E. 42 St., New York, N. Y. 10017; telephone: 212-867-3700.)

First stand in front of a mirror and view your breasts with your hands at your sides; then with hands raised above your head; with hands pushing firmly on your hips or with both palms pressed against each other. Good lighting will make the examination easier. You should look for differences in shape (not size) in both breasts: for a flattening or bulging in one, but not the other; for puckering of the skin; for a discharge from a nipple when it is gently squeezed; and for a reddening or scaly crust on a nipple. You should also be suspicious when one nipple is particularly hard or inelastic, or when the two nipples point in asymmetric directions. Many nipple asymmetries are not due to cancer, but it is better to check. Make sure a sore on a nipple is investigated for cancer before assuming it is merely a skin disorder.

Next, lie down on a bed or couch. (Or you may want to perform this part of the exam in a bathtub, with soapy fingers.) Examine each breast with the arm on that side raised above your head or with the corresponding hand under your head and the elbow lying flat. A small pillow or large folded towel placed under your shoulder will distribute the breast tissue more evenly. Also examine each breast with the arm lying along your side or hanging over the edge of the bed.

Feel your breast gently and systematically with the flat of the fingers of the opposite hand. Move your fingers in small circles or with a slight back-and-forth motion, covering the entire breast with a broader motion. The most common location of tumors is between the nipple and armpit, so give special attention to that area.

The indication that should lead you to consult a doctor is anything that seems abnormal compared with how your breast usually looks and feels at that time of the month. (General thickening, pain, or tenderness are likely to occur normally just before or during your periods.) Cancer often causes a thickening in a specific area. A discrete, round, hard lump might be a noncancerous cyst but should still be checked by a doctor.

Treatment of breast cancer. Cancer of the breast usually spreads into the lymphatic system before it reaches the bloodstream. Lymphatics are thin-walled vessels that form a network from the breast to certain glands called lymph nodes. These vessels drain tissue fluids from the breast, including fluids which may contain cancerous cells. The lymph nodes which are first affected by cancerous cells are near the armpit, under the sternum, or along the upper spine. Until recently, only metastasis in the armpit nodes was considered important. However, it has become clear that the nodes under the sternum and along the spine are also important places for metastasis to occur. Adequate treatment of breast cancer must consider all three areas.

The traditional policy, and still most common procedure, when a breast tumor is detected is to send a woman into surgery as soon as possible, obtain a piece of the tumor (an open biopsy), examine it while the woman is still asleep on the table, and then, if it is malignant, remove the entire breast, and sometimes tissue in the armpits or under the chest wall (a radical mastectomy: removal of arm muscles may make physical therapy necessary). The biopsy is now one of the most common operations performed on women, but only a small proportion of the lumps turn out to be malignant.

Though standard procedure for many surgeons, a radical mastectomy is not the only and not always the best treatment for breast cancer. In cases where the lump is very small (less than one inch in diameter), it is sometimes sufficient to perform a lumpectomy (removal of the lump and some surrounding tissue). This operation is most likely to be successful when the lump is on the inside of the breast, thereby reducing the possibility that the cancer has spread to the lymph nodes by the armpit. Another procedure used to remove small lumps is the "simple" mastectomy (removal of the breast alone). During this operation, after the breast is removed the surgeon can feel the armpit nodes and remove whichever ones are enlarged (and, therefore, possibly cancerous). Just to be safe, some surgeons remove whatever nodes they can reach whether or not they are enlarged (called a modified radical mastectomy). This is a very useful practice, since the nodes can then be examined for cancerous cells and, if necessary, further treatment can be considered (for example, radiation therapy of the nodes and surrounding tissue). An important drawback of a lumpectomy or simple mastectomy is that you never know for sure if metastasis has occurred in the armpit nodes. To know this, at least a section of the nodes must be removed and examined.

In cases where the lump is fairly large, there are a number of possible treatments. Some doctors recommend a radical mastectomy. Others recommend a superradical mastectomy, which involves removal of the breast, all the armpit glands, the underlying muscles of the chest wall, and the nodes under the sternum. (This operation is fairly risky, since the chest wall must be opened.) Still other doctors prefer to do a lumpectomy followed by radiation therapy. They argue that if the cancer has probably spread to the nodes along the spine (and this is more likely with a very large malignant lump), then any kind of mastectomy still will not eliminate all the cancer.

There are other kinds of treatments, including hormones and anti-cancer drugs. But the important thing to remember is that breast cancer is still not very well understood, that probably no one treatment is clearly the best one, and that your feelings about losing a breast or receiving radiation or taking general anesthesia are all important considerations in making any decision.

Remember, also, that the doctor must have your permission for anything s/he does to you. If s/he refuses to consider alternative treatments or you do not feel that you can trust him or her, don't hesitate to change doctors. Speed is important, however, so if you change doctors, do it fast and get as much information as you can from local health groups, hospitals, and other women.

* * *

I discovered a lump in my breast and went to my doctor.

He wanted me to go into surgery within three days and wanted my permission to remove the breast if the tumor was found malignant. I found the whole process frightening and decided to find out if another procedure would be possible for me. I went to another doctor, who first did a needle biopsy* that proved inconclusive. Then he did a diagnostic lumpectomy with local anesthetic at the hospital, while my daughter was in for something minor. I was able to leave in three hours with my daughter and was saved the whole agonizing performance of going into surgery not knowing what was going to happen to me. The lump was found benign, and I have since had a lump in the other breast similarly removed.

* * *

Remember: you have a choice about having your breast removed. You don't have to choose between immediate, painful death and breastlessness when you first discover a lump. It is probably not malignant, but if it is, you will have a better chance, whatever treatment you elect, if you seek help at once. Also, the earlier you get help, the less tissue will need to be removed. Don't be afraid to examine your breasts, and consult a doctor if you find something unusual.

Cervical Cancer

Cervical cancer is the second most common cancer in women. About one woman in a hundred will get it, and half of these will die from it. It may occur at any age, but is most common between the ages of forty-five and fifty. Women who get cervical cancer tend to have begun having intercourse earlier than women who don't get it, but these women generally belong to lower socioeconomic groups, so they may not have been getting as good medical care throughout their lives. Women with chronic vaginal and cervical infections get cervical cancer more often than others. Women whose husbands were circumcised in childhood get it less often than other women. Nuns and other virgins rarely get it.

Cancer of the cervix can be detected by a Pap smear (see p. 259). Since it does not progress as rapidly as breast cancer, a Pap test once or twice a year is adequate. Make this a habit by the time you are twenty-five. A biopsy should be performed on all abnormal areas of the cervix.

Treatment may involve removal of the uterus (hysterectomy, see p. 267), the ovaries, and the fallopian tubes. Radiation and drugs are also used.

Other Female Cancers

Postmenopausal women who are diabetic or obese are

*In fact, this was not a true needle biopsy, but just a test to see whether or not the lump contained any fluid. If it had, then it clearly would have been nonmalignant. Some doctors object to this procedure because of the possibility of spreading cancerous cells.

especially prone to cancer of the body of the uterus. This condition tends to run in families, and delayed menopause, with irregular bleeding, is sometimes associated with it. These women should watch closely for abnormal bleeding, since a Pap smear often fails to detect this form of cancer.

Cancer can affect the vagina and vulva, but both such cancers are rare. They are usually the result of the spreading of cervical cancer, and mostly occur in women over sixty.

Cancer of the ovaries is hard to find until it becomes a lump that can be felt. It is more often fatal than the other cancers. Ovarian cancer can occur at any age, but it is a fairly rare occurrence. Ovarian tumors are often not malignant. They may produce either male or female hormones, which can cause physical changes in your body. Once a tumor is detected, it is either removed or watched to see if it gets bigger. Some just go away. If a tumor is malignant, many doctors consider it safest to remove the ovaries, tubes, and womb, just in case the cancer has spread. If it is not malignant, as little as possible of the affected ovary should be removed.

The Gynecological Exam

Early detection of cancer greatly increases the chances of successful treatment, so it is important to get a check-up every year until you are forty, then every six months thereafter. Exams twice a year are sometimes recommended for women taking birth-control pills. Routine exams are also important to discover many other unusual conditions. A gynecological exam may also be in order if you have abnormal bleeding. Any passed blood

PLACEMENT OF SPECULUM FOR A PELVIC EXAM. Spatula scrapes cervix for Pap smear (this is painless).

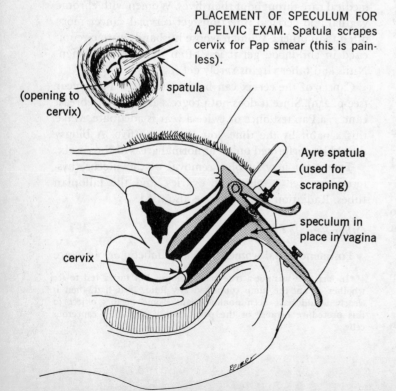

(opening to cervix)

spatula

Ayre spatula (used for scraping)

speculum in place in vagina

cervix

clots and tissues should be saved and taken to the doctor for examination. Do not douche before having the exam, and it is a good idea for you to empty the rectum before you go for it, so that the organs may be palpated (felt) more easily. You should be asked for a urine sample, so drink before you go to the appointment, and empty the bladder when you give the sample.

A good exam should include: (1) temperature-, weight-, and pulse-taking, and blood-pressure measurements; (2) a general medical history (on a first visit), including a review of past and present diseases, allergies, unusual symptoms, and so on; (3) a gynecological history, including information about menstruation, pregnancy, abortions, birth-control methods, previous infections, diseases, and operations; (4) a physical exam, including an examination of the heart, eyes, ears, throat, lungs, breasts, and abdominal organs; and (5) a pelvic, or internal, exam. Samples should be taken for: (1) a Pap test; (2) an examination of any unusual discharge; (3) a test for gonorrhea, which should be part of your routine check-up—a culture is more accurate than a simple "gram stain"; (4) blood analysis for white- and red-cell counts, and blood sugar (to detect anemia, mononucleosis, and diabetes), and a special test in case you have been exposed to syphilis; (5) urine tests (for a urinary infection and diabetes: urine test is often done only if you report some symptoms).

If you will be more at ease during the exam, ask a friend to accompany you. You may also ask for a nurse, receptionist, or another woman to be present during the exam. For the pelvic exam the doctor will ask you to lie on a table with your feet up in stirrups. All parts of the genitals should be checked for growths, damage, and signs of infection. After examining the external parts, the doctor will insert a speculum (see diagram) in the vagina. It holds the walls of the vagina open so that the inside is easily seen. Breathing deeply to relax may make you more comfortable. The vagina and cervix can now be examined for any discharge and other abnormalities. The doctor should then put on sterile rubber gloves and insert two fingers into your vagina. With the other hand on your abdomen, s/he will gently feel the various organs for any abnormalities. You should be told if your uterus is tipped or tilted. This is not unhealthy, but some people think it can cause problems in pregnancy or abortion. A similar exam, with one finger in the rectum, may be performed on a virgin. However, one finger can usually be inserted into the vagina of a virgin without pain. A special speculum is used for a virgin. You may also be examined with one finger in the rectum and one in the vagina. If you are relaxed, a pelvic exam should not hurt.

You may feel that there is something unpleasant, or "dirty," about a pelvic exam, but there is nothing "dirty" about doing everything you can to maintain your health. Being examined by a doctor who is brusque and insensi-

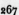

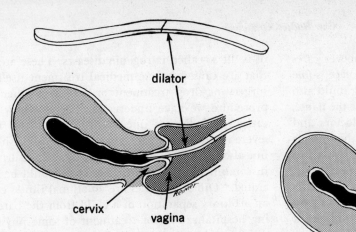

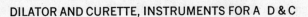

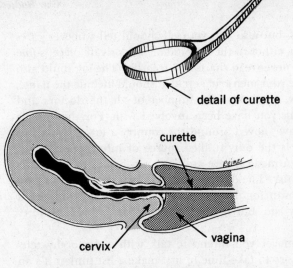

DILATOR AND CURETTE, INSTRUMENTS FOR A D & C

tive, or who acts disapproving of your sex life, *can* be unpleasant. For your first pelvic exam especially, try to go to a doctor who has been recommended to you as careful, accepting and gentle. Your feeling tense about the exam can tighten the entrance to your vagina and make the exam painful, so be sure to relax. (When you find yourself in that unfamiliar spread-knee position at the end of the examining table, remember that your gynecologist sees many, many vaginas every day.) The doctor should tell you everything s/he is doing. If not, asking questions will teach you about your body and also help you to relax.

DILATATION AND CURETTAGE (D & C)

A D & C may be performed for many reasons. As a method of abortion, it has been largely replaced by the suction method. It may be performed for infertility (some doctors question its usefulness) and to prevent the spread of infection following an incomplete abortion or delivery. Some doctors perform one routinely before most major gynecological operations. It is also used to diagnose cancer of the uterus and fallopian tubes, the cause of abnormal uterine bleeding or discharge, or a pregnancy outside the uterus. Sometimes a cone of tissue from

the cervix is also removed (conization). This may lead to complications in future pregnancies.

In a D & C the cervical opening is first increased in size (dilated) by inserting several probes of increasing size. Care must be taken to prevent puncturing the uterus. The womb is then gently scraped with a curette, a metal loop on the end of a long, thin handle. The patient is totally anesthetized and requires from six hours to two days to recuperate. During this time there may be some bleeding.

HYSTERECTOMY

A hysterectomy is the removal of the uterus, but it is often used as a quick way of referring to removal of the ovaries, fallopian tubes, and cervix as well (a pan-hystero-salpingo-oophorectomy). An oophorectomy is removal of the ovaries. A salpingectomy is removal of the fallopian tubes. Most hysterectomies are performed because of the presence of uterine fibroids. Fibroids are benign tumors and are not dangerous as long as they remain small. Most of your estrogen is produced by the ovaries, so if they are removed, estrogen may be prescribed for you. (See chapter on "Menopause" for estrogen-deficiency symptoms and treatment.)

SECTION FOUR:
HOW TO COPE AND ORGANIZE

From all that we've said it can be seen that the way for women to begin getting better care is to learn to negotiate this nonsystem while they are still reasonably well and healthy. One reason for choosing a doctor before you really need one is to be in contact with someone who can refer to your medical record (if not to a relationship) when you are ill, someone who can also get you into a hospital in a hurry if you need one. But that someone should be as close to a generalist as possible; someone who understands as much about the entire body system

and its interrelationships as possible, and not a doctor with a narrow interest in one body part or system.

It is very useful to keep a kind of log, or dated record book, on yourself, making entries whenever there are unusual physical events, or symptoms, or visits to a doctor, or course of medication started, or any other facts relating to your body worth marking down. Any unusual reactions to drugs should be noted, with the time sequences. (Especially if you are allergic to any drug, you should make sure it is entered into all your medical records, but also you yourself should tell whoever cares for you, either in the hospital or in a private office; some people never read charts and records.) The log could also include your menstrual cycle. It should include the name, address, and telephone number of all the doctors and hospitals you have been involved with. For those of us who have moved around the country a lot, this kind of record is the only unified source of information about our own medical care and our own bodies that has any continuity. The doctor's record is still sacrosanct. There was reason for this in a small-town or rural practice a century ago, but it can be a real barrier to continuity today.

Whenever you intend to talk with a doctor by telephone, try to take time to first make a list (unless it's an emergency) of what you want to ask him or report to him—and keep a record of his answers. Also take a list with you when you make office visits and refer to all the points on it no matter how trivial the questions or symptoms may suddenly seem to you when you get there. Remember, you are paying for the doctor's time. As we have said earlier, far too many doctors have varying standards of health for us and may be likely to dismiss serious symptoms as "neurotic complaints." Ask the doctor why certain procedures are done if you don't understand.

If this is true for office visits and phone calls, it is doubly important for a hospital stay. The blood tests may have been ordered but not actually done before they wheel you off to surgery, and only you may know this. Also, when you go to the hospital, be sure to have with you a lightweight robe or wrapper and a roll of dimes, so you can get to the phone and the outside world or your doctor, if you need or want to, without being embarrassed by a hospital johnny open all the way up the back. (See "What to Expect from Your Hospital," p. 258).

If medications are prescribed, ask doctors to be sure to write down the generic rather than the brand name of a drug whenever possible; and if you are told it isn't possible, ask the reason. Many doctors often cannot give a valid reason why the more expensive, elaborately advertised drug "seems better." Request that the name of the drug and clear instructions be written on the label, because of the risk to others who may take it in error, and also because when traveling you may be challenged at times for possession of pills. Whenever you can, insist on being billed for care, and if you do pay in cash, always insist on having a receipt.

"Shop" drugstores too. Studies have shown that many drugstores in poorer neighborhoods charge more than those in better neighborhoods.*

Another area in medical care we all need to be aware

of is the so-called iatrogenic diseases. These are diseases that are caused by the medical treatment itself, by the surgery or drug treatment or whatever other kind of procedure we have undergone. There is now a whole category of diseases due to drug treatment, not only severe reactions to a particular drug, so-called side-effects, but also diseases that are caused by certain drugs given in combination which in themselves would be well tolerated.* Other examples are emotional illness caused by an arbitrary separation of a child from the parents during hospitalization for treatment of some physical condition; violent or even fatal reactions to an anesthetic given for a surgical procedure that would otherwise be safely tolerated; and many, many of the obstetrical procedures that are either routine or unnecessarily interfering, causing problems from which the mother or the baby then has to be rescued. The average woman and consumer is quite insulated from this kind of information.

The failure of so many doctors to communicate even on a barely adequate and honest level with their patients is partly responsible for the recent reported upsurge in malpractice suits; a lawsuit is literally the only form of communication some doctors seem capable of responding to. One expert has even suggested that without the legal process medical-practice standards would deteriorate.† This statement implies, of course, that other existing mechanisms for keeping a man on his toes and making him justify his actions and decisions are not working very well. The much-touted "peer review" is clearly not reaching the issues concerning the patient. We know that there are many, many women whose stories make it clear that they had ample grounds for suing their doctors and should have done so. They either didn't know how, didn't have records, or didn't want to, but most of all they couldn't afford it; a lawsuit is a recourse of the affluent, who know how to negotiate the system. There is now a presidential commission to investigate the rise in malpractice suits,‡ largely because they increase the cost of malpractice-insurance premiums—a cost that the doctor predictably passes on to his patients, thus driving up the cost of medical care for all of us. Women everywhere can improve their chances of satisfaction through the courts by keeping better personal medical records and working with women lawyers to set up better guidelines for suits.

We are saying this: Knowledge is power. To get control of your own life and your own destiny is the first and most important task, which can also be the effort of a whole lifetime. But it begins with getting control of

*Alex Gerber, *The Gerber Report* (New York: David McKay Co., Inc., 1971), pp. 158-59.

*Robert H. Moser, "Diseases Due to Drug Treatment," in "The Medicated Society" (Lowell Lectures, Boston, March 1967).

†"Injury Prevention a Steady Concern," *ACOG Bulletin*, Vol. 15, No. 5, May 1971, pp. 6-7.

‡HEW News Release (A86), U.S. Department of Health, Education and Welfare, Office of Public Affairs, August 22, 1971.

your own body everywhere in your life. Demand answers and explanations from the people you come in contact with for medical care; know your right to refuse treatment with or without these answers and explanations; and insist on enough information to negotiate the system instead of allowing the system to negotiate you.

There are some other ways of approaching the situation. One is to make a concerted effort with your friends to tackle the common problems you may have with particular doctors or hospitals, and also the problems that you may need resolved that perhaps a doctor will not or cannot help you with.

Keep records of everything that happens to you and also to other women you know. Form groups to learn facts and share experiences. If you find when you go to a doctor or a clinic that you are always left with a sense of confusion about what was said or how you were really being treated, bring a friend with you the next time, someone who can support you and be strong in demanding your rights.

The only other method available is to organize on the community level—form women's groups, welfare-rights groups, church groups, students' associations, and so on—and agree to form subgroups based on the common denominator of being patients at the same hospital or clinic or even of the same group of physicians. In no other way can women get any kind of reasonable grip on what is really rotten in the system that claims it is serving them. Even now there are some new health-care plans that purport to give a single standard of care to a whole population, but almost none of them have provided any mechanisms for the consumers to take action as consumers or as members of a community. There is no way of knowing whether the care is single-standard or not, since the recipients are purposely kept isolated from one another and are represented by token consumers, selected by the care-givers rather than by the consumers themselves. Under this system there is no mechanism whatever whereby consumers can either rate or affect the quality of the care they receive.

One of the large national insurance companies that was asked to pay for clinic care sent young women into some of the "best" gyn teaching clinics in one city with tiny, concealed tape recorders in order to try to verify the reports they were receiving about degrading treatment by the young residents. They were shocked by what they learned. No one knows what use was made of the reports, but in the hands of a patients' association or a health-care consumer group such evidence might be the basis of a suit, or at least a means of bringing recognition of the problem to both the public and the institution. These are just some of the possibilities for a beginning toward bringing changes for yourself and the women who come after you.

But there are very few patients' associations as yet, and clearly these are not much geared to the level of clinic patients on welfare, although welfare-rights groups and neighborhood health associations have made some efforts. As long as the system encourages people to make the decision to seek health care essentially a private one, there is no real mechanism whereby patients can collectivize or organize. Hospitals and doctors will not release the names of patients for reasons of "confidentiality" (except for such commercial interests as diaper services or baby photographers), although they are notoriously poor at protecting patients' privacy and records. (See Appendix B, p. 273, for one plan that has worked in some communities.)

FUTURE DEMANDS

Lots of changes are coming, and women's clinics and health centers will probably be part of them, but for most of us for a long time doctors and hospitals as they are now will be part of our lives. Just being enraged with the system shouldn't keep us from trying to get the very best medical care that money can buy right now, for the very least that we can pay, whenever we need it. But there is at present almost no way that we can get perspective on the system or the care we receive, even in a women's clinic, without study. Which doesn't mean, as the doctors are fond of interpreting, that we all want to learn to become nurses or doctors or amateur specialists. For some of us that may be what we really want, but for others of us it is another matter, first of all that of having something to say about what happens to our bodies. Also, it is a hunger after those approaches and understandings that preserve health and prevent disease rather than a fascination with the drama of emergency curative care.

Medicine in the United States has been for too long arrested at the level of symptoms and mechanisms and chemical tinkering, when it should be pushing on for causes, which will require integration and coordination of all of the fragmented specialties, now so disparate and competitive. Health is more than just the mere absence of disease, whether physical or mental or a blend of both, and the concept of homeostasis, which is still operating in the minds of most men of medicine, is not enough of a goal anymore in this age of knowledge explosion, instant communication, and virtually unlimited technological capability. Attaining a broader goal, however, will require an altogether new responsibility from the patient, and a partnership between patient and doctor that bears almost no resemblance to the romanticized model still held in the hearts of so many doctors and perhaps patients too. Health will be the full-time responsibility of the patient, but not health as it is identified today, which is really synonymous with disease. The

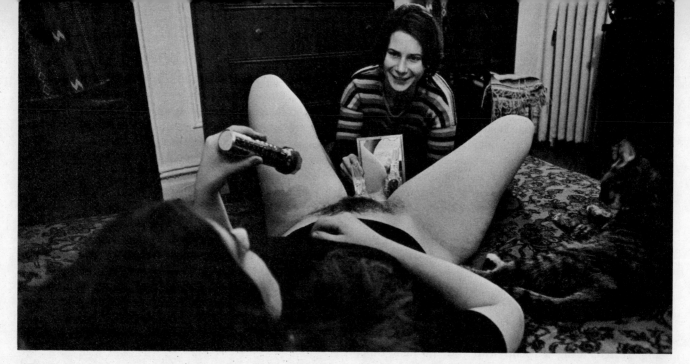

tools for prevention belong in the hands of the patients, as the tools for management of disease belong with the doctors. There should be programs in health information and education—even whole centers devoted to this purpose—as well as instruction in repairing your own automobile engine and re-covering a sofa, in all adult and school-age educational systems. But what passes for health education today has little value. Courses taught by people who are part of the "health" system have rarely given really honest consumer information or unbiased weighing of advantages and disadvantages. For the most part they are highly partisan offerings designed to defend the system and frighten you. Most of these programs are concerned with several factors: what the disease or problem is, how to recognize it, how widespread it is, and how much money is still needed for research. And they usually offer one over-all answer: trust your hospital and get regular check-ups from your doctor.

Only when health education is based in the community and run by the community will women be able to get completely truthful information about the risks they take and the decisions they are making concerning everything from nutrition to surgery. And if they are well run, these centers will offer all kinds of people the resources and the sense of initiative to keep up with their own health education instead of waiting to be told what the experts consider fit for them to know. Never at any other time has the responsibility for maintaining health and avoiding disease been so squarely up to the women in our society. Therefore, our need for the tools of genuine health care and prevention will remain the greatest.

In fantasy we jump to a Yellow Pages for doctors, hospitals, and clinics, compiled by both women and men, rating people and institutions on their humaneness, efficiency, medical excellence, openness and responsiveness to the surrounding community. And we envision medical "clearing houses" in each community, run by and com-

posed of community people, doctors, medical students, and nurses to match up peoples' needs and medical services, to handle complaints and more severe cases of malpractice, to educate community people from childhood up in preventive commonsense medicine, to fight for equal medical care, and finally to keep doctors and nurses really in touch with the people they are caring for.

SOME NEW BEGINNINGS

The belief that women should have basic knowledge about their own bodies seems to be one of the last heresies in a world that otherwise claims to believe so much in knowledge and freedom of knowledge. This book is one way of breaking down that taboo; for some women this kind of knowledge is a step toward action.

The following is a discussion by some women who have made a beginning toward a health skill and a health-education center.

* * *

P.: The women from the regular clinic questioned whether we had enough legitimately trained personnel, and strongly questioned the use of paramedics.

R.: Did the idea of being paramedics come out of this challenge?

P.: I remember talking about it. I think it had something to do with how many nurses we had. We realized we didn't have enough nurses and some of us would have to be trained by the nurses. . . . It was just that we were all feeling that we were taking this on ourselves, and we would have to learn, and that we had a right to the knowledge, and nobody else was going to do it for us, so why not?

R.: In fact, we were talking about whether or not we should have a pelvic party. (A pelvic party is an excellent way to let paramedics in training learn to do pelvic exams by practicing on each other.)

S.: *Wow. I remember when I worked in the clinic that first night with Steve Jones. There was a woman on the table, and we'd had one class, and he said, "Well, here, I'll assist you," and he started handing me the speculum. And I was terrified, and I said, "Wait a minute, I've never even seen one of these exams before." [Laughter] And so he did it, but he always pushed us to go ahead and do it ourselves, and as soon as we had practiced on each other some we started to do it for patients, and since then we've just assumed that we do the basic speculum exam, and all the other doctors just had to get used to the idea.*

G.: *Well, this is where we learn by doing instead of by talking. We'd been talking, and everybody's words sounded so neat, but when you actually get around to making it work, and the doctor steps aside and hands you this speculum. . . . But that's what we learned by having a clinic, that it's so different from anything else I've ever done, because I've never done anything else besides talk my whole life. [Laughter] I mean, have you?*

J.: *Well, whose idea was it to have paramedics?*

S.: *Well, we were talking about a lot of things, like the importance of doctors being teachers, and of all the women, patients as well as us, learning as much as they could. We wanted to break down professionalism, and medical rules that say, "A nurse does this, but only a doctor ever does that." At first I don't think we realized how far we could go, or how far our ideas would go.*

R.: *Now the doctors operate as a backup for us, explain things we don't understand yet, and check the patient after we've done the speculum exam and the test for vaginitis and VD, and the Pap smears. At first we worried about the patient's reactions, but we decided that if we talked to the women and included them in the learning process, both politically and medically, they would really like it. And, in fact, many women have told us that they prefer having the exam done by a woman, whether she's a doctor or not.*

K.: *We have tried to set up the clinic so the patient can participate in every part of it. When she first comes in, the receptionist can answer her medical questions because she's been a paramedic too.*

N.: *In the beginning was the clinic set up the way it is now, with everyone rotating through all the jobs, being receptionist, paramedic, lab assistant, and doing the educational?*

R.: *Well, there were so few of us that we had to take turns.*

H.: *Right. Everybody wanted to have a chance to do the medical work, and nobody wanted to be just a receptionist, so we just started rotating every job.*

G.: *We started out with two doctors and two paramedics who happened to have some medical background.*

Two more people trotted behind the paras, so we started calling the paras-in-training "trotters."

K.: *The paramedic explains the origin of the clinic and some of the ideas about medicine and feminism to each new patient. In the educational we try to get the patients to really rap to each other about their experiences, as well as teaching them a lot about medicine and demonstrating a pelvic exam. In the exam with the doctors the paramedic not only does the basic part of the exam but also acts as a patient advocate, making sure that the woman understands anything the doctor has to say about her medical problems. If the patient wants to, she may look at her own cervix in a mirror. Most patients prefer to do away with the paper drape between them and the doctor. If lab tests are needed, the patient goes to the lab with the paramedic to look through the microscope, so the whole clinic experience is an education.*

L.: *The educational became the most popular part of the clinic, and we suddenly found that many patients started joining our group every week.*

R.: *We really progressed, because every week we held business meetings, where we summed up what we had done, tried to see what mistakes we had made, and how we could do better.*

S.: *That's true. But at the beginning we were only discussing how we could make the clinic better medically. We had to gain a lot of confidence in running a good medical clinic before we could tackle the political problems.*

APPENDIX A: PREAMBLE TO THE 1970 EDITION OF THE ACCREDITATION MANUAL FOR HOSPITALS*

The objective of clinicians and of the institutions in which they work always has been to implement the findings of research in the natural sciences and to bring their fruits to the direct and immediate service of the sick, the injured, the disabled and the handicapped. Their concern with continuing improvement in patient care led to the formulation of the original standard for the accreditation of hospitals. For some fifty years, the standards faithfully reflected the emphasis upon developments in the support of clinical care which have characterized the pursuit of excellence in medicine.

It seems appropriate at the outset to call attention to a shift in emphasis over the years within the body of the standards. The new standards are free of all direct demands upon the physician's clinical judgment and decision. Current standards relate entirely to the supporting elements of hospital life and the environment of medical practice.

*Joint Commission on the Accreditation of Hospitals, Chicago, Illinois.

Environmental factors, physical and other, serve to create the climate within which patient care takes place. Further, it has long been recognized that the patient's perception of and his response to his environment are important factors in his progress and recovery. Environmental considerations are reflected in the standards in certain general principles which may be said to represent a set of rights accruing to the patient, the consumer of health care services, the protection of which is one of the goals of the Joint Commission.

Equitable and humane treatment at all times and under all circumstances is such a right. This principle entails an obligation on the part of all those involved in the care of the patient to recognize and to respect his individuality and his dignity. This means creating and fostering relationships founded on mutual acceptance and trust. In practical terms, it means that no person should be denied impartial access to treatment or accommodations which are available and medically indicated, on the basis of such considerations as race, color, creed, national origin or the nature of the source of payment for his care.

Every individual who enters a hospital or other health facility for treatment retains certain rights to privacy, which should be protected by the hospital without respect to the patient's economic status or the source of payment for his care. Thus, representatives of agencies not connected with the hospital, and who are not directly or indirectly involved in the patient's care, should not be permitted access to the patient for the purpose of interviewing, interrogating or observing him, without his express consent given on each occasion when such access is sought. This protection should be provided in the emergency department and outpatient facilities as well as on the floors of the hospital. The hospital, like the church of old, must impart at least some sense of sanctuary.

The individual's dignity is reflected in the respect accorded by others to his need to maintain the privacy of his body. To the extent possible, given the inescapable exposure entailed in the provision of needed care, the patient should be aided in maintaining this privacy. The design and furnishings of examination and treatment areas, in the emergency department and outpatient facilities as well as in other parts of the hospital, should be so planned as to facilitate the maintenance of the patient's privacy, and, as far as possible, to shield him from the view of others.

Another important aspect of the patient's right to privacy relates to the preservation of the confidentiality of his disclosures. The setting in which the patient's history is taken, for example, should be such that he can communicate with the physician in confidence. This is true of the emergency department as well as of other parts of the hospital.

In many teaching hospitals, and particularly in those which are closely affiliated with medical schools, all patients, regardless of their economic status, may be expected to participate to some extent in clinical training programs or in the gathering of data for research purposes. For all patients, regardless of the source of payment for their care, this should be a voluntary matter. The level of the patient's participation in such activities should in no way be related to the nature of the source of payment for his care.

In many large hospitals, the patient may be seen by several physicians during the course of his treatment. He has the right to know the identity of the physician who is primarily responsible for his care. In addition, the patient has the right to be informed as to the nature and purpose of any technical procedures which are to be performed upon him, as well as to know by whom such procedures are to be carried out.

The patient has the right to communicate with those responsible for his care, and to receive from them adequate information concerning the nature and extent of his medical problem, the planned course of treatment and the prognosis. In addition, he has a right to expect adequate instruction in self care in the interim between visits to the hospital or to the physician. In the matter of communication, ethnic and cultural considerations are highly significant, and should be taken into account by providing interpreters where language barriers are a continuing problem.

It should also be borne in mind that, even among people who ostensibly speak the same language, cultural variations may have the effect of obstructing effective communication. Where this is a likely possibility, the hospital should employ individuals who will be able to facilitate meaningful communication among hospital staff and patients.

What has been said of the obligation of the hospital, its personnel and its physicians, to observe the human rights of the individual patient is equally true of their obligation to all patients, to the community served. Communication, mutual respect and trust, a matching of achievable resources to observable needs, all of these are inherent in the attitude and spirit of the true hospital. Whatever its community, the hospital is there to serve it, governed by scientific rule and logic, but imbued primarily with the sense of service, of compassion, of the fellowship of man.

The spirit and intent expressed in this preamble relative to the hospital patient's rights and needs and the observance of these in practice will be considered as a persuasive factor in the determination of a hospital's accreditation, in the same manner as are any of the standards of this volume.

APPENDIX B:

Guidelines for NEIGHBORS*

Although it is obvious that we are people who are fed up -- even angrily fed up -- with medical care as it is, our policies are essentially positive and cooperative. Only indirectly,
if at all, do we demonstrate, blacklist or boycott. Our major concern is in finding ways to
help one another. Self-help means non-professionals organized to provide services (including
referral services) for one another.

Probably 15 to 25 people is the best size for a NEIGHBORS group. Local groups operate independently of one another although they may cooperate by sharing information, recommending or
providing speakers, or holding occasional joint meetings. NEIGHBORS is not a national organization, but a spreading idea.

NEIGHBORS saves money but does not cost money. Meetings can be held in members homes, the few
forms that need to be duplicated can often be obtained from a community center, church, or other
free or low-cost way. The group's resource library consists of items owned and loaned by members.
When you enter a group, you contribute your item. When you leave, you take it with you to a new
NEIGHBORS group. This way, a certain amount of circulation takes place. Members who are unable
to contribute to the library are not required to, and they may still enjoy the services.

Certain forms are important:
        1. Resumes for all doctors known to members. The group keeps a file of these forms which
include age, schools attended, medical specialties, publications, hospital privileges, membership
in professional and other organizations, etc. Some of this information can be obtained by examining the walls of the office, other information can be obtained at the library, and some from the
hospitals and doctors themselves. This information is used to help with decisions as to which
doctors to visit or to recommend to others. Reactions of patients with experience with the doctors
is also included.

        2. Medical Services Records. Each member should have a supply of these available so that
a report can be made after each and every medical experience by the member and family and friends
willing to supply the information. Members may wish to keep a copy for themselves, but should
always send one in to the group's file so that the information will be available to others. (See
sample on facing page.)

        3. Descriptions of each member, including physicians and hospitals known, illnesses
experienced, medical or other skills, times available, etc.

The central files and library can either be kept in the same place all the time or rotate among
members' homes. The important thing is that each member have access to it when needed -- 24 hours
a day, if emergencies arise. Among important items for the library are the Physician's Desk
Reference, a good medical dictionary, a basic medical text, descriptions of laboratory tests, and
any other books that can be obtained which you feel might be helpful. Highly recommended for all
groups is Medical Terminology: A Programmed Text, by Genevieve Love Smith and Phyllis E. Davis (2nd
edition, 1967, John Wiley & Sons). Written for nurses and medical students, this book enables you
to "speak medicine" almost instantly. It also enables you to read the medical books.

NEIGHBORS keep their own Life Charts in which they write out as full a medical history as they can
remember. They include vaccinations, surgical operations, physicians and clinics visited, hospitali-
zations, copies of prescriptions, effects and side effects of medications, etc.

The relationship of NEIGHBORS with the medical profession is likely to be strained at first, but our
positive and informed approach will gain respect as medical practitioners come to recognize the seri-
ousness of our intent, the power in our numbers, and, most of all, our willingness to use a positive
approach in which we withhold our blame and seek out things to praise.

*Copyright © 1972 by Dorothy Tennov (reproduced by permission).

MEDICAL SERVICES RECORD (NEIGHBORS)   Date received_____ #_____

Name_____ Address_____ Tel._____
Type of service: Office visit____Clinic visit____ Other (specify)_____
                                                   Date of Service_____
Reason:_____
_____
Names & Titles of all medical persons involved:_____
_____
_____
_____
Location(s):_____
_____
Time of appointment_____ Time of arrival of patient_____Time seen_____ By whom:
_____ Total time spent by patient_____ Time with doc-
tor_____ Time with other medical personnel_____ Comment_____
_____
Information given by patient_____
_____
_____
By whom_____
Services (e.g., X-ray, blood tests, blood pressure, etc.) List below:

SERVICE	PERFORMED BY WHOM	REASON (if known)

Medication (Indicate precisely and whether given or prescribed):_____
_____
_____
Diagnosis?_____ By whom?_____ Did patient have
to ask for it? Yes____ No____ Comment_____
Fee(s) charged (List each and by whom)_____
_____
Cost of medication_____ Where obtained_____
Other costs (specify)_____ Total cost_____
Use reverse for additional comment. Indicate what particularly pleased or displeased the
patient about the treatment.

FURTHER READINGS

I. Books About Medicine for the Nonmedical Reader

GENERAL WORKS

Burack, Richard. *New Handbook of Prescription Drugs.* rev. ed. New York: Pantheon Books, 1970.
> Good guide to prescription drugs and prices.

Cook, Fred J. *The Plot Against the Patient.* Englewood Cliffs, N. J.: Prentice-Hall, Inc., 1967.
> Excellent reporting of the way things are and why. Should have become a classic.

Cope, Oliver. *Man, Mind and Medicine.* Philadelphia: J. B. Lippincott Co., 1968.
> Good analysis of lack of humanism and awareness of emotions in medical education.

Di Cyan, Erwin, and Lawrence Hessman. *Without Prescription.* New York: Simon and Schuster, 1972.
> Gives basic information about ingredients and about cautions indicated, and lists side-effects of cedtain ingredients of medicines sold over-the-counter without prescription.

Duff, Raymond S., and August B. Hollingshead. *Sickness and Society.* New York: Harper & Row Publishers, Inc., 1968.
> Thorough analysis and documentation of mismanagement of medical care, including sociological and mental health considerations. Yale's best effort.

Ehrenreich, Barbara, and Deirdre English. *Witches, Midwives, and Nurses—A History of Women Healers.* Oyster Bay, N. Y.: Glass Mountain Pamphlets, 1972.
> A provocative and important pamphlet on the rise of male medical professionals and the suppression of women healers since the 14th century. You can order it from Glass Mountain Pamphlets, P.O. Box 238, Oyster Bay, N. Y. 11771. Prices: $1.00 first class, $.75 third class, $.70 twenty or more.

The Health Policy Advisory Committee (Health-PAC). *American Health Empire: Power, Profit and Politics.* New York: Random House, Inc., 1970.
> A strong analysis of who controls American medicine today; excellent and important.

Kennedy, Edward M. *In Critical Condition: The Crisis in America's Health Care.* New York: Simon and Schuster, 1972.
> Elegant exposé via subcommittee testimony of the nonsystem and its excesses. Especially good picture of the medical consumer's financial problems, particularly the failure of health insurance, and some courageous suggestions for change.

Knowles, John, ed. *Views of Medical Education and Medical Care.* Cambridge, Mass.: Harvard University Press, 1968.
> The academic medical establishment's own critique of the nonsystem, with practical recommendations for change, which are closer to some of ours than you might expect.

Kunnes, Richard. *Your Money or Your Life.* New York: Dodd, Mead & Co., 1971.
> Young radical psychiatrist takes on his profession for its lack of social and political responsibility.

Lewis, Howard and Martha. *The Medical Offenders.* New York: Simon and Schuster, 1970.
> Malpractice and its difficulties.

Mintz, Morton. *By Prescription Only* (formerly *The Therapeutic Nightmare*). Boston: Beacon Press, 1967.
> Report on how the drug industry controls the FDA and AMA and knowingly markets worthless, injurious, and even lethal drugs.

The Politics of Health Care (a bibliography). Medical Committee for Human Rights, 1151 Massachusetts Ave., Cambridge, Mass. 02138.
> Detailed subheadings on all aspects of health. Can be ordered from New England Free Press, 791 Tremont St., Boston 02118 (30¢ plus 15¢ postage each).

Sanders, Marion K., ed. *The Crisis in American Medicine.* New York: Harper & Row Publishers, Inc., 1961.
> A more professional view of some basic problems in health care.

ESPECIALLY FOR WOMEN

Llewellyn-Jones, Derek. *Everywoman and Her Body.* New York: Taplinger Publishing Co., Inc., 1971. (In Britain, *Everywoman: A Gynaecological Guide for Life.* London: Faber & Faber, 1971.)

The Report of the Women's Action Program. U. S. Department of Health, Education and Welfare, Washington, D.C. GPO-922-425, January 1972 (116 pages). Foreword by Eliot Richardson.
> HEW's women staffers' own report on how bad things are for women seeking health care, physical and mental. Exposes the "double standard" for men and women. Suppressed by HEW. Hard to get! Ask for it!

MAGAZINES AND POPULAR PERIODICALS

Campion, Rosamond. "The Right to Choose," *McCall's Magazine* (February 1972).

Fortune (January 1971).
> Four articles on medicine as a fast-growing, profitable big business.

Health-PAC Bulletin (HPB), 17 Murray Street, New York, N. Y. 10007.
> "The only radical publication on health statistics." Should be read regularly by anyone who considers herself a health activist.

Health Rights News (HRN). Medical Committee for Human Rights, 1520 Naudain Street, Philadelphia, Pa. 19146.
> Informative news items and articles by the counter-AMA group of medical professionals.

Maynard, Fredelle. "Breast Cancer: Is There an Alternative to Surgery?" *Woman's Day* (November 1970).

Nolen, William, M. D. "The Operation Women Fear Most," *McCall's Magazine* (April 1971).

II. Books About Medicine for Doctors and Other Professionals

GENERAL WORKS

Becker, H. S., B. Geer, E. C. Hughes, and A. L. Straus. *Boys in White.* Chicago: University of Chicago Press, 1961.
> Sociological profile of the doctor as student in medical school and residency.

The Graduate Education of Physicians. Report of the Citizen's Commission on Graduate Medical Education of the AMA (1966). Council on Medical Education, AMA, 535 North Dearborn Avenue, Chicago, Ill. 60610.
> Succinct guide to the problem of the specialists and strong suggestions for change.

Hodgkin, Keith. *Towards Earlier Diagnosis.* London: E & S Livingstone, Ltd., 1966.
> Valuable aid for making diagnoses without hospitalization or expensive laboratory tests.

Hollingshead, A. B., and F. C. Redlich. *Social Class and Mental Illness.* New York: John Wiley & Sons, Inc., 1958.

Classic work revealing the way social class affects both diagnosis, treatment and stigma in mental illness.

O'Grady, Francis, ed. *Urinary Tract Infection*. New York and London: Oxford University Press, 1968.
    See especially chapters 20 and 23.

Stetler, C. Joseph, and Alan R. Moritz. *Doctor and Patient and the Law*. 4th ed. St. Louis: The C. V. Mosby Co., 1962.
    A book about malpractice written for doctors but helpful to laywomen.

ABOUT WOMEN AND WOMEN'S CONDITIONS

Breast Cancer: Early and Late. Chicago: Yearbook Medical Publishers, Inc., 1970.
    A collection of papers presented at the 13th Annual Conference on Cancer (1968), at Texas University, Houston, Texas. The current controversy is presented here.

Gardner, Herman L., and Raymond H. Kaufman. *Benign Diseases of the Vulva and Vagina*. St. Louis: The C. V. Mosby Co., 1969.
    Technical information on vaginitis, and color photos.

Greenhill, J. P. *Office Gynecology*. 9th ed. Chicago: Yearbook Medical Publishers, Inc., 1971.
    Easy-to-understand guide to common diseases and problems.

Moore, Francis D., *et al.* "Carcinoma of the Breast," *New England Journal of Medicine* (August 1967).

Nash, Ethel M. "Divorce, Marriage Counselling," in Allan C. Barnes, ed. *The Social Responsibility of Obstetrics and Gynecology*. Baltimore: Johns Hopkins University Press, 1965.
    Role and training of ob-gyn for counselling on sexual adjustments.

Scott, C. Russell. *The World of a Gynecologist*. London: Oliver and Boyd, 1968.
    Marvelous portrait of the gynecologist's view of his importance to women.

N. B.: See bibliography of chapter on "Childbearing" for books on obstetrics and gynecology and on infant care.

JOURNALS

Hospital Medicine. Hospital Publications, 18 E. 48 Street, New York, N. Y. 10017.
    Issues up to 1968 contain much basic, still valid information. Clearly written, well illustrated. Now has subheading "A Pictorial Review of Medicine." Little text in current issues. Not as useful.

Postgraduate Medicine, issue on preventive medicine (January 1972).
    Interesting straight view of the need and the hope.